Hypothalamus and Endocrine Functions

CURRENT TOPICS IN MOLECULAR ENDOCRINOLOGY

Series Editors: Bert W. O'Malley and Anthony R. Means
Department of Cell Biology
Baylor College of Medicine
Houston, Texas

Volume 1:   *Hormone Binding and Target Cell Activation in the Testis*
Edited by Maria L. Dufau and Anthony R. Means

Volume 2:   *Hormonal Regulation of Spermatogenesis*
Edited by Frank S. French, Vidar Hansson,
E. Martin Ritzen, and Shihadeh N. Nayfeh

Volume 3:   *Hypothalamus and Endocrine Functions*
Edited by Fernand Labrie, Joseph Meites,
and Georges Pelletier

A Continuation Order Plan is available for this series. A continuation order will bring delivery of each new volume immediately upon publication. Volumes are billed only upon actual shipment. For further information please contact the publisher.

INTERNATIONAL SYMPOSIUM ON

Hypothalamus and Endocrine Functions

Edited by

Fernand Labrie
Centre Hospitalier de l'Université Laval
Quebec, Canada

Joseph Meites
Michigan State University
East Lansing, Michigan

and

Georges Pelletier
Centre Hospitalier de l'Université Laval
Quebec, Canada

PLENUM PRESS · NEW YORK AND LONDON

Library of Congress Cataloging in Publication Data

International Symposium on Hypothalamus and Endocrine Functions, Quebec, 1975.
  Hypothalamus and endocrine functions.

  (Current topics in molecular endocrinology; v. 3)
  Includes bibliographies and index.
    1. Hypothalamic hormones–Congresses. I. Labrie, Fernard, 1937-   II. Meites,
  Joseph, 1913-   III. Pelletier, Georges, 1939-   IV. Title V. Series. [DNLM:
  1. Hypothalamus–Physiology–Congresses. 2. Pituitary hormone releasing factors–
  Congresses. W1 CU82M v. 3/WL312 I594h 1975]
  QP572.H9I58 1975   599'.01'927   76-13912
  ISBN 0-306-34003-8

Proceedings of the International Symposium on Hypothalamus and
Endocrine Functions held in Quebec City, September 21-24, 1975

© 1976 Plenum Press, New York
A Division of Plenum Publishing Corporation
227 West 17th Street, New York, N.Y. 10011

United Kingdom edition published by Plenum Press, London
A Division of Plenum Publishing Company, Ltd.
Davis House (4th Floor), 8 Scrubs Lane, Harlesden, London, NW10 6SE, England

Printed in the United States of America

Preface

Although physiological and anatomical evidence had
clearly indicated for many years that the secretion of
anterior pituitary hormones is under control by the
central nervous system, it is only recently that the
isolation and determination of structure of three hypothalamic hypophysiotropic hormones have been accomplished.
This has brought the concept of neurohormonal control
of adenohypophyseal function into precise biochemical
and chemical terms. The relative ease of synthesis of
TRH (thyrotropin-releasing hormone), LH-RH (luteinizing
hormone-releasing hormone), somatostatin and their
analogues has opened a new era in the field of endocrinology and has led to a rapid expansion of our knowledge of the control of anterior pituitary function.

The rapid evolution of fundamental and clinical
research on hypothalamic hormones and the many potential
clinical applications indicate the importance of inte-
grating the knowledge gained in recent years. This is
well illustrated in the Proceedings of the International
Symposium on Hypothalamus and Endocrine Functions held
in Quebec City on September 21-24th, 1975, which indicates that impressive progress has been made in large
variety of aspects of hypothalamic hormone research. In
fact, attempts were made to review the recent achieve-
ments in the localization of hypothalamic hormones using
immunohistochemical methods, chemistry and assays of hypothalamic hormones, control of hypothalamic hormone secretion by neurotransmitters, prostaglandins and cyclic
nucleotides, mechanisms of action of hypothalamic hormones, clinical studies with TRH, LH-RH and somatostatin,
effect of somatostatin on glucagon and insulin secretion, control of growth hormone and prolactin secretion,
and mechanisms of steroid feedback on gonadotropin secretion in laboratory animal and man.

Although many important aspects of the current research in neuroendocrinology were not discussed at this
Symposium, the text of the main lectures as well as the
abstracts of poster sessions contained in this book should
offer a useful and stimulating review of the current
trends of investigation in this fast-moving field.

                              Fernand Labrie
                              Joseph Meites
                              Georges Pelletier

Contents

Preface... 1

    F. Labrie, J. Meites and G. Pelletier

CONTROL OF HYPOTHALAMIC HORMONE SECRETION

Relation of the Hypothalamo-Pituitary-Gonadal System to
    Decline of Reproductive Functions in Aging Female
    Rats.. 3

    J. Meites, H.H. Huang and G.D. Riegle

Role of Prostaglandins (PGs) in the Control of Adenohy-
    pophyseal Hormone Secretion....................... 21

    S.M. McCann, S.R. Ojeda, P.G. Harms, J.E. Wheaton,
    D.K. Sundberg and G.P. Fawcett

Adrenergic and Cholinergic Inputs to the Amygdala: Role
    in Gonadotropin Secretion......................... 37

    J. Borrell, F. Piva and L. Martini

Neurotransmitters and Control of Pituitary Function..... 51

    C. Kordon, M. Hery and A. Enjalbert

CLINICAL APPLICATIONS OF LH-RH and TRH

Studies on the Diagnostic Use of LH-RH................... 65

J.G. Rochefort, A. Chapdelaine, G. Tolis and J.
Van Campenhout

Diagnostic and Therapeutic Use of LH-RH in the Infertile
Man... 73

L. Schwarzstein

Therapeutic Use of Luteinizing Hormone-Releasing Hormone
in the Human Female................................... 93

S.J. Nillius

SOMATOSTATIN

Clinical Implications of Growth Hormone Release-Inhibiting Hormone (GH-RIH) 115

G.M. Besser

Somatostatin and the Endocrine Pancreas................. 127

J.E. Gerich

MECHANISM OF ACTION OF HYPOTHALAMIC HORMONES
AND STEROID FEEDBACK

New Aspects of the Mechanism of Action of Hypothalamic
Regulatory Hormones................................. 147

F. Labrie, A. De Lean, N. Barden, L. Ferland, J.
Drouin, P. Borgeat, M. Beaulieu and O. Morin

Steroid Binding in the Hypothalamus and Pituitary.......   171

    J.-P. Raynaud, M.-M. Bouton, D. Philibert and
    B. Vannier

Role of Sex Steroids on LH and FSH secretion in the Rat..   191

    L. Ferland, J. Drouin and F. Labrie

The Role of Estradiol in Modulating LH and FSH Response   211
    to Gonadotropin Releasing Hormone.................

    R.B. Jaffe, W.R. Keye, Jr. and J.R. Young

CONTROL OF PRL AND GH SECRETION AND ACTION

Control of Prolactin Secretion in Man...................   257

    H.G. Bohnet and H.G. Friesen

Neuropharmacological Aspects of the Neural Control of   283
    Prolactin Secretion..............................

    J.A. Clemens

Episodic GH Secretion: Evidence for a Hypothalamic Dopa-   303
    minergic Mechanism..............................

    J.O. Willoughby and J.B. Martin

Hormonal Control of Liver Prolactin Receptors............   321

    P.A. Kelly, L. Ferland, F. Labrie and A. De Lean

CHEMISTRY AND ASSAY OF HYPOTHALAMIC HORMONES

Suppression of Gonadotropin Release and Ovulation in
Animals by Inhibitory Analogs of Luteinizing
Hormone-Releasing Hormone........................   339

D.H. Coy, E.J. Coy, J.A. Vilchez-Martinez, A. de
la Cruz, A. Arimura and A.V. Schally

Isolation and Characterization of Hypothalamic Peptide
Hormones..   355

R. Burgus, M. Amoss, P. Brazeau, M. Brown,
N. Ling, C. Rivier, J. Rivier, W. Vale
and J. Villarreal

Analogs of Somatostatin Part A. Chemistry and In Vitro Results.......................................   373

H. Immer, N.A. Abraham, V. Nelson, K. Sestanj, M.
Götz, P. Brazeau and J.B. Martin

Part B. In Vivo Activities:
Prolongation of Action with Protamine Zinc   379

P. Brazeau and J.B. Martin

In Vivo Methods for Studying the Action of Hypothalamic
Hormones with Special Reference to their Antisera
as Tools for Investigation........................   387

A. Arimura

Applications of Adenohypophyseal Cell Cultures to Neuroendocrine Studies.................................   397

W. Vale, C. Rivier, M. Brown, L. Chan, N. Ling and
J. Rivier

LOCALIZATION OF HYPOTHALAMIC HORMONES

Immunohistochemical Localization of Hypothalamic Hormones at the Electron Microscope Level.......... 433

    G. Pelletier

Immunohistochemical Localization of Hypothalamic Hormones (especially LRF) at the Light Microscopy Level...... 451

    J. Barry

ABSTRACTS.. 475

CONTRIBUTORS... 501

INDEX... 506

Control of Hypothalamic Hormone Secretion

Relation of the Hypothalamo-Pituitary-Gonadal System to Decline

of Reproductive Functions in Aging Female Rats

Joseph Meites[1], H.H. Huang and G.D. Riegle[2]

Department of Physiology, Michigan State University

East Lansing, Michigan 48824

Introduction

In mammalian species, reproductive functions decline with
aging and the capacity to produce live offspring by the female
usually ceases well before death of the individual. Many neuroendocrine and other mechanisms involved in these changes remain
to be investigated. In women, menstrual cycles generally cease
between 40-50 years of age, but for 2-3 years prior to the menopause,they tend to become irregular and there is an increase in
the number of anovulatory cycles (Timeras and Meisami, 1972),
suggesting a possible decrease in LH secretion. The ovaries
tend to form large or cystic follicles and there is inadequate
development and often early involution of the corpus luteum
leading to shortening of the cycle. Both estrogen and progesterone secretion appear to decline in women approaching the
menopause and the ovaries show a reduced capacity to respond to
gonadotropins. In the postmenopausal period, ovulation rarely
occurs, the ovaries loose their follicles and become fibrotic,
and the pituitary responds to loss of inhibitory gonadal feedback
by increasing release of gonadotropins, particularly FSH. However, a sharp fall in gonadotropin release has been observed in
women after 80 years of age (Albert et al., 1956).

For the past 10 years, we have used the rat as a model for
the study of reproductive changes with aging, and there appears
to be a number of similarities as well as differences between
the rat and human species. Rats have a lifespan of about 3
years, but beginning about 8 months of age or even earlier, the
cycles of some rats become irregular and show a gradual reduction

3

in the number of eggs ovulated. We (Clemens and Meites, 1971; Huang and Meites, 1975) have observed a progression in vaginal smear patterns from regular to irregular cycles, the latter characterized by prolonged estrous phases. This is then followed by a constant estrous syndrome characterized by ovaries with well developed or even cystic follicles but no corpora lutea. The latter in turn changes to a series of pseudopregnancies of irregular length ranging from 8-30 days duration, with ovaries containing corpora lutea that apparently secrete progesterone (Aschheim, 1961). The anestrous state usually is the final stage seen in rats 2-3 years of age, and the ovaries generally are atrophic and contain but few small follicles; the uterus is atrophic in these animals (Meites and Huang, 1975). It must be emphasized that not all aging rats necessarily follow the above sequence nor is each stage of similar duration. Thus regular or irregular cycles, or constant estrus, may continue in some rats for even up to 2 years of age or longer; others may revert from the constant estrous or pseudopregnant state to irregular cycles; and some rats may go directly from cycling to the pseudopregnant state. We have not observed that any of the old anestrous rats return to the earlier patterns.

Our approach has been to try to determine changes in the hypothalamus, pituitary, ovaries and reproductive tract that may contribute to the reproductive decline in old female rats. We therefore have measured pituitary hormone content of FSH, LH and prolactin, and also have assayed these hormones in the serum. We have tested the ability of the pituitary to respond to synthetic LRH and more recently to TRH. We have measured the response of the hypothalamo-pituitary system to many stimuli that normally result in release of or inhibition of release of FSH, LH and prolactin, and also have directly stimulated hypothalamic areas electrochemically to determine the effects on hormone release. In addition, we have attempted to reinitiate cycling (and even pregnancies) by administering treatments that attempt to correct neuroendocrine deficiencies in old female rats. We shall describe some of these experiments and discuss their possible significance.

Serum LH, FSH and Prolactin in Intact Young and Old Female Rats, and After Castration and Estrogen Administration

Previously, we reported that in old Sprague-Dawley constant estrous rats (20-24 months old), pituitary concentration of FSH and prolactin were higher and LH was lower than in young (3 to 4 months old) rats on their day of estrus (Clemens and Meites, 1971). A comparison of serum concentration of LH and prolactin in old Long-Evans (23-30 months) and young (4 to 6 months) female rats, without regard to their reproductive states, showed that LH values were about the same in both groups but serum prolactin levels were about 6-fold greater in the old rats (Shaar et al.,

1975). Serum concentrations of LH and prolactin in old constant estrous rats were found to be higher than in old pseudopregnant rats (Wuttke and Meites, 1973).

In the present study,a comparison was made on blood levels of FSH, LH and prolactin in 4-5 month old female rats on their day of estrus or 2nd day of diestrus, 24 month old constant estrous or pseudopregnant rats and 26-30 month old anestrous rats. All rats were of the Long-Evans strain (Blue Spruce Farms, Altamont, NY) and were approximately of the same weight (325-375 grams). Only healthy, non-diseased rats were used in this study. They were maintained under standard conditions of temperature (75$\pm$2°F), lighting (14 hours of light daily) and nutrition. Blood samples for NIAMDD double antibody radioimmuno-assays were collected by orbital sinus puncture under light ether anesthesia. Blood samples were taken before, 7 weeks after ovariectomy and 8 days after injecting subcutaneously 0.5 ug of estradiol benzoate (EB) per 100 gm body weight daily. The reference standards used were NIAMDD rat prolactin-RP-1, LH-RP-1 and FSH-RP-1. The serum values and their standard errors are given in Table 1.

It can be seen that in intact young rats,serum LH was higher on the day of estrus than on diestrous day 2. Seven weeks after ovariectomy of both groups of young rats, serum LH rose about <u>26-fold</u>. Eight days after daily injection of EB, serum LH felt to about 1/8 of its initial ovariectomy value. In intact old con-stant estrous rats serum LH was slightly higher than in young rats on the day of estrus, and in intact old pseudopregnant rats serum LH was about the same as in young rats in diestrus. After ovariectomy, serum LH rose only about <u>3 fold</u> in the old constant estrous rats and about 14-fold in the old pseudopregnant rats, but the absolute LH values were much lower than in the young rats. After EB injections,the relative fall in serum LH in both old groups of rats was less than in the young rats. In the old an-estrous rats, serum LH was <u>not detectable</u> under any condition of treatment, and did not rise after ovariectomy.

Serum FSH values in the young and old rats appeared to parallel the LH values except in the old anestrous rats. In the young rats, serum FSH was much higher on the day of estrus than on diestrus, rose after ovariectomy and felt after EB treat-ment. The intact old constant estrous and pseudopregnant rats showed about the same serum FSH values as in young estrous rats, but exhibited a smaller FSH rise after ovariectomy and a smaller FSH fall after EB administration. The old anestrous rats showed only a <u>small rise</u> in serum FSH after ovariectomy and <u>no fall</u> after EB injections.

Table 1. Serum LH, FSH and Prolactin in Young and Old Female Rats

Group, Age, No.	AP wt. (mg)	LH (ng/ml)			FSH (ng/ml)			Prolactin (ng/ml)		
		Intact	Ovx[1]	EB[2]	Intact	Ovx	EB[2]	Intact	Ovx	EB[2]
Young, 4-5 mths										
Estrus (6)	15.3 ±0.8	34.8 ±4.0	736.1 ±14.4	84.2 ±4.2	124.0 ±11.5	485.0 ±18.8	140.3 ±12.3	175.1 ±27.8	66.5 ±9.4	338.5 ±16.8
Diestrus (6)		20.7 ±3.2			26.5 ±3.9			108.7 ±18.8		
Old Constant Estrus										
24 mths (8)	19.6 ±2.9	52.4 ±6.3	169.3 ±18.4	40.5 ±7.6	121.5 ±8.1	250.8 ±41.5	137.0 ±9.8	395.0 ±34.1	127.6 ±28.8	487.7 ±56.1
Old Pseudopreg.,										
24 mths (6)	29.0 ±9.8	20.8 ±2.7	291.3 ±32.4	49.2 ±2.1	83.7 ±25.7	300.5 ±30.4	116.8 ±13.3	188.4 ±42.7	165.0 ±25.3	665.2 ±55.4
Old Anestrus										
26-30 mths (6)	227.5 ±46.6	Not detectable			47.6 ±9.9	70.0 ±2.9	72.8 ±3.9	807.8 ±135.5	870.2 ±107.3	1116.9 ±51.7

1 Seven weeks after ovariectomy
2 Eight days after injecting 0.5 ug estradiol benzoate (EB)/100 gm BW daily

(from Huang and Meites, unpublished)

Serum prolactin concentration in the intact young estrous rats were higher than in diestrous rats. These basal prolactin values are several fold higher than we have usually found in intact mature female rats except on the afternoon of proestrus, and may be due to the stress of blood collection. Serum prolactin levels felt after ovariectomy and rose after EB administration, in agreement with previous observations by us and others. The intact old constant estrous rats had significantly higher serum prolactin than the young rats, in agreement with other reports by us (Shaar et al., 1975; Meites and Huang, 1975). Ovariectomy and estrogen administration appeared to produce effects comparable to those in young rats. The old pseudopregnant rats had less serum prolactin than the old constant estrous rats, confirming the observation of Wuttke and Meites (1973), and showed only a small fall after ovariectomy and a marked rise after EB treatment. The intact old anestrous rats showed much higher serum prolactin values than any of the other groups, and interestingly, no fall in serum prolactin after ovariectomy reflecting lack of estrogen stimulation from the ovaries. Estrogen administration was able to increase serum prolactin in these rats.

The pituitaries of the old constant estrous and pseudopregnant rats were heavier than those of the young rats and those of the old anestrous rats were tumorous in every case. We previously have described these differences in pituitary size among the different categories of old rats and have compared them with young rats (Huang and Meites, 1975). We occasionally have observed small pituitary tumors in old pseudopregnant rats.

Effects of Synthetic LRH on Pituitary Release of LH in Old and Young Rats

Old (23-30 months) and young adult (4-6 months) female Long-Evans rats were maintained in a temperature ($75\pm2^{o}F$) and light-controlled (14 hours light daily) room under identical conditions and fed a standard rat pellet diet. The experimental groups were aged constant estrous or pseudopregnant rats, each showing persistent cornified (constant estrus) or leucocytic vaginal smears with epithelial cells (pseudopregnant) for at least 10 days duration, and young rats during proestrus, estrus or diestrus day 2 of their estrous cycle. All experiments were begun at 1000 hours and completed by 1100 hours. Rats were injected iv with 0, 5, 50 or 500 ng synthetic LRH in 0.5 ml of 0.85% NaCl (LRH was obtained through the courtesy of Dr. J. A. Clemens, Eli Lilly & Co., Indianapolis, IN). Blood samples were collected by orbital sinus puncture 15 minutes before and 15, 30 and 60 minutes after LRH injection. Serum LH was measured by a standard double antibody radioimmunoassay (Monroe et al., 1969) and the reference hormone was NIAMDD rat LH-RP-1.

Table 2. Effects of LRH on Serum LH Levels in Young and Aged Female Rats

Reproductive State	No.	Serum LH (ng/ml)[a] Time (minutes)			
		-15	15	30	60
Young proestrus					
Control	9	38.4 + 6.8[b]	51.0 + 7.5	47.5 + 6.5	68.0 + 10.0
5 ng LRH	9		41.4 + 9.0	48.7 + 15.5	69.0 + 16.9
50 ng LRH	12		104.8 + 14.8	73.0 + 8.4	70.0 + 11.5
500 ng LRH	9		611.0 + 112.0	421.0 + 66.6	250.0 + 72.0
Young estrus					
Control	10	22.6 + 1.6	33.1 + 8.8	35.8 + 11.5	50.0 + 12.1
5 ng LRH	10		47.2 + 13.2	28.1 + 7.4	15.4 + 4.9
50 ng LRH	10		87.8 + 12.8	64.6 + 13.0	22.8 + 7.1
500 ng LRH	9		800.0 + 196.0	433.0 + 67.5	334.0 + 85.8
Young diestrus					
Control	10	18.1 +5.2	8.8 + 3.0	4.9 + 0.3	9.5 + 2.2
5 ng LRH	10		6.3 + 0.5	7.5 + 1.2	8.3 + 1.7
50 ng LRH	10		26.0 + 5.8	11.5 + 4.2	9.7 + 2.6
500 ng LRH	10		292.0 + 44.7	236.0 + 68.5	135.0 + 29.8
Old constant estrus					
Control	9	37.9 + 2.3	25.7 + 4.9	40.6 + 16.1	57.4 + 18.3
5 ng LRH	9		41.4 + 15.4	15.9 + 5.0	13.3 + 3.7
50 ng LRH	9		59.4 + 12.6	38.6 + 16.2	35.3 + 16.1
500 ng LRH	10		172.0 + 21.5	174.0 + 13.6	171.0 + 41.8
Old pseudopregnant					
Control	10	22.0 + 3.7	17.5 + 7.6	12.2 + 6.6	22.2 + 10.0
5 ng LRH	10		7.8 + 1.4	14.0 + 7.0	16.7 + 6.6
50 ng LRH	10		41.0 + 18.5	25.8 + 6.1	18.7 + 7.0
500 ng LRH	10		83.6 + 6.3	83.9 + 14.5	66.0 + 12.8

a Hormone concentrations are shown as mean + S.E.M.
b Pretreatment control values were pooled for all treatments in a given reproductive state

(from Watkins, Meites and Riegle, unpublished)

The results are shown in Table 2. It can be seen that young
proestrous and old constant estrous rats had about the same serum
LH values in the pretreatment period, and these were somewhat
greater than in any of the other groups. A dose of 5 ng LRH had
no significant effect on serum LH in any of the groups, but 50
and 500 ng LRH increased serum LH in all groups. Serum LH elevations produced by LRH were much higher in the young than in the
old rats, particularly in the young proestrous and estrous rats
as compared to the old constant estrous and pseudopregnant rats.
The increase in serum LH evoked by 500 ng LRH at 15 minutes were
approximately 16-fold in the young proestrous rats, only about
4.5-fold in the old constant estrous rats and about 4-fold in
the old pseudopregnant rats. The old pseudopregnant rats were
the least responsive of any of the groups to LRH. The relative
decline in serum LH at 30 and 60 minutes after LRH injection was
greater in the young than in the old groups, although absolute
serum LH values at 60 minutes remained higher in the young
proestrous and estrous rats than the old rats. These results
demonstrate that the anterior pituitary of old female rats shows
much less capacity to respond to LRH with release of LH than the
anterior pituitary of young mature female rats.

Reinitiation of Estrous Cycles in Old Rats by Different Methods
     Although old female rats usually cease to cycle, their
ovaries are capable of responding to gonadotropic stimulation.
Thus transfer of ovaries from old to young ovariectomized rats
was reported to result in resumption of cycling (Peng and Huang,
1972). Aschheim (1965) reported that LH administration produced
ovulation in old constant estrous rats. We observed induction of
ovulation in old constant estrous rats after administration of
progesterone or epinephrine or after electric stimulation of the
preoptic area of the hypothalamus (Clemens et al., 1969). Reinitiation of regular or irregular estrous cycles was induced in
old constant estrous rats by injections of epinephrine, a catecholamine (Clemens et al., 1969) or by injections of L-dopa or
iproniazid (Quadri et al., 1973), drugs that increase brain catecholamines.

     The present study compared the abilities of progesterone,
ACTH, ether stress and L-dopa to induce cycling in old constant
estrous rats. Multiparous female Long-Evans rats, 10-12 months
old, were maintained under standard temperature ($75\pm2^{\circ}F$) and
light (6 AM to 8 PM) conditions, and fed a complete pellet diet.
When the rats reached 16 months of age, daily vaginal smears were
taken and only rats exhibiting vaginal cornification for 20 days
or more were used. Progesterone (0.5 mg in 0.1 ml corn oil) was
injected sc twice daily, ACTH (porcine, grade II, Sigma Chemical
Co., St. Louis, MO), was injected sc twice daily at a dose of
2.2 I.U./rat, L-dopa (30 mg) was injected sc twice daily, and

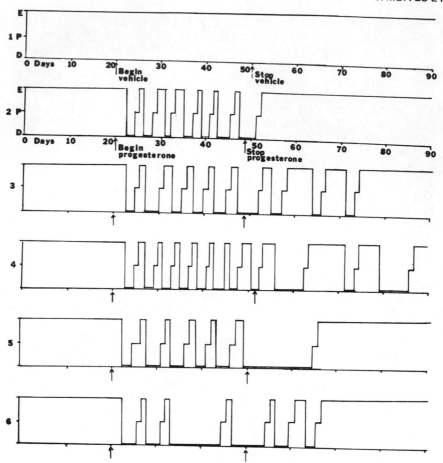

Fig. 1   Vaginal smear patterns in 6 representative old constant estrous rats induced to cycle by progesterone: (1) control rat injected with vehicle alone, showing constant estrus (2) rat given progesterone, showing regular cycles during the treatment period and constant estrus after termination of treatment (3) rat given progesterone, showing regular cycles during treatment, and irregular cycles followed by constant estrus during post-treatment (4) rat given progesterone, showing regular cycles during treatment and irregular cycles throughout post-treatment period (5) rat given progesterone, showing regular cycles during treatment and one period of pseudopregnancy followed by constant estrus during post-treatment period (6) rat given progesterone, showing two regular cycles and 1 period of pseudopregnancy during treatment, followed by irregular cycles and constant estrus during post-treatment. E = estrus, P = proestrus, D = diestrus.

rats were placed in an atmosphere of saturated ether for about 3 minutes twice daily. Daily monitoring of vaginal smears continued during the treatment period of 30 days and during a post-treatment period of 30-40 days.

Twenty-six control rats given daily injections of corn oil or physiological saline continued in constant estrus during and after treatment. When 26 constant estrous rats were given progesterone twice daily, 23 showed regular 4 or 5 day cycles during treatment, 2 showed regular 4 or 5 day cycles during treatment, 2 showed 2 regular cycles followed by pseudopregnancy, and one remained in

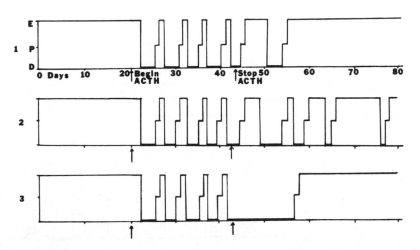

Fig. 2 Vaginal smear patterns in 3 representative constant estrous rats treated with ACTH showing (1) regular estrous cycles during treatment period, followed by 1 irregular estrous cycle and constant estrus during post-treatment (2) regular estrous cycles during the treatment period, and irregular estrous cycles throughout the post-treatment period (3) regular cycles during the treatment period, and 1 period of pseudopregnancy early in the post-treatment period followed by constant estrus.

constant estrus. After treatment was terminated, most of these rats exhibited a few irregular cycles and then returned to the constant estrous state. Representative vaginal patterns before, during and after treatment with progesterone are shown in Fig. 1. ACTH elicited regular estrous cycles in 10 of 12 treated rats and 2 remained in constant estrus. After termination of treatment, these rats showed a few irregular cycles followed by constant estrus. Representative vaginal patterns in the ACTH-treated rats are shown in Fig. 2.

L-dopa induced regular cycling in only 3 of 12 treated rats, irregular cycles in 5 rats, pseudopregnancies followed by irregular cycles in 2 rats, and no change in 2 rats. These rats showed a few irregular cycles and then a return to the constant estrous state after treatment was terminated. Representative vaginal patterns from the L-dopa treated rats are shown in Fig. 3. In the 22 ether-stressed animals, only 8 exhibited regular estrous cycles, 10 had irregular cycles, 2 showed a single pseudopregnancy followed by irregular cycles, and 2 remained in constant estrus. After treatment was terminated, most of these rats showed a few irregular cy-

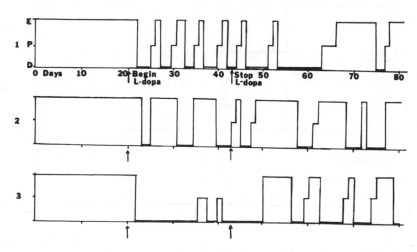

Fig. 3 Vaginal smear patterns in 3 representative constant estrous rats treated with L-dopa, showing (1) regular estrous cycles during the treatment period, and irregular estrous cycles during post-treatment period (2) irregular estrous cycles throughout the treatment and the post-treatment periods (3) 1 period of pseudopregnancy during treatment period, and irregular estrous cycles during post-treatment period.

cles followed by a return to the constant estrous state. Representative vaginal patterns from the ether-stressed animals are shown
in Fig. 4.

Laparotomies showed that corpora lutea were present in the
ovaries of 25 of 26 progesterone-treated rats, 10 of 12 ACTH-treated rats, 5 of 12 L-dopa-treated rats, and 10 of 12 ether-stressed
rats. Serum LH peaks were observed at variable times on the afternoon of proestrus in 14 of 20 rats given progesterone, in 6 of
10 rats given ACTH, in 2 of 10 rats given L-dopa and in 6 of 20
rats given ether stress. Thus progesterone and ACTH were the most
effective of any of the treatments used for inducing regular cycling
and LH surges in old constant estrous rats.

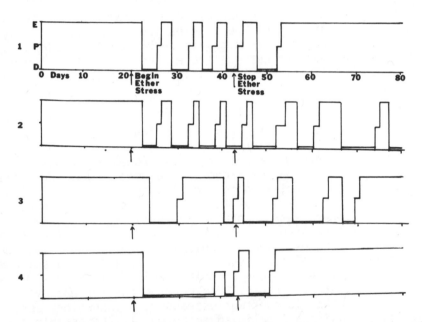

Fig. 4 Vaginal smear patterns in 4 representative constant estrous
rats treated with ether stress showing (1) regular estrous cycles
during the treatment period, followed by 1 irregular estrous cycle
early in the post-treatment period and constant estrus thereafter
(2) regular estrous cycles during the treatment period, followed by
irregular estrous cycles throughout the post-treatment period (3)
irregular estrous cycles throughout the treatment and the post-
treatment periods (4) 1 period of pseudopregnancy during the treatment period, followed by 1 irregular estrous cycle early in the
post-treatment period and constant estrus.

Discussion

The experimental studies reported here, as well as earlier reports by us, indicate that significant changes occur in hypothalamic, pituitary and ovarian function in aging female rats. Preliminary studies suggest that important changes also occur in the neuroendocrine system of the aging male rat. It is apparent that the capacity to secrete FSH and LH is profoundly reduced in all categories of old rats, and prolactin secretion is increased. When subjected to ovariectomy and thereby loss of inhibitory feedback from the ovaries, there was only a relatively small rise in serum LH and FSH in the old constant-estrous and pseudopregnant as compared to the young rats. In the intact anestrous rats LH was not detectable and FSH was lower than in any of the other old or yound rats. LH remained undetectable after ovariectomy or estrogen administration and FSH was little altered, indicating that the atrophic ovaries of the anestrous rats were producing little or no estrogen. However, we have observed that transplantation of the ovaries from anestrous old rats to young ovariectomized rats resulted in development of follicles and appearance of a constant estrous state, indicating that these ovaries are capable of being activated by adequate secretion of gonadotropins (Huang and Meites, unpublished).

The constant estrous state in the old rats can be attributed in large part to failure of the LH surge mechanism, suggesting a functional change in the anterior hypothalamus (preoptic area?), but it is apparent that inadequate secretion of progesterone also may be involved since injections of progesterone were almost 100% effective in reinitiating regular estrous cycles in these rats. It was notable that the few rats that failed to respond had cystic follicles. The prolonged estrous phases in the irregular cycling rats that precede the constant estrous state can be attributed to similar neuroendocrine changes. The mechanisms responsible for the repeated series of usually prolonged pseudopregnancies in old rats are more difficult to explain. It can be seen (Table 1) that these rats apparently have a greater capacity to respond to ovariectomy with a rise in LH than the old constant estrous rats. However, serum prolactin levels, which are believed to be mainly responsible for the maintenance of the corpora lutea of pseudopregnancy in rats, were higher than in young rats during the diestrous phase of the cycle and as high as on the day of estrus. It is possible therefore, that the relatively high prolactin levels in these pseudopregnant rats are sufficient to maintain active corpora lutea for relatively prolonged periods, interspersed by occasional surges of LH release and ovulation. The reasons for the anestrous state in the oldest rats appears to be more obvious. These animals show a profound deficiency in secretion of gonadotropins by their tumorous pituitaries, and hence the ovaries are atrophic and contain only a few small follicles. A lack of estrogen secretion is indicated by the atrophic uterus in these rats (Huang and Meites, 1975).

The mechanisms responsible for the considerable increase in prolactin release by all categories of old rats are not entirely clear at this time. A reciprocal relationship between secretion of prolactin and gonadotropins has been observed under many physiological states, i.e. after ovariectomy or estrogen administration, during suckling, etc. PIF activity in the hypothalamus was reported to be unchanged in old constant estrous rats (Clemens and Meites, 1971), but PRF activity may be increased. Serum prolactin was highest by far in the old anestrous rats and next highest in the constant estrous rats. These elevated serum prolactin levels undoubtedly account to a large degree for the increase in spontaneous mammary tumors commonly seen in old female rats. We reported earlier that experimentally induced increases in prolactin release can hasten the onset of spontaneous mammary tumors in rats, whereas reductions in prolactin release can inhibit development of these tumors (Welsch and Meites, 1974). The development of prolactin secreting pituitary tumors in old rats of both sexes has been described previously (Furth, 1975), and apparently is not due to estrogen secretion by the ovaries. In fact the pituitary tumors appear at a time when the ovaries show minimal function. It is more likely that a central mechanism is responsible for the increase in prolactin secretion and development of pituitary tumors in aging rats.

It is apparent that changes occur in the pituitary itself as well as in the hypothalamus of old rats. The pituitary of old female rats responded less to LRH administration with release of LH than young female rats. We have observed a similar reduction in pituitary release of LH in response to LRH injection in old as compared to young male rats (Riegle and Meites, unpublished). In addition, we have recently found that TSH release in response to TRH administration is decreased significantly in old as compared to young rats (Chen, Huang and Meites, unpublished). The cause of the decline in the capacity of the anterior pituitary of old rats to respond to LRH administration is not clear. Our earlier study on anterior pituitary content of old constant estrous rats showed that significantly less LH was present in the pituitary of old constant estrous than in young estrous rats (Clemens and Meites, 1971). Thus less LH may be available for release in the pituitary of old female rats. Another possibility is that fewer LRH receptors are present in the anterior pituitary of old as compared to young rats, and hence LRH is less effective in stimulating LH release. These and other possibilities remain to be investigated.

There is now considerable evidence to indicate that the hypothalamus of aging female rats exhibits functional (and perhaps anatomical) changes that are at least partially if not mainly responsible for the decline in reproductive functions and the increase in prolactin secretion in old female rats. We previously have reported a decrease in LRF content in the hypothalamus of old constant estrous rats (Clemens and Meites, 1971), but these observations were based on crude extraction and indirect bioassay of LRF activity. Direct radioimmunoassay of hypothalamic LRH content in old female rats should be more rewarding. Old constant estrous rats can respond directly to electrochemical stimulation of the preoptic area with release of LH and ovulation (Clemens et al., 1969; Wuttke and Meites, 1973), suggesting that LRH is present in sufficient quantities to induce rapid release of LH. It is possible therefore, that signals from other areas of the CNS are inadequate to induce release of ovulatory quantities of LH in the old rats. In this respect, the feedback by estrogen on the hypothalamus may be important. Peng and Peng (1973) observed decreased uptake of tritiated estradiol by the anterior hypothalamus of old constant estrous and anestrous rats. This may explain in part the inability of old constant estrous rats to show a preovulatory surge in LH and FSH release, since estrogen is believed to stimulate this surge. The absence of active corpora lutea in the ovaries of constant estrous old rats suggests that progesterone secretion also is deficient. Another indication that the hypothalamus of old female rats is less responsive to stimuli that normally release gonadotropins is that electrical or mechanical stimulation of the cervix of old constant estrous rats did not induce LH release or ovulation in contrast to the effects of similar stimulation of young female rats on the day of estrus (Clemens et al., 1969; Huang and Meites, unpublished). However, when mated with young mature male rats, many old constant estrous rats became pseudopregnant and a few even became pregnant (Huang and Meites, unpublished). Further details of these experiments will be published elsewhere.

We have reinitiated regular or irregular cycling in old constant estrous but not in old pseudopregnant or anestrous rats by injections of epinephrine (Clemens et al., 1969), L-dopa or iproniazid (Quadri et al., 1973), or as seen here, by progesterone, ACTH or ether stress. Progesterone has been shown to hasten ovulation in normal cycling rats and to induce cycling in constant estrous rats (Everett, 1948). Kalra et al. (1972) reported that anti-adrenergic drugs block LH release by progesterone, indicating that this action of progesterone requires the mediation of hypothalamic catecholamines. ACTH has been reported to increase progesterone secretion on the day of proestrus and to facilitate release of ovulatory amounts of LH (Feder and Ruf, 1969; Nequin and Schwartz, 1971; Barraclough et al., 1971). In addition, ACTH also may act centrally to induce LH release (Baldwin et al., 1974). Ether stress also has been shown to stimulate ACTH release (Cook et al., 1973), which could then promote progesterone release from the adrenals. L-dopa is the precursor of the catecholamines, and there is increasing evidence that hypothalamic catecholamine stimulation, particularly by norepinephrine, is necessary for LH release (Sawyer et al., 1974). Thus all the agents that we have used to induce cycling in old constant estrous rats may act by increasing hypothalamic catecholamine activity, which in turn activate LRH release. We have previously hypothesized that a major cause for the failure of ovulation in old constant estrous rats was low hypothalamic catecholamine activity (Clemens et al., 1969; Clemens and Meites, 1971). Preliminary evidence from our laboratory indicates that old male rats have significantly less norepinephrine and dopamine in the hypothalamus than young mature male rats (Miller, Riegle, Shaar and Meites, unpublished). Finch (1973) also has reported that old male mice have less catecholamine turnover than young male mice. However, other brain neurotransmitters, such as serotonin, acetylcholine and possibly GABA, also may be involved since these too have been reported to influence gonadotropin and prolactin secretion (Kamberi et al., 1971; Meites et al., 1972; Grandison et al., 1974; Ondo, 1974, Mioduszewski et al., 1975).

The implications of these studies in aging female rats and their possible relation to problems of reproductive aging in women are difficult to assess at this time because of the many gaps in our knowledge. The primary cause for reproductive failure in the old female rats appears to be due to functional and perhaps morphological changes in the hypothalamus and pituitary. Both appear to be less reactive to stimuli that normally result in release of gonadotropins, and more responsive to stimuli that release prolactin. Further work is necessary to determine the role of neurotransmitters and releasing factors in the hypothalamus and perhaps in other portions of the brain, and functional changes in the pituitary. The ovaries of aging female rats apparently are capable of normal or nearly normal function throughout the lifespan of the individual, as indicated by the use of drugs and by transplantation of the ovaries to young female rats. Although we have produced a few pregnancies in old constant estrous rats by mating them with young mature males, we have not yet seen any live births, perhaps due to the functional and anatomical regression of the reproductive tract (Talbert and Krohn, 1966).

There appear to be some parallels in reproductive functions between women approaching the menopause and in aging female rats. In both species as they near the end of reproductive life, the cycles tend to become irregular, follicles develop but often become cystic, and there is decreased frequency of ovulation. In women there is reduced secretion of estrogen and progesterone

by the ovaries; in rats progesterone secretion appears to be deficient and estrogen secretion also may be reduced. The ability of
the pituitary to release ovulatory amounts of LH may be low in both
species during these periods. It is possible that menstrual cycles
can be prolonged and normalized in pre-menopausal women, as the estrous cycles of aging female rats. However, it has been demonstrated that there is an increased frequency of abnormal births in older women, perhaps due to defects in the ova and reproductive tract
(Timeras and Meisami, 1972). In the postmenopausal state, the differences in reproductive functions between women and old female rats
appear to be more evident than any similarities. The ovaries of postmenopausal women apparently lose all their follicles, atrophy and become non-responsive to gonadotropins. The ovaries of old anestrous
rats similarly lose most of their follicles and atrophy, but are capable of respondinf to gonadotropins (Huang and Meites, unpublished).
Thus the primary cause of cessation of menstrual cycles in aging
women appears to lie in the ovaries rather than in the hypothalamo-
pituitary system. These problems require further examination.

References

Albert, A., Randal, R.V., Smith, R.A., and Johnson, C.E. (1956)
     In: Hormones and the Aging Process, Academic Press, Inc.,
     New York, N.Y. pp.

Aschheim, P. (1961). Compt. Rend. Acad. Sci., Paris 253, 1988-1990.

Aschheim, P. (1965). Compt. Rend. Acad. Sci., Paris 260, 5627-5630.

Baldwin, D.M., Huan, C.K., and Sawyer, C.H. (1974). Brain Research
     80, 291-301.

Barraclough, C.A., Collu, R., Massa, R., and Martini, L. (1971).
     Endocrinology 88, 1437-1447.

Clemens, J.A., Amenomori, Y., Jenkins, T., and Meites, J. (1969)
     Proc. Soc. Exp. Biol. Med. 132, 561-563.

Clemens, J.A., and Meites, J. (1971). Neuroendocrinology 7, 247-
     256.

Cook, D.M., Kendal, J.W., Greer, M.A., and Kramer, R.M. (1973).
     Endocrinology 93, 1019-1024.

Everett, J.W. (1948). Endocrinology 43, 389-405.

Feder, H.H., and Ruf, K.B. (1969). Endocrinology 84, 171-174.

Finch, C.E. (1973). Brain Research 52, 261-276.

Furth, J. (1975). In: Cancer (F.F. Becker, ed.), Plenum Press,
    New York, pp. 75-120.

Grandison, L., Gelato, M., and Meites, J. (1974). Proc. Soc. Exp.
    Biol. Med. 145, 1236-1239.

Huang, H.H., and Meites, J. (1975). Neuroendocrinology 17, 289-295.

Kalra, P.S., Kalra, S.P., Krulich, L., Fawcett, C.P., and McCann,
    S.M. 91972). Endocrinology 90, 1168-1176.

Kamberi, I.A., Mical, R.S., and Porter, J.C. (1971). Endocrinology
    88, 1288-

Meites, J., Lu, K.H., Wuttke, W., Welsch, C.W., Nagasawa, H., and
    Quadri, S.K. (1972). Recent Progr. Hormone Res. 28, 471-516.

Mioduszewski, R., Grandison, L., and Meites, J. (1975). Proc. Soc.
    Exp. Biol. Med., in press.

Nequin, L.G., and Schwartz, N.B. (1971). Endocrinology 88, 323-325.

Ondo, J.G. (1974). Science 186, 738-739.

Peng, M.T., and Huang, H.H. (1973). Fertility and Sterility 24, 534-
    539.

Peng, M.T., and Huang, H.H. (1972). Fertility and Sterility 23, 535-
    542.

Quadri, S.K., Kledzik, G.S., and Meites, J. (1973). Neuroendocrino-
    logy 11, 248-255.

Sawyer, C.H., Hilliard, J., Kanematsu, S., Scaramuzzi, R., and Bla-
    ke, C.A. (1974). Neuroendocrinology 15, 328-337.

Shaar, C.J., Euker, J.S., Riegle, G.D., and Meites, J. (1975) J.
    Endocrinol. 66, in press.

Talbert, G.B., and Krohn, P.L. (1966). J. Reprod. Fert. 11, 399-
    406.

Timeras, P.S., and Meisami, E. (1972). In: Developemntal Physiol-
    ogy and Aging (P.S. Timeras, ed.), MacMillan, New Yord, pp.
    527-541.

Welsch, C.W., and Meites, J. (1974). In: Mammary Cancer and Neuro-
    endocrine Therapy (B.A. Stoll, ed.), Butterworths, London, pp.
    25-26.

Wuttke, W., and Meites, J. (1973). Pflügers Arc. 341, 1-6.

Acknowledgements

[1] Aided in part by NIH grant HD 09184 from the National Institute of Child Health and Human Development, AM 04784 from the National Institute of Arthritis, Metabolic Diseases and Diabetes, and CA 10771 from the National Cancer Institute.

[2] Also affiliated with Endocrine Research Unit and Department of Animal Husbandry. Aided in part by NIH grant HD 06223 from the National Institute of Child Health and Human Development.

ROLE OF PROSTAGLANDINS (PGs) IN THE CONTROL OF ADENOHYPOPHYSEAL HORMONE SECRETION*

S.M. McCann, S.R. Ojeda, P.G. Harms, J.E. Wheaton,
D.K. Sundberg, and C.P. Fawcett

The University of Texas Health Science Center at Dallas
Southwestern Medical School, Dallas, Texas 75235

INTRODUCTION

With the realization of the wide-spread distribution and biological action of the prostaglandins, it was natural to search for possible effects of these agents on the hypothalamic-pituitary unit. In this communication we will review the evidence which indicates that prostaglandins can act both on the pituitary and on the hypothalamus to alter the release of adenohypophyseal hormones. The review will summarize the present status with respect to ACTH, TSH and growth hormone but will concentrate on the role of the prostaglandins on the secretion of FSH, LH and prolactin with which we have been particularly concerned in this laboratory.

Perhaps the first evidence for a role of prostaglandins to alter the function of the anterior pituitary was provided by the findings of Zor et al. (1969, 1970) that prostaglandins could increase the adenylate cyclase and cyclic AMP levels in the adenohypophysis incubated in vitro; however, in these studies none of the prostaglandins increased the release of LH. Subsequent studies have shown that the systemic administration of prostaglandins is accompanied by alterations in adenohypophyseal hormone release and that these actions are exerted not only directly on the pituitary itself but also, at least in some instances, on the hypothalamus which in turn alters the release of pituitary hormones.

In this review we will first examine the effects of systemic

*Supported by grants from NIH (AM 10073 and HD 05151) and the Ford Foundation.

administration of prostaglandins on the release of the various
pituitary hormones and then turn to the studies in which the prostaglandins have been incubated with pituitaries in vitro or injected
into the gland in vivo. Next we will consider the studies in which
the prostaglandins have been injected into hypothalamic tissue or
into the ventricular system to study their possible effects on the
CNS. Finally, the possible physiological role of prostaglandins in
pituitary hormone release will be considered by examining the results
of experiments in which inhibitors of prostaglandin synthesis have
been used.

The Effects of Systemic Administration of Prostaglandins on Adenohypophyseal Hormone Release

In the initial experiments of this type, PGE_1 was shown to
increase ACTH secretion (Peng et al., 1970). Since the response
could be blocked by treatment with Nembutal plus morphine, the action
was thought to be via an effect on the CNS. Similarly, PGE_1 and PGE_2
are the most potent prostaglandins in releasing GH (Ito et al., 1971;
Hertelendy et al., 1972). In the case of gonadotropins, both PGE_2
and E_1 injected intravenously can stimulate gonadotropin release in
either male or female rats (Tsafrini et al., 1973; Harms et al.,
1974; Sato et al., 1974). Although PGE_1 or E_2 failed to increase
plasma prolactin titers in ovariectomized rats following their intravenous injection (Ojeda et al., 1974a),larger doses of PGEs or PGFs
induced prolactin release in ovariectomized, estrogen-primed rats
(Sato et al., 1974). $PGF_{2\alpha}$ has recently been reported to be a potent
stimulus for prolactin release in the cow (Louis et al., 1974; Tucker
et al., 1975) and in the human female (Yue et al., 1974). TSH release
was not altered by the systemic administration of prostaglandins in
the experiments of Brown and Hedge (1974). The problem with all of
these experiments with systemic administration of prostaglandins is
that the wide-spread physiological effects of the compounds may produce nonspecific stress which could then produce an alteration in
hormone release via the CNS. In order to localize the action of
prostaglandins in the hypothalamic pituitary unit, it was essential
to perform experiments in which the drugs were applied directly to
tissue. This has been accomplished by both in vivo and in vitro studies.

Effects of Prostaglandins on the Release of Anterior Pituitary Hormones from Pituitaries Incubated In Vitro

In most of these studies, hemipituitaries have been used, but
in a few cases experiments have been carried out on pituitary cells
in tissue culture. It was first shown that pituitary ACTH secretion
could be enhanced in vitro by several prostaglandins (DeWied et al.,
1969). Vale et al. (1972) observed increased TSH release from cultured anterior pituitary cells after addition of PGE_2 to the

incubation fluids. Dupont and Chavancy (1972) similarly found that PGE$_1$ increased TSH release from hemipituitaries incubated in vitro, but Tal et al. (1974) and Sundberg et al. (1975) found no effects of prostaglandins on release of TSH by pituitaries incubated in vitro. However, Sundberg et al. did observe that prostaglandins could potentiate the stimulatory effect of thyrotropin-releasing hormone (TRH) on TSH secretion. None of the prostaglandins examined affected either basal or hypothalamic extract-altered release of LH, FSH or prolactin (Sundberg et al., 1975), but Makino (1973), Ratner et al. (1974) and Sato et al. (1975a) did report increased LH release following incubation of pituitaries with prostaglandins.

Standing in contrast to the relative lack of effect of prostaglandins on the in vitro release of gonadotropins and prolactin is their dramatic stimulation of the release and synthesis of growth hormone in vitro (Schofield, 1970; MacLeod and Leymeyer, 1970; Hertelendy, 1971; Sundberg et al., 1975). It is possible that the effect of prostaglandins, particularly of the E series, in releasing growth hormone is mediated by adenylate cyclase since the prostaglandins increased not only adenylate cyclase but also cyclic AMP levels in the pituitary (Zor et al., 1970) and this increase was correlated with their effectiveness in increasing GH release (Sundberg et al., 1975). Furthermore, an increase in cyclic AMP levels has been found to precede the release of GH stimulated by prostaglandins (MacLeod and Leymeyer, 1970).

TABLE 1

Effect of Prostaglandins E_1, E_2, $F_{1\alpha}$ and $F_{2\alpha}$ on
Basal Hormone Release In Vitro[1]

	LH	FSH	PRL	TSH	GH
			µg hormone/ml/4 hr		
Experiment 1:					
Control	0.21 ± 0.03	5.5 ± 0.2	16.4 ± 1.1	30 ± 5	50 ± 4
PGE$_1$ 0.03 mM	0.18 ± 0.01	5.8 ± 0.2	16.4 ± 0.9	30 ± 7	173 ± 15**
Experiment 2:					
Control	0.17 ± 0.02	6.1 ± 0.3	14.4 ± 0.5	27 ± 1	34 ± 3
PGE$_2$ 0.015 mM	0.18 ± 0.01	6.3 ± 0.5	16.3 ± 0.7	26 ± 1	166 ± 12**
PGF$_{1\alpha}$ 0.015 mM	0.20 ± 0.02	6.9 ± 0.3	15.2 ± 1.5	24 ± 1	88 ± 14*
PGF$_{2\alpha}$ 0.015 mM	0.19 ± 0.02	6.2 ± 0.4	15.6 ± 1.3	24 ± 3	84 ± 3**

[1] Each value represents the mean ± S.E. of four flasks per experimental group.

* = P<0.05; ** = P<0.01 vs the respective control.
(From Sundberg et al., Proc. Soc. Exp. Biol. Med. 148:56, 1975, p. 55)

The Effects of Prostaglandins on Hormone Release Following Their
Injection Directly into the Anterior Pituitary or Their
Injection into Cannulated Portal Vessels

Hedge (1972) reported that injection of prostaglandins directly
into the anterior pituitary had no effect on ACTH secretion in the
rat as measured by changes in plasma corticosterone titers. Intrapituitary injection of prostaglandin E_2 produced a slight increase
in prolactin release in ovariectomized but not in ovariectomized,
estrogen-primed rats (Ojeda et al., 1974a). This prostaglandin had
no effect on prolactin release when injected into a cannulated portal vessel in male rats (Eskay et al., 1975). Prostaglandin E_2 and
E_1 had no effect on LH release following intrapituitary injection in
ovariectomized animals but PGE_2 produced a small increase in plasma
LH in ovariectomized, estrogen-primed rats (Harms et al., 1974).
Infusion of PGE_2 into cannulated portal vessels in male rats had no
influence on FSH and LH titers (Eskay et al., 1975). From these
in vivo studies it would appear that there is little action of prostaglandins on the anterior pituitary itself except for a slight
action in the case of gonadotropins and prolactin (Figs. 1 and 2).

The in vivo effects on growth hormone secretion of prostaglandins applied directly to the anterior pituitary have yet to be evaluated. In view of the earlier cited in vitro studies, it is probable
that GH release would be elicited by the application of prostaglandins to the pituitary directly in vivo.

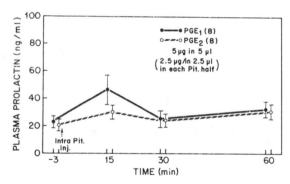

Fig. 1: Effect on plasma prolactin of intrapituitary injection of
PGE_1 or PGE_2 in ovariectomized rats. 2.5 µg in 2.5 µl of each prostaglandin were injected into each lobe.
(From Ojeda et al., Endocrinology 96:613, 1974, p. 616.)

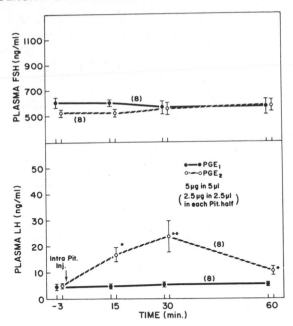

Fig. 2:   Concentration of plasma LH and FSH before and after intrapituitary injections of PGE_1 or PGE_2 in ovariectomized rats treated
with estrogen.
(From Harms et al., Endocrinology 94:1459, 1974, p. 1463.)

Effects of Injection of Prostaglandins into Hypothalamic Tissue
or the Ventricular System on Pituitary Hormone Release

     Hedge (1972) was the first to inject prostaglandins into hypo-
thalamic tissue. He observed that PGE_1, $PGF_{1\alpha}$ and $PGF_{2\alpha}$ stimulated
ACTH secretion when microinjected into the median eminence but not
into neighboring portions of the basal hypothalamus or into the
anterior lobe. On the other hand, Brown and Hedge (1974) failed to
observe any effect of intrahypothalamic prostaglandin injection on
TSH release.

     The intraventricular injection of PGE_1, but not PGE_2, $PGF_{1\alpha}$ or
$PGF_{2\alpha}$ evoked release of prolactin in ovariectomized rats whether or
not they were primed with estrogen (Ojeda et al., 1974a) (Fig. 3).
The response to PGE_1 was directly related to the dose injected.
Injection of PGE_2 into the lateral ventricle released prolactin in
intact male rats (Eskay et al., 1975).

     Dopamine exerts an inhibitory action on prolactin release as
exemplified by the ability of intraventricular injection of dopamine
to lower plasma prolactin. This action of intraventricular dopamine

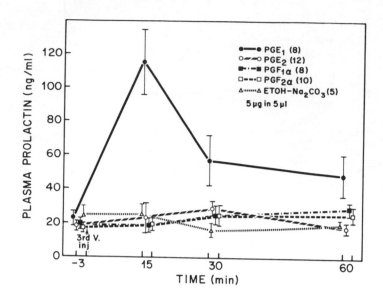

Fig. 3:   Effect of third ventricular injections of prostaglandins
on plasma prolactin in ovariectomized rats. Controls (injected with
5 µl, 95% ethanol:0.02% Na$_2$CO$_3$, 1:9) are also represented. Vertical
lines represent the standard error of the mean and figures in parentheses indicate the number of animals used.
(From Ojeda et al., Endocrinology 96:613, 1974, p. 615.)

was completely blocked by the injection of PGE$_1$ which suggests that
PGE$_1$ may elevate prolactin by blocking the stimulatory effect of
dopamine on the release of prolactin-inhibiting factor (PIF); however, a stimulatory effect of PGE$_1$ on prolactin-releasing factor
discharge cannot be ruled out (Ojeda et al., 1974b).

     The PIF-releasing action of dopamine is thought to be mediated
by cyclic AMP. Intraventricular PGE$_1$ had no effect on the lowering
of prolactin induced by intraventricular injection of dibutyryl cyclic
AMP, which suggests that prostaglandins act prior to the cyclic AMP
step in the sequence (Ojeda et al., 1974b) (Fig. 4).

     A stimulatory effect of prostaglandins on the release of LH-
releasing hormone (LHRH) has been established. In ovariectomized
animals, prostaglandin E$_2$ evoked a dramatic increase in plasma LH
concentrations and a slight increase in plasma FSH following its
injection into the third ventricle (Harms et al., 1973). The effect
could be accounted for by a presumed release of the decapeptide LHRH
since LHRH has a greater effect on LH than FSH release. In ovariectomized, estrogen-primed rats the effect was even more pronounced

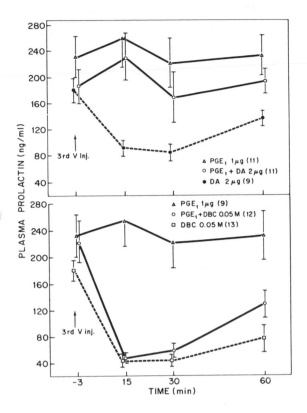

Fig. 4: Effect of intraventricular injection of PGE$_1$ on the decrease in plasma prolactin induced by dopamine (DA) (upper panel) or dibutyryl cyclic AMP (DBC) (lower panel) in ovariectomized, estrogen-treated rats. PGE$_1$ was administered 5 min before in a 2 μl volume. (From Ojeda et al., Endocrinology 95:1694, 1974, p. 1698.)

and in this situation, PGE$_1$ was also effective (Harms et al., 1974). The response to PGE$_2$ was dose-related. Similar results were observed in conscious male rats with only prostaglandin E$_2$ effective in castrate males, but PGE$_1$ exerting a small effect in intact animals as well (Ojeda et al., 1974c). PGF$_{1\alpha}$ and PGF$_{2\alpha}$ were ineffective in altering gonadotropin release in these studies (Figs. 5 and 6).

The intraventricular injection of PGE$_2$ in conscious, ovariectomized rats increased peripheral plasma LHRH titers as measured by radioimmunoassay (Ojeda et al., 1975)(Fig. 7). Similarly, PGE$_2$ increased the titer of LHRH in hypophyseal portal blood of anesthetized male

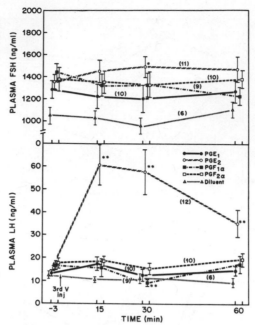

Fig. 5:   Concentrations of plasma LH and FSH before and after 3rd V
injection of PGs in ovariectomized rats.   Values are means ± S.E.,
with number of animals in parenthesis. Arrow indicates time of injection.   Statistical significance: * = P<0.05; ** = P<0.01; *** =
P<0.001.
(From Harms et al., Endocrinology 94:1459, 1974, p. 1461.)

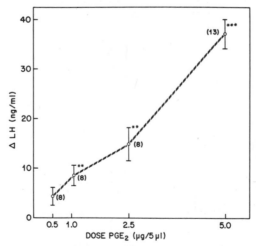

Fig. 6:   Increases in plasma LH 30 min following 3rd V injections of
varying doses of PGE_2 in ovariectomized estrogen-primed rats.
(From Harms et al., Endocrinology 94:1459, 1974, p. 1462.)

rats (Eskay et al., 1975). Sato et al. (1975b) detected a decrease
in hypothalamic LHRH content within 5 min after a massive intravenous
injection of PGE_2 which markedly increased plasma LH in ovariectomized, estrogen progesterone-treated rats. Further support for the
concept that prostaglandins act primarily via a release of LHRH is
provided by the findings of Chobsieng et al. (1975) who observed
that an antiserum to LHRH completely blocked the effect of systemic
PGE_2 on LH release.

PGE$_2$ is thought to act within the LHRH-secreting neuron to stimulate release of the neurohormone since a variety of receptor blocking
drugs failed to modify the LH release induced by intraventricularly
injected PGE_2 (Harms et al., 1975). Thus, phentolamine, an alpha
blocker, Pimozide, a dopamine receptor blocker, methysergide and
Cinanserin, serotonin receptor blockers, and atropine, a cholinergic
receptor blocker, were all ineffective in altering PGE_2-induced LH
release.

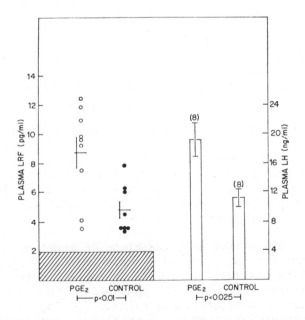

Fig. 7: Effect of 3rd V injection of PGE_2 on plasma LRF and LH
concentrations of ovariectomized rats decapitated 5 min after injection. The shaded area represents the limit of sensitivity of the
LRF assay. The numbers in parentheses indicate the numbers of animals used. Vertical lines are the SEM.
(From Ojeda et al., Neuroendocrinology 17:283, 1975, p. 285.)

Effects of Inhibitors of Prostaglandin Synthesis on
Pituitary Hormone Release

To determine the importance of prostaglandins in releasing
pituitary hormones, inhibitors of prostaglandin synthesis, such as
aspirin and indomethacin, have either been injected systemically,
implanted into the hypothalamus or added to media for incubation of
pituitary glands to observe their effects on pituitary hormone
release.   In the case of growth hormone, 7-oxa-13 prostanoic acid,
a prostaglandin antagonist, and indomethacin have suppressed release
of this hormone from pituitaries incubated in vitro (Ratner et al.,
1973; Sundberg et al., 1975).

In initial studies, it was shown that indomethacin could block
ovulation in the absence of a suppression of LH release (Tsafrini
et al., 1973; Carlson et al., 1973); however, in recent studies it
has been found that there is a latency of more than 8 hours before
systemic injection of indomethacin can suppress LH release (Ojeda et
al., in press). After this latent period, indomethacin was found to
depress LH levels in ovariectomized rats, to inhibit the circhoral
rhythm of LH release in these animals and to prevent the post-castration rise of plasma LH titers in males.   Indomethacin could also
block the progesterone-induced LH release in estrogen-primed, ovariectomized rats (Ojeda et al., in press)and estrogen-induced LH release
in sheep (Carlson et al., 1974).   In contrast to the suppression of
the release of LH by indomethacin was the lack of effect of the drug
on FSH release except for the progesterone-induced release of FSH in
ovariectomized, estrogen-primed rats which was partly suppressed
(Fig. 8).

The action of indomethacin appeared to be exerted on the CNS
since the drug did not inhibit the LH release in response to synthetic LHRH in ovariectomized rats and only partially blocked the
response in estrogen, progesterone-treated animals (Ojeda et al., in
press; Sato et al., 1975a).   Surprisingly, in this latter situation,
indomethacin actually potentiated the FSH release in response to
LHRH (Ojeda et al., in press) (Fig. 9).

Further evidence that this inhibitor of prostaglandin synthesis
was acting centrally was provided by experiments in which the drug
was injected into the third ventricle or implanted into the medial
basal hypothalamus.   In this situation, plasma LH was suppressed
within 1-6 hours in ovariectomized animals.   Using this experimental design, another inhibitor of prostaglandin synthesis, 5,8,11,14-
eicosatetraynoic acid, also suppressed plasma LH in ovariectomized
rats following its injection into the third ventricle.   Since the
doses of indomethacin used in these studies were higher than the
minimal dose required to lower prostaglandin levels in tissue, it
is still conceivable that these effects were exerted by another
action of the drug; however, they provide evidence that prostaglandins

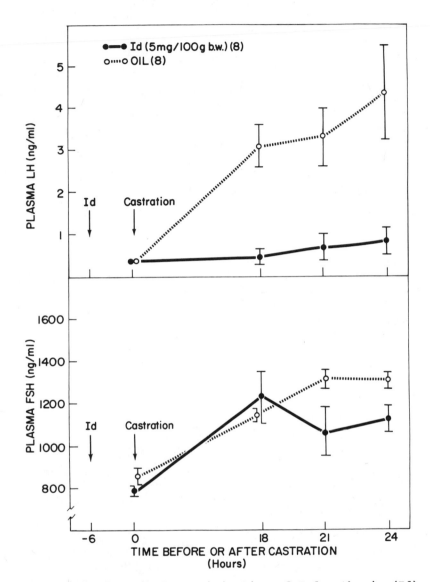

Fig. 8: Effect of a single sc injection of Indomethacin (Id) (5 mg/100 g body weight) on the post-castration rise in plasma gonadotropins of male rats.
(From Ojeda, S.R., Harms, P.G., and McCann, S.M., Endocrinology, in press.)

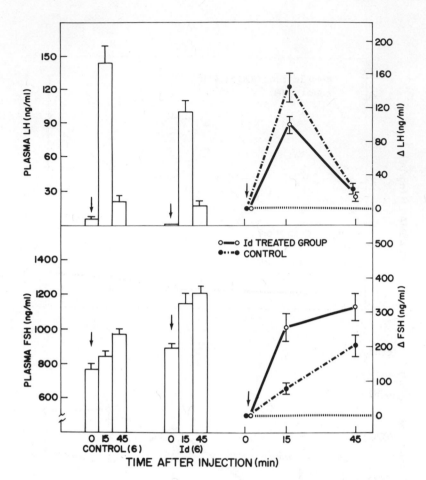

Fig. 9:   Release of gonadotropins in response to an injection of
synthetic LHRH (100 ng/rat, iv) in ovariectomized, estrogen,
progesterone-treated rats injected with a single sc dose of indomethacin (Id) (5 mg/100 g body weight) 28 hr before LHRH.   Arrows
indicate time of LHRH injection.
(From Ojeda, S.R., Harms, P.G., and McCann, S.M., Endocrinology,
in press.)

may play an essential role in control of LH release (Ojeda et al., 1975).

Clearly, there was no inhibitory effect of indomethacin directly on gonadotropin release from the pituitary since incubation of glands with this inhibitor of prostaglandin synthetase did not affect either basal or LHRH-stimulated release of gonadotropins (Sundberg et al., 1975). High doses of the drug even augmented responses to LHRH, an altered response similar to that encountered for FSH release in the living animal.

CONCLUSIONS

It is obvious from the results presented above that prostaglandins have wide-spread effects on the release of pituitary hormones. In the case of ACTH, they appear to be capable of acting centrally to cause corticotropin-releasing factor release which in turn stimulates secretion of adrenocorticotropin. In the case of TSH release, there appears to be an action at the pituitary to increase responsiveness to TRH. On the basis of in vitro studies only, it appears apparent that prostaglandins can increase growth hormone release from the pituitary directly and that this effect is accompanied by and may be causally related to an increase in cyclic AMP within the gland. In the case of prolactin, PGE_1 appears to have an action on the hypothalamus to stimulate prolactin release. This action may be via an inhibition of dopamine-induced PIF discharge. In the case of the gonadotropins, the primary action appears to be on the hypothalamus, probably directly on the LHRH-secreting neurons to stimulate the discharge of LHRH. Both in the case of growth hormone and LH, inhibitors of prostaglandin synthesis can reduce release of the pituitary tropins at least under certain conditions which suggests that the prostaglandins may play an essential role in the release process; however, additional work is necessary to substantiate this hypothesis.

REFERENCES

Brown, M., and Hedge, G.A. (1974) Endocrinology 95, 1392-1397.
Carlson, J.C., Barcikowski, B., and McCracken, J.A. (1973) J. Reprod. Fert. 34, 357-361.
Carlson, J.C., Barcikowski, B., Cargill, U., and McCracken, J.A. (1974) J. Clin. Endocrinol. Metab. 39, 399-
Chobsieng, P., Naor, Z., Zor, U., and Lindner, H.R. (1975) Neuro-endocrinology 17, 12-17.
DeWied, D., Witter, A., Versteeg, D.H.G., and Mulder, A.H. (1969) Endocrinology 85, 561-569.
Dupont, A., and Chavancy, G. (1972) Prog IV Interntl. Cong. Endo., p. 84.
Eskay, R.L., Warberg, J., Mical, R.S., and Porter, J.C. (in press), Endocrinology.
Harms, P.G., Ojeda, S.R., and McCann, S.M. (1973) Science 181, 760-761.
Harms, P.G., Ojeda, S.R., and McCann, S.M. (1974) Endocrinology 94, 1459-1464.
Harms, P.G., Ojeda, S.R., and McCann, S.M. (in press) Endocrinology.
Hedge, G.A. (1972) Endocrinology 91, 925-933.
Hertelendy, F. (1971) Acta Endocrinol. 68, 355-362.
Hertelendy, F., Todd, H., Ehrhart, K., and Blute, R. (1972) Pros-taglandins 2, 79-
Ito, H., Momse, G., Katayama, T., Takagishi, H., Ito, L., Nakajima, H., and Takei, Y. (1971) J. Clin. Endocrinol. Metab. 32, 857-859.
Louis, T.M., Stellflug, J.N., Tucker, H.A., and Hafs, H.D. (1974) Proc. Soc. Exp. Biol. Med. 147, 128-133.
MacLeod, R.M., and Lehmeyer, J.E. (1970) Proc. Natl. Acad. Sci. U.S.A. 67, 1172-1179.
Makino, T. (1973) Am. J. Obstet. Gynecol. 115, 606-614.
Ojeda, S.R., Harms, P.G., and McCann, S.M. (1974a) Endocrinology 95, 613-618.
Ojeda, S.R., Harms, P.G., and McCann, S.M. (1974b) Endocrinology 95, 1694-1703.
Ojeda, S.R., Harms, P.G., and McCann, S.M. (1974c) Prostaglandins 8, 545-552.
Ojeda, S.R., Harms, P.G., and McCann, S.M. (in press) Endocrinology.
Ojeda, S.R., Wheaton, J.E., and McCann, S.M. (1975) Neuroendocrin-ology 17, 283-287.
Peng, T.C., Six, K.M., and Munson, P.L. (1970) Endocrinology 86, 561-569.
Ratner, A., Wilson, M.C., Srivastava, L., and Peake, G.T. (1974) Prostaglandins 5, 165-
Sato, T., Jyujo, T., Iesaka, T., Ishikawa, J., and Igarashi, M. (1974) Prostaglandins 5, 483-490.
Sato, T., Hirono, M., Jyujo, T., Iesaka, T., Taya, K., and Igarashi, M. (1975a) Endocrinology 96, 45-49.

Sato, T., Jyujo, T., Kawarai, Y., and Asai, T. (1975b) Am. J.
     Obstet. Gynecol. 122, 637-641.
Schofield, J.C. (1970) Nature 228, 179-180.
Sundberg, D.K., Fawcett, C.P., Illner, P., and McCann, S.M. (1975)
     Proc. Soc. Exp. Biol. Med. 148, 54-59.
Tal, E., Szabo, M., and Burke, G. (1974) Prostaglandins 5, 175-182.
Tsafrini, A., Koch, Y., and Lindner, H.R. (1973) Prostaglandins 3,
     461-467.
Tucker, H.A., Vines, D.T., Stellflug, J.N., and Convey, E.M. (1975)
     Proc. Soc. Exp. Biol. Med. 149, 462-469.
Vale, W., Grant, G., Amoss, M., Blackwell, R., and Guillemin, R.
     (1972) Endocrinology 91, 562-572.
Yue, D.K., Smith, I.D., Turtle, J.R., and Shearman, R.P. (1974)
     Prostaglandins 8, 387-395.
Zor, U., Kaneko, T., Schneider, H.P.G., McCann, S.M., Lowe, I.P.,
     Bloom, G., Borland, B., and Field, J.B. (1969) Proc. Nat.
     Acad. Sci. U.S.A. 63, 918-925.
Zor, U., Kaneko, T., Schneider, H.P.G., McCann, S.M., and Field,
     J.B. (1970) J. Biol. Chem. 245 2883-2888.

ADRENERGIC AND CHOLINERGIC INPUTS TO THE AMYGDALA:

ROLE IN GONADOTROPIN SECRETION

J. Borrell,[x] F. Piva and L. Martini

Departments of Endocrinology and Pharmacology
University of Milano
21, Via Andrea Del Sarto, 20129 - Milano, Italy

Several data suggest that the limbic structures in general and the amygdala in particular may be involved in the regulation of LH and FSH secretion. On the basis of lesion and stimulation experiments, it has been postulated that, in adult animals, the amygdala may exert either stimulatory or inhibitory influences on gonadotropin release (for references, see: Schiaffini and Martini, 1972; Smith and Lawton, 1972; Kawakami and Terasawa, 1972; Karakami et al., 1973; Ellendorf et al., 1973; Kanematsu et al., 1974). A participation of the amygdala in the development of puberty has also been suggested (Critchlow and Bar-Sela, 1967), but this has been denied by others (Bloch and Ganong, 1971; Relkin, 1971 a and b). In addition, the hypothesis has been put forward that the amygdala might participate in the feedback mechanisms through which sex steroids control LH and FSH output (for references, see: Piva et al., 1973; McEwen and Pfaff, 1973; Terasawa and Kawakami, 1974; Parvizi and Ellendorf, 1975). Finally, it has been reported that the oxydative metabolism of the amygdala may be influenced by castration as well as by the administration of sex steroids and of anterior pituitary hormones (Schiaffini and Martini, 1972).

It is presently accepted that the amygdala receives adrenergic as well as cholinergic inputs from other parts of the brain (Ungerstedt, 1971; Eidelberg and Woodbury, 1972; Brownstein et al., 1974; Palkovits et al., 1974). Moreover, this structure is rich in choline acetyltransferase (Palkovits et al., 1974), and in monoamine oxydase; the activity of this enzyme fluctuates during the different phases of the estrous cycle (Kamberi, 1973). Adrenergic inputs

x Fellow of the March Foundation, Madrid, Spain

reaching the amygdala have been shown to play a role in the control of behavioral phemonena. Leaf et al. (1969) have found that norepinephrine placed in the amygdala inhibits the neurons mediating punishing behavior in the rat, and that this inhibitory activity disappears when the α-adrenergic receptor blocker phentolamine is implanted into this structure. Propranolol, a β-adrenergic receptor blocker, has been reported to be ineffective in this study.

The experiments to be described here have been planned in order to elucidate whether adrenergic and cholinergic signals arriving to the basomedial portion of the amygdala might take part in the control of gonadotropin secretion in the rat. The approach selected for these studies has been that of implanting bilaterally into the basomedial region of the amygdala of adult castrated female rats drugs known to affect adrenergic and cholinergic transmission. Serum levels of LH and FSH have been measured in the implanted animals at different intervals after the correct placement of the various drugs, and compared to those found, at similar intervals, in sham-implanted animals.

MATERIALS AND METHODS

Adult female rats of the Sprague-Dawley strain were used in all the experiments. They were castrated when weighing 160-170 g. Castrated animals have been preferred to normals in order to avoid the interference of the fluctuations of serum gonadotropin levels which are present in normally cycling females. However, it is recognized that the selection of this type of animal model might not be ideal, because the elevated serum levels of LH and FSH present in castrated animals (Zanisi and Martini, 1975 a and b) might mask the possible stimulatory effects on gonadotropin release possessed by some of the drugs used. The animals were caged under standard conditions, in rooms with controlled temperature and humidity. Lights were on for 14 hours per day, from 6.30 a m to 8.30 p m. The rats were fed a standard pellet diet: water was allowed ad libitum.

Cannulae bearing crystals of the different drugs were prepared by tamping 26-gauge stainless tubings into a mixture of the drug to be studied and cocoa butter (ratio 1:1) as reported previously (David et al., 1966). Excess material reamining on the external surface of the tubings was carefully removed. The cannulae were implanted bilaterally into the basomedial portion of the amygdala under pentobarbital anesthesia 4 weeks after castration. To this purpose the animals were mounted on a Stoelting stereotaxic instrument. The appropriate coordinates were selected according to the rat forebrain atlas of De Groot (1959). The needles were subsequently fixed to the skull with dental cement and remained in place until the animals were sacrificed. For sham-implantations, similar cannulae filled with cocoa butter alone were used.

Control and experimental animals were killed with a guillotine 3, 6, 12, 24, 48 and 72 hours after the end of the implantation procedure. At the moment of sacrifice, blood from the trunk vessels was collected. The sera were separated by centrifugation, and stored frozen until the moment of assay. Serum LH and FSH levels were measured using respectively the radiommunoassay procedures of Niswender et al., (1968) and of Daane and Parlow (1971). Each value given in the figures is the mean of at least 8 observations.

DRUG	PHARMACOLOGICAL EFFECT
PHENOXYBENZAMINE	α-Adrenergic blocker
PROPRANOLOL	β-Adrenergic blocker
CLONIDINE	α-Receptor stimulant
PIMOZIDE	Dopamine receptor blocker
2-BROMO-α-ERGOCRYPTINE (CB-154)	Dopamine receptor stimulant
PROSTIGMINE	Acetylcholinesterase inhibitor

Fig. 1

After sacrifice, the location of the tips of the cannulae was verified histologically. Only animals in which the cannulae were correctly placed in the basomedial region of the amygdala were retained.

The drugs which have been used in the present experiments and their more prominent pharmacological effect are summarized in Figure 1.

RESULTS AND DISCUSSION

In all figures the results are expressed in terms of the differences between the serum LH and FSH values found (at each time inter-

val considered). in the animals implanted with the different drugs
and those detected in the respective sham-implanted control
groups. The LH results are represented by the dark columns in the
upper panels, and the FSH values are represented by the stripped
columns in the lower panels. The white "boxes" around the "zero"
line represent the standard errors of the means of the values of
serum LH and FSH found in sham-implanted animals. The time intervals at which both sham- and drug-implanted animals have been killed are indicated on the abscissa. This procedure has been selected for expressing the results in order to facilitate their read-
ing in view of the fact that the anesthesia, the surgical manipu-
lations and the permanence of the cannulae in the amygdala have
induced a decrease of serum levels of the two gonadotropins (mainly
of LH) in sham-implanted animals.

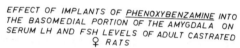

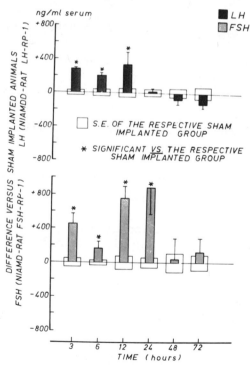

Fig. 2

Figure 2 summarizes the results obtained when the α-adrenergic receptor blocker phenoxybenzamine was implanted into the baso-medial portion of the amygdala. Animals killed 3, 5 and 12 hours after the placement of the drug have serum levels of LH significantly higher than those found in the respective controls. The effect of the drug was no more apparent 24, 48 and 72 hours after implantation. Phenoxybenzamine induced also an enhancement of serum titers of FSH which was already evident 3 hours after implantation of the drug into the basomedial region of the amygdala. In the implanted animals, serum levels of TSH were significantly higher than in controls also 6, 12 and 24 hours after implantation. The effect of the drug on FSH disappeared at later intervals. It is evident from a comparison of the upper and lower panels of Figure 2 that phenoxybenzamine placed in the basomedial portion of the amygdala seems to stimulate more the release of FSH than that of LH. From these results, one may infer that there are α-adrenergic receptors located in the basomedial portion of the amygdala. Since the blockade of these receptors brings about a stimulation of LH and of FSH release, one may argue that their physiological activation through adrenergic inputs arriving at the amygdala from other brain structures may exert an inhibitory influence on gonadotropin secretion.

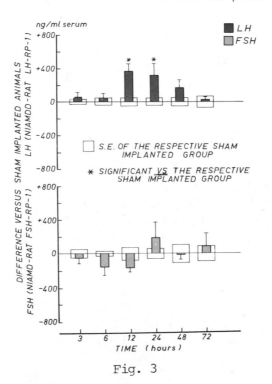

EFFECT OF IMPLANTS OF PROPRANOLOL INTO THE BASOMEDIAL PORTION OF THE AMYGDALA ON SERUM LH AND FSH LEVELS OF ADULT CASTRATED ♀ RATS

Fig. 3

Figure 3 shows the results obtained when propranolol, a blocker of β-adrenergic receptors, was implanted into the basomedial portion of the amygdala. It is clear that this drug induces a significant increase of LH release 12 and 24 hours after implantation, without influencing serum concentrations of FSH at any interval studied. These results may suggest that the basomedial region of the amygdala contains, in addition to α-adrenergic receptors, also β-adrenergic receptors. The physiological activation of these receptors appears to exert an inhibitory role on the release of LH.

The results of experiments in which an opposite type of approach was used are summarized in Figure 4. Clonidine, a compound known to stimulate selectively the α-adrenergic receptors, has been implanted into the basomedial region of the amygdala. It is apparent that this drug does not modify serum levels of either LH or FSH at any time considered. The results are not believed to contradict the hypothesis that α-adrenergic receptors located in the basomedial portion of the amygdala might play a role in the control

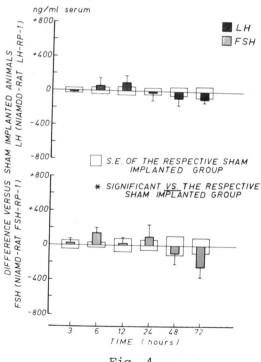

EFFECT OF IMPLANTS OF <u>CLONIDINE</u> INTO THE BASOMEDIAL PORTION OF THE AMYGDALA ON SERUM LH AND FSH LEVELS OF ADULT CASTRATED ♀ RATS

Fig. 4

of gonadotropin secretion. If one postulates that these α-adrenergic receptors are maximally activated, in normal conditions, by adrenergic inputs arriving to the amygdala, a negative result with the implantation of additional quantities of receptor stimulants is what one expects.

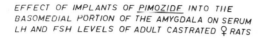

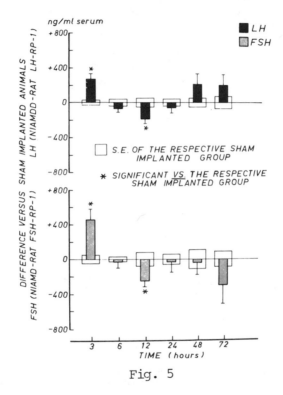

Fig. 5

The next series of esperiments has been devoted to analyse whether the basomedial region of the amygdala might possess also dopaminergic receptors involved in the control of gonadotropin secretion. To this purpose, the effects of intraamygdalar implants of the dopamine receptor blocker pimozide have been studied (Figure 5). The drug increases significantly the release of both LH and FSH 3 hours after implantation. On the contrary, serum levels of both gonadotropins are depressed 12 hours after the local placement of the drug. At any other time considered, serum levels of LH and FSH were not significantly different in the experimental and in the sham-operated animals. From these results, one may conclude that pimozide placed into the amygdala exerts a biphasic effect on gonadotropin output. This biphasic effect does not permit to derive firm conclusions on the possible role played by dopaminergic receptors located in the basomedial region of the amygdala in the control of gonadotropin release. It is possible that the biphasic effect of pimozide shown by the present experiments might be due to the fact that the drug does not act exclusively as a blocker of dopaminergic receptors. Pimozide has been shown to increase the turnover of both dopamine and norepinephrine (Anden <u>et al</u>., 1970).

In the hope of clarifying the role of intraamygdalar dopaminergic receptors, additional experiments were performed with 2-bromo-α-ergocryptine (CB-154), a specific, clean, and long-lasting dopaminergic receptor stimulant. Figure 6 shows that animals implanted in bhe basomedial portion of the amygdala with CB-154 have serum levels of LH significantly elevated above those of sham-implanted animals 24 and 72 hours after implantation. At all other

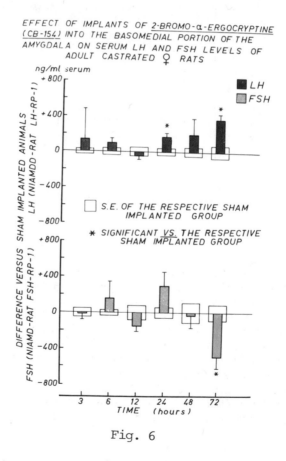

Fig. 6

intervals, serum LH titers were not different from those of the proper controls. CB-154 induced a significant decrease of serum FSH levels only when the hormone was measured 72 hours after the intra-amygdalar placement of the drug. The results obtained with CB-154, like those obtained with pimozide, show then some ambiguity. However, the two groups of results seem to suggest that also dopaminergic receptors important for the control of gonadotropin secretion might be present in the basomedial region of the amygdala.

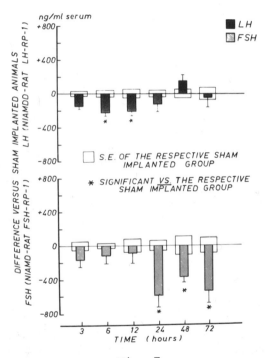

EFFECT OF IMPLANTS OF <u>PROSTIGMINE</u> INTO THE BASOMEDIAL PORTION OF THE AMYGDALA ON SERUM LH AND FSH LEVELS OF ADULT CASTRATED ♀ RATS

Fig. 7

The following figure (Figure 7) shows the results obtained after the implantation into the basomedial portion of the amygdala of prostigmine, a drug which inhibits the cholinesterases and which consequently acts as a cholinergic agonist. Prostigmine reduced significantly serum levels of LH 6 and 12 hours after implantation. FSH release was also inhibited 24, 48 and 72 hours after implantation. A comparison of the upper and the lower panels of Figure 7 suggests

that intraamygdalar implants of prostigmine might inhibit more effi-
ciently the release of FSH than that of LH. This series of experiments, alhtough preliminary in nature, suggests that also cholinergic
receptors present in the basomedial region of the amygdala might in-
tervene in the modulation of donadotropin release. The stimulation
of these receptors seems to inhibit the output of both LH and FSH.

CONCLUSIONS

     It emerges from the data that the basomedial portion of the
amygdala possesses several types of receptors which are involved
in the control of the secretion of anterior pituitary gonadotropins:
1) α-adrenergic receptors which seem to keep under an inhibitory
   tone LH and FSH release
2) β-adrenergic receptors which seem to exert an inhibitory influence on LH release.
3) dopaminergic receptors whose physiological role remains to be
   determined.
4) cholinergic receptors which seem to exert an inhibitory influence on the release of both gonadotropins.
Further studies are obviously needed in order to definitely assess
the physiological role played by each type of these receptors in
the mechanisms controlling gonadotropin secretion. In particular,
mechanisms controlling gonadotropin secretion. In particular, experiments similar to the ones here reportes should be performed in
normally cycling females, in prepuberal animals of both sexes, and
in adult male rats. These experiments are presently underway in
the Milano laboratory. Additional studies are also needed in order
to ascertain whether similar receptors might be present in other
districts of the amygdala.

     The results here reported indicated that an additional "sta-
tion" must be considered when interpreting the effects on gonadotropin secretion of the systemic administration of drugs which interfere with acetylcholine and catecholamines biosynthetis, action
and catabolism (Donoso et al., 1971; Kalra et al., 1972; Choudhury
et al., 1973; Ojeda and McCann, 1973; Kalra and McCann, 1974; Libertun and McCann, 1973, 1974; Ojeda et al., 1974; Justo et al.,
1975).

     It is interesting to note that the results here reported have
shown that, in several instances, the release of LH diverges from
the release of FSH (intraamygdalar implants of propranolol increase
LH release without affecting FSH release; CB-154 enhances LH release while diminishing FSH secretion, etc.). These results, like several other previously reported (Kalra et al., 1971; Motta et al.
1971, 1975; Zanisi et al, 1973; Zanisi and Martini, 1975 a and b),
are difficult to reconcile with the hypothesis that one single hy-

pothalamic releasing hormone might be responsible of the control of the two gonadotropins (Schally et al., 1971; Matsuo et al., 1971 a and b).

ACKNOWLEDGEMENTS

The experiments described in this paper have been supported by grants of the Ford Foundation, New York, of the Population Council, New York, and of the Consiglio Nazionale delle Richerche, Roma. All such support is gratefully acknowledged. Kits for LH and for FSH radioimmunoassay have been kindly provided by the Rat Pituitary Hormone Distribution Program of the National Institutes of Arthritis, Metabolism and Digestive Diseases of the National Institutes of Health. Thanks are also due to Mrs. Paola Assi Brunone for her skilful technical assistance.

REFERENCES

Anden, N.-E., Butcher, S.G., Corrodi, H., Fuxe, K. and Ungerstedt, U. (1970) Eur. J. Pharmacol. 11, 303-314.

Bloch, G.J. and Ganong, W.F. (1971) Endocrinology 89, 898-901.

Bronstein, M., Saavedra, J.M. and Palkovits, M. (1974) Brain Res. 79, 431-436.

Choudhury, S.A.R., Sharpe, R.M. and Brown, P.S. (1973) Neuroendocrinology 12, 272-283.

Critchlow, V. and Bar-Sela, M.E. (1967) In: Neuroendocrinology (L. Martini and W.F. Ganong, eds), vol. 2, Academic Press, New York, pp. 101-162.

Daane, T.A. and Parlow, A.F. (1971) Endocrinology 88, 653-663.

David, M.A., Fraschini, F. and Martini, (1966) Endocrinology 78, 55-60.

De Groot, J. (1959) Trans. Roy. Neth. Acad. Sci. 52, 1-40.

Donoso, A.O., Bishop, W., Fawcett, C.P., Krulich, L. and McCann, S.M. (1971) Endocrinology 89, 774-784.

Eidelberg, E. and Woodbury, C.M. (1972) In: The Neurobiology of the Amygdala (B.E. Eleftheriou, ed.) Plenum Press, New York.

Ellendorff, F., Colombo, J.A., Blake, C.A., Whitmoyer, D.I. and Sawyer, C.H. (1973) Proc. Soc. Exp. Biol. Med. 142, 417-420.

Justo, G., Motta, M. and Martini, L. (1975) Experientia 31, 598-599.

Kalra, P.S., Kalra, S.P., Krulich, L., Fawcett, C.P. and McCann, S.M. (1972) Endocrinology 90, 1168-1176.

Kalra, S.P. and McCann, S.M. (1974) Neuroendocrinology 15, 79-91.

Kalra, S.P., Ajika, K., Krulich, L., Fawcett, C.P., Quijada, M. (1971) Endocrinology 88, 1150-1158.

Kamberi, I.A. (1973) Progr. Brain Res. 39, 261-280.

Kanematsu, S., Scaramuzzi, R.J., Hilliard, J. and Sawyer, C.H. (1974) Endocrinology 95, 247-252.

Kawakami, M. and Terasawa, E. (1972) Endocrinol. Japon. 19, 335-347.

Kawakami, M., Terasawa, E., Kimura, F. and Wakabayashi, K. (1973) Neuroendocrinology 12, 1-16.

Leaf, R.C., Lerner, L. and Horovitz, J.P. (1969) In: Aggressive Behavior (S. Garattini and E.B. Siggs, eds.) Excerpta Medica, Amsterdam, pp. 120-131.

Libertun, C. and McCann, S.M. (1973) Endocrinology 92, 1714-1724.

Libertun, C. and McCann, S.M. (1974) Proc. Soc. Exp. Biol. Med. 147, 498-504.

Margules, D.L. (1971) Eur. J. Pharmacol. 16, 21-26.

Matsuo, H., Baba, Y., Nair, R.M.G., Arimura, A. and Schally, A.V. (1971 a) Biochem. Biophys. Res. Commun. 43, 1334-1344.

Matsuo, H., Arimura, A., Nair, R.M.G. and Schally, A.V. (1971 b) Biochem. Biophys. Res. Commun. 45, 822-827.

McEwen, B.S. and Pfaff, D.W. (1973) In: Frontiers in Neuroendocrinology (W.F. Ganong and L. Martini, eds.) vol. 3, Oxford University Press, New York, pp. 267-335.

Motta, M., Piva, F., Tima, L., Zanisi, M. and Martini, L. (1971) J. Neuro-Visc. Relat. Suppl. X, 32-40.

Motta, M., Daniels, E.L. and Martini, L. (1975) Endocr. Exp. 9, 3-9.

Niswender, G.D., Midgley, A.R., Jr., Monroe, S.E. and Reichert, L.E., Jr. (1968) Proc. Soc. Exp. Biol. Med. 128, 807-811.

Ojeda, S.R. and McCann, S.M. (1973) Neuroendocrinology 12, 295-315.

Ojeda, S.R., Harms, P.G. and McCann, S.M. (1974) Endocrinology 94, 1650-1657.

Palkovits, M., Saavedra, J.M., Kobayashi, R.M. and Brownstein, M. (1974) Brain Res. 79, 443-450.

Parvizi, N. and Ellendorff, F. (1975) Exp. Brain Res. 23, (Suppl.), 156.

Piva, F., Kalra, P.S. and Martini, L. (1973) Neuroendocrinology 11, 229-239.

Relkin, R. (1971 a) Endocrinology 88, 415-418.

Relkin, R. (1971 b) Endocrinology 88, 1272-1274.

Schally, A.V., Arimura, A., Baba, Y., Nair, R.M.G., Matsuo, H., Redding, T.W., Debeljuk, L. and White, W.F. (1971) Biochem. Biophys. Res. Commun. 43, 393-399.

Schiaffini, O. and Martini, L. (1972) Acta Endocr. 70, 209-219.

Smith, S.W. and Lawton, I.E. (1972) Neuroendocrinology 9, 228-234.

Terasawa, E. and Kawakami, M. (1974) Endocrinol. Japon. 21, 51-60.

Ungerstedt, U. (1971) Acta Physiol. Scand. Suppl. 367, 1-48.

Zanisi, M. and Martini, L. (1975 a) Acta Endocr. 78, 683-688.

Zanisi, M. and Martini, L. (1975 b) Acta Endocr. 78, 689-694.

Zanisi, M., Motta, M. and Martini, L. (1973) In: Hypothalamic Hypophysiotropic Hormones (C. Gual and E. Rosemberg, eds.) Excerpta Medica, Amsterdam, pp. 24-32.

NEUROTRANSMITTERS AND CONTROL OF PITUITARY FUNCTION

Claude Kordon, Micheline Hery and Alain Enjalbert

Unité de Neurobiologie, I.N.S.E.R.M., 2ter, rue

d'Alésia, 75014 Paris, France

In recent years, interaction of neurotransmitters with the release of neurohormones controlling anterior pituitary secretion has mainly been studied by histophysiological and pharmacological tools. The first approach led to the observation that neurotransmitter content of discrete aminergic tracts, particularly dopaminergic tubero-infundibular neurons, correlates with changes in neuroendocrine activity (Fuxe and Hokfelt, 1967; Luchtensteiger, 1969). Pharmacological studies then confirmed that experimental modulation of dopamine (DA) and also of noradrenalin (NA), serotonin (5-HT) and acetylcholine can affect pituitary hormone output (see reviews in Wurtman, 1971; Kordon and Glowinsky, 1972; Sawyer, 1975).

The most clear-cut involvement of an amine in adenohypophyseal regulation is represented by the DA-prolactin interaction. There is a general agreement that the amine is inhibitory to prolactin release under all conditions tested (Lu et al., 1973; Ojeda et al., 1973), and that this action can partly be accounted for by a direct impact on the pituitary itself (McLeod and Lehmwyer, 1974; Clemens et al., 1975).

The other effects of DA on hormone secretion, as derived from pharmacological experiments, are still controversial. Specificity of the pharmacological tools available for such studies is not entirely satisfactory, and the drugs used affect amine metabolism in the entire nervous system. This makes it almost impossible to distinguish primary neuroendocrine effects from indirect ones elicited by overall changes in neural activity. Such methodological limitations explain, for instance, why, in spite of extensive

research, the action of DA on gonadotropic secretion (Fuxe and Hokfelt, 1967; Luchtensteiger, 1969; Kordon et al., 1969; Rubinstein
and Sawyer, 1975), is still open to discussion. With these reser-
vations in mind, proposed DA effects can be summarized as being
likely to inhibit the release of growth hormone (Martin et al.,1973;
Muller et al., 1963) and ACTH (Ganong et al., 1972; Scapanini et
al., 1972). NA is also postulated to facilitate FSH and LH release
(Rubinstein and Sawyer, 1970). However, most of these conclusions
are still based on indirect pharmacological evidence and do not yet
meet general agreement.

In the present paper, we will concentrate on specific interactions between 5-HT and the phasic release of three pituitary hormones FSH, LH and prolactin.

Interaction of central 5-HT on the phasic release of FSH and LH

Inhibitory effects of 5-HT on LH release and ovulation have
been described by several authors, in particular after direct infusion of the amine into the cerebro-spinal fluid (Schneider and
McCann, 1970). A similar conclusion was obtained from experiments
on ovulation induced in immature female rats by pretreatment with
seric gonadotropins. Under these conditions, a pharmacological
increase of endogenous serotonin, but not of catecholamines, inhibits ovulation (Kordon et al., 1968). The impact of this effect
is very likely to occur at the level of the arcuate-median eminence
region.   This is suggested by reports that systemic injections
of 5-HT can block LH release (O'Steen, 1965), since the median eminence is the only neuroendocrine structure which lies outside the
blood brain barrier. Furthermore, micro-injection of drugs resulting in elevating the synaptic concentration of 5-HT are only effective when localized within the median basal hypothalamus (Kordon,
1971).

In contrast to this inhibitory action of 5-HT, long-term pharmacological inhibition of the biosynthesis of the amine has also
been shown to result in ovulation blockade (Hery et al., 1975a).
The possibility that this paradoxical effect could result from non
specific effects of the drugs used in such studies call for more
careful evaluation of this interaction. In particular, it is necessary to check whether this inhibition is really correlated with
changes in 5-HT extraneuronal release, and to investigate whether
other methods which deplete 5-HT content in nerve terminals (like
destruction of central serotoninergic cell bodies) would be equally
effective in blocking the phasic release of gonadotropic hormones.

Changes in pituitary sensitivity resulting from variations in
endogenous steroid circulating levels have been shown to play an
important role in the ovulatory release of gonadotropins in the

rat estrous cycle (Legan et al., 1973). In order to test elective effects of 5-HT on the neural mechanisms triggering pituitary
secretion, a preparation recently described by Chazal et al.,
(1974) and Legan et al. (1975) was used. It consists of castrated
females receiving a silastic implant of crystalline estradiol.
Under these conditions, circulating levels of the steroid have been
shown to remain constant over a prolonged period of time. Under
these conditions, the pituitary sensitivity to exogenous LH-RH no
longer varies as a function of time. As soon as 3 days after the
implantation of estradiol, there appears a circadian rhythm of FSH
and LH which lasts for at least 40 days.

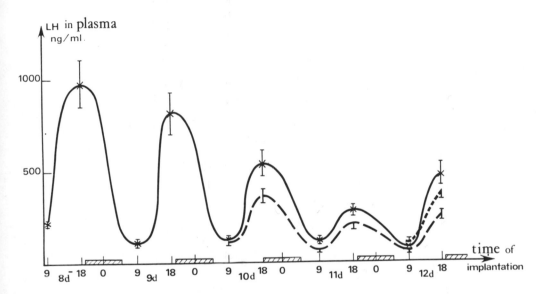

Figure 1:   Circadian release of LH in castrated estradiol
implanted females.

In the absence of changes in pituitary feedback sensitivity, such
changes can thus be assumed to depend only upon changes in the release rate of endogenous LH-RH (Chazal et al., 1974).

     The circadian FSH and LH release in castrated estradiol-implan-
ted female rats is abolished by treatment with the 5-HT synthesis
inhibitor p-chlorophenyl-alanine (PCPA), provided the drug is given
24 hours prior to the first expected hormonal surge (Hery et al.,
1975b). The inhibition remains as long as the synthesis of the
neurotransmitter is blocked (Koe and Weissman, 1966) and parallels
the depletion of the amine and of its oxydized metabolite, 5-hydro-
xy-indole acetic acid (5 HIAA). Restoration of normal concentrations

of the transmitter and metabolite by administration of the immediate precursor of 5-HT, 5 hydroxytryptophane (5-HTP), induces a paral-
le restoration of the capacity of the hypothalamo-hypophyseal
system to release FSH and LH. In this case, the effects of the
precursor on hypothalamic endogenous levels of 5-HT and 5-HIAA, on
one hand, and on the amplitude of the phasic gonadotropic variations, are well correlated (fig. 2) (Hery et al., 1975b).

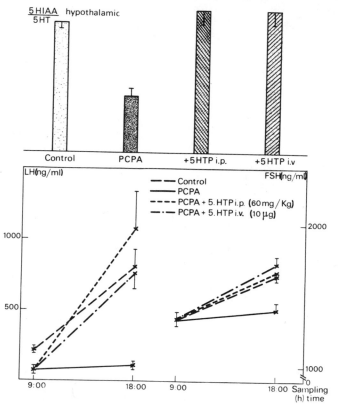

Figure 2: Effect of inhibition of serotonin by PCPA and of
its restoration by 5 HTP, on turnover of the amine, LH and
FSH secretion.

Destruction of serotoninergic neurons by two different methods ,
electrolytic lesion of the ventral and central Raphé nuclei or
transection of ascending serotoninergic projections in the mediobasal pontine region (Palkovits, unpublished data) - induced a very
marked depletion of hypothalamic 5-HT. However, the depletion of
the metabolite of the amine is greater after deafferentation than

after electrolytic lesion of the cell bodies. After such treatment,
the degree of 5-HIAA depletion also correlates well with the inhibition of FSH and LH circadian variations. Raphé lesions significantly reduce the afternoon rise in both hormones, while not completely abolishing the cycle itself. In contrast, a significant
rhythmical variation is no longer seen after baso-pontine transection (Fig. 3).

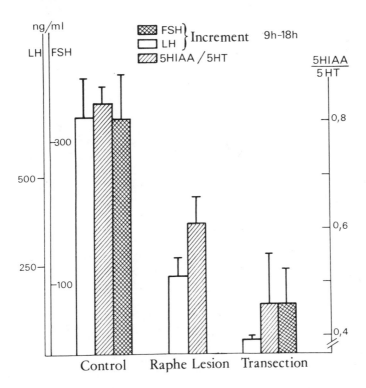

Figure 3: Effect of raphé nucleus lesion, and transection
of serotoninergic projections in the mediobasal pontine
region, on turnover of serotonin, LH and FSH secretion.

The concentration of 5-HIAA has been shown to be a reliable
index of 5-HT release, in particular under conditions where endogenous stores of the amine itself remain constant (Héry et al.,
1972). Thus, the fact that level of the metabolite is slightly
more elevated after Raphé lesions than after either pontine tran-
sections or pharmacological synthesis inhibition is suggestive
than some 5-HT-containing fibers projecting to the hypothalamus could
be spared by the lesion, and exhibit compensatory hyperactivity.
In this respect, it is of interest to observe that phasic gonado-

tropic release is totally abolished only when the levels of the metabolite are maximally inhibited. The fact that the hormonal release is better correlated with the release index of the transmitter than to the endogenous stores of the amine is a fair indication
that serotoninergic synaptic transmission is involved in the hormonal response. This is further substantiated by the parallelism
of 5-HT and 5-HIAA and phasic gonadotropic release in the pharmacological experiments.

It thus seems that the neural trigger which phasically activa-
tes neurosecretory effector neurons to release FSH/LH-RH under stea-
dy state conditions of steroid circulating levels depends upon a
facilitatory influence of serotoninergic neurons. The site of this
regulation differs from that of the inhibitory action of the amine,
which, as seen above, acts on the final common pathway of gonadotropin release-regulating structures. In view of the fact that
the delay at which serotonin inhibition has to be applied in order
to effectively block ovulation coincides well with the spontaneous
elevation of estradiol circulating levels within the estrous cycle,
it was hypothesized that 5-HT might interfere with estradiol receptors in the hypothalamus or the pituitary. However, this possibility could be ruled out on the basis of experiments showing that
the nuclear retention of [^{3}H] estradiol was not affected by experimental modulation of the neurotransmitters (Gogan and Rotsztejn,
1972). Since the suprachiasmatic nucleus is very rich in 5-HT terminals (Fuxe and Jonsson, 1974) and this structure is important for
the regulation of a number of circadian rhythms (like those affecting motor activity), it is tempting to speculate that 5-HT may
interact at that level with the circadian inputs to neuroendocrine
effector systems. However, this hypothesis awaits further confirmation.

Interaction of central 5-HT with phasic prolactin regulation

As demonstrated by several studies which have been referred
to above, tuberoinfundibular dopamine (DA) plays an important
role in the regulation of prolactin secretion. In addition, pharmacological data suggest that prolactin control also involves a
serotoninergic component; direct infusion of the amine into the
third ventricle has been reported to elevate plasma levels of the
hormone (Kamberi et al., 1971b).

The role of neurotransmitters in the hypothalamo-hypophyseal
response to nerve impulses which trigger the release of prolactin
has also been investigated. It is well known that the suckling stimulus induces a very rapid depletion of pituitary stores of the
hormone (Grosvenor et al., 1967) At the same time, it markedly
elevates plasma prolactin concentration. In this experimental
model, inhibition of the biosynthesis of 5-HT is able to block the
prolactin response to suckling (Kordon et al., 1973). As observed

in the case of LH regulation which was reported in the preceding section, administration of the immediate precursor of the transmitter restores the ability of lactating animals to respond to suckling by increased prolactin release. This observation suggests that 5-HT has a positive effect upon the response to this neural input.

In order to check whether this interaction of 5-HT with prolactin secretion is of physiological significance, the turnover of the neuro-transmitter was investigated in different brain structures at various time intervals after a suckling stimulus was applied to lactating rats. Two groups of lactating rats were used: in the first, mothers were separated from their pups for 8 hours, an interval after which prolactin release has been shown to be maximally stimulated by suckling. In the second, mothers were separated for 24 hours, a delay after which suckling no longer determines significant increases in plasma prolactin (Table 1).

Under conditions which permit prolactin release as a response to suckling, hypothalamic levels of 5-HT are decreased and 5-HIAA concentrations are increased in the hypothalamus 15 minutes after the onset of the stimulus. The ratio 5-HIAA/5-HT, which has been shown under experimental conditions to be a good index of the release rate of the transmitter, increases steadily over the first 15 minutes of suckling and remains elevated as long as the stimulus is applied (Fig. 4). No change in 5-HT or 5-HIAA can be observed in other brain structures under the same conditions. Moreover, the effect of suckling on release of the amine can no longer be observed under weaning conditions (after removing the pups for 24 hours) (Fig. 4). It thus seems that an increased turnover in serotinergic neurons correlates well with the prolactin response to suckling.

Surgical experiments suggest that the neural pathways which convey the information released by mammary stimulation involves two distinct neuronal systems. There are likely to be wired in parallel since destruction of either the bundle of Schütz (Beyer and Mena, 1965) or the median forebrain bundle (which carries most aminergic ascending projections) (Averill and Purves, 1966) do block evoked electrical responses following mammary stimulation within the pituitary stalk and the subsequent release of oxytocin. These experiments suggest that nerve impulses travelling across either one of these tracts are not sufficient in themselves to elicit the response of the neurosecretory neurons involved in prolactin control.

The respective contributions of these two neuronal systems is still a matter of speculation. The observation that pharmacological stimulation of serotoninergic afferents does not per se induce pro-

lactin release unless the suckling stimulus is concomitantly applied
makes it tempting to consider that 5-HT- containing projections to
the hypothalamus act by sensitizing hypothalamic neurons to specific information delivered by mammary stimulation. In the absence

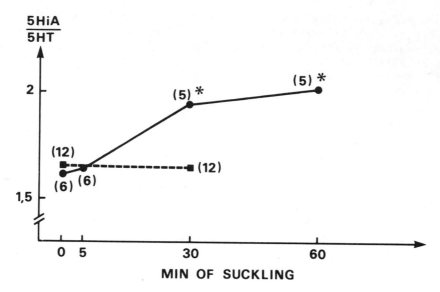

Figure 4:   Hypothalamic 5 HIAA/5 HT ratio at avrious intervals of suckling in mothers separated from their pups for
8 hours (fall line or 24 hours (dotted line). A significantly different from 0 time values. Nb. of animals in
( ).

of such sensitization, as for instance after pharmacological blockade of 5-HT biosynthesis or under weaning conditions, stimuli of
comparable intensity would no longer be able to reach threshold levels of prolactin stimulation.

CONCLUSIONS

In both examples presented, serotonin seems to play an important role in facilitating the response of hypothalamic neurons
responsible for triggering pituitary hormone release. In the first
case, the amine facilitates the transfer of a circadian input leading to gonadotropin release. A similar role of serotonin has
also been described in the case of the circadian variation of corti-
cotropic control. 5-HT synthesis inhibition blocks the daily fluctuation of ACTH and of corticosterone (Scapanini et al., 1972).

In the lactating rat, 5-HT facilitates the transfer of information of a different nature generated by activation of a well-defined neural pathway.

The precise sites of such interactions between synaptic 5-HT and neuroendocrine effector structures are still unclear. In the case of prolactin regulation, it will first be necessary to find out whether the amine exerts its effects by activating positive triggers of pituitary secretion (for instance, the release of TRH or a still hypothetical prolactin releasing factor) or alternately, by removing inhibitory influences which may involve dopamine or another factor antagonistic to the secretion of prolactin. In the case of gonadotropin control, the role of anterior hypothalamic structures, and particularly the supra-chiasmatic nucleus which has well defined regulatory influences on the determinism of the estrous cycle will have to be reassessed in the light of serotonergic innervation. Whatever answers will finally be offered, serotonin appears to have an important modulatory effect on hypothalamic sensitivity towards inputs which affect its neuroendocrine set point. This may be of interest in view of the suggestions that 5-HT may play an important role in synchronizing several centrally neuroal processes.

Table 1 - Effect of suckling on plasma prolactin levels

after various times of pup separation

Time of pup separation	8 hours		24 hours	
	Control	30'suckled	Control	30'sucked
Plasma Prolactin levels (ng/ml)	27 ± 6 (10)	405 ± 55(10)	35 ± 5(8)	30 ± 5(8)

Nb animals in parenthesis

REFERENCES

Averill, R.L. W. and M.D. Purves (1966) J. Endocr. 26, 463.

Beyer, C. and F. Mena (1965) Amer. J. Physiol. 208, 585.

Chazal, G., M. Faudon, F. Gogan, M. Hery and E. Laplante (1974) J. de Physiol. 68, 18b.

Clemens, J.A. (1975) In "Hypothalamus and Endocrine Functions" (F. Labrie, J. Meites and G. Pelletier, eds), Plenum Press, New York, in press.

Fuxe, K. and Hokfelt, H. (1967) In "Neurosecretion" (S. Sutinskyn, ed), Springer Verlag, p. 277.

Fuxe, K. and Jonsson, Y. (1974) Adv. in Biochem. Psychopharmacol. Vol. 10, Raven Press, New York.

Ganong, W.F. (1970) In "The Hypothalamus" (F. Fruschini, F. Mata and L. Martini, eds), Academic Press, New York, p. 313.

Gogan, F. and W. Rotsztejn (1972) Lille Médical 17, 1355.

Grosvenor, C.E., F. Mena and D.A. Schafgen (1967) Endocrinology 81, 449.

Hery, F., E. Rouer and J. Glowinski (1972) Brain Research 43, 445.

Hery, M., E. Laplante, E. Pattou and C. Kordon (1975a) Annales d'Endocrinologie 36, 123.

Hery, M., E. Laplante, and C. Kordon (1975b) Endocrinology, in press.

Kamberi, I.A., R.S. Mical and J.C. Porter (1971b) Endocrinology 88, 1288.

Koe, B.K. and A. Weissman (1966) The J. of Pharmacol. and Exp. Therapeutics 154, 499.

Kordon, C., F. Javoy, G. Vassent and J. Glowinski (1968) Europ. J. Pharmacol. 4, 169.

Kordon, C., and J. Glowinsky (1969) Endocrinology 85, 924.

Kordon, C. (1971) Neuroendocrinology 7, 202.

Kordon, C. and J. Glowinsky (1972) J. Neuropharmacol. 11, 153.

Kordon, C., C.A. Blake, J. Terkel and C.H. Sawyer (1973) Neuroendocrinology 13, 213.

Legan, S.J., L. Gay and A.R. Midgley (1973) Endocrinol. 93, 781.

Legan, S.J, G. Allyn Coon and F.J. Karsch (1975) Endocrinology 96, 50.

Luchtensteiger, W. (1969) 165, 204.

Lu, K.H. and Meites, J. (1973) Endocrinology 93, 152.

Martin, J.B., J. Counter and P. Mead (1973) Endocrinology 92, 1354.

McLeod, R., Lehmeyer, J.E. (1974) Endocrinology 94, 1077.

Muller, E.E., P. Dal Pra and A. Pecile (1963) Endocrinology 83, 893.

Ojeda, J.R. and S.M. McCann (1973) Neuroendocrinology 12, 295.

O'Steen, W.K. (1965) Endocrinology 77, 937.

Rubinstein, L. and Sawyer, C.H. (1970) Endocrinology 86, 988.

Sawyer, C.H. (1975) Neuroendocrinology 17, 97.

Scapanini, V., M.P. Van Loan, M.D., G.P. Moberg, P. Preziosi, and W.F. Ganong (1972) 10, E-155.

Schneider, H.P.G. and S.M. McCann (1970) Endocrinology 86, 1127.

Wurtman, R.J. (1971) Rec. Prog. Brit. 9, 172.

Clinical Applications of LH—RH and TRH

STUDIES ON THE DIAGNOSTIC USE OF LH-RH

J. Guy Rochefort, A. Chapdelaine, G. Tolis and
J. Van Campenhout

Department of Clinical Pharmacology, Ayerst Laboratories;
Section Endocrinologie, Département de Médecine, Hôpital
Maisonneuve; Endocrinology Section, Department of
Gynecology and Obstetrics, Royal Victoria Hospital;
Départment d'Obstétrique-gynécologie, Hôpital Notre-
Dame; Montreal, Quebec, Canada

Numerous studies involving the administration of
natural or synthetic HL-RH to normal subjects and to patients with
various endocrinopathies have been published in the past few years.
A recent review summarizes some of the available data (Yen, 1975).

Amongst others, it had been a hope that the parenteral administration of LH-RH to hypogonadal patients would function as a
diagnostic test to delineate between hypothalamic and anterior
pituitary dysfunction, as well as to demonstrate the presence of
a pituitary gonadotropic reserve (Schally et al., 1971). The
demonstration of functional gonadotropic tissue and of gonadotropic
reserve can be satisfactorily established with the use of the
LH-RH test (Besser et al., 1972; Harsoulis et al., 1973; Antaki
et al., 1974; Taymor, 1974). Although there is now general agreement that the LH-RH test cannot per se distinguish between a pituitary and hypothalamic disorder (Mortimer et al., 1973), nonethe-
less, utilized concomittantly to clinical observations and other
diagnostic procedures, it can provide very valuable information as
to identification of the disorder and the choice of proper therapeutic measures (Lunenfeld, 1973; Ginsberg et al., 1975; Wentz et
al., 1975).

Recent data have indicated that in patients with a negative
response to the standard 100 mcg diagnostic test, the chronic
administration of larger doses of LH-RH induced over time a positive
response of pituitary secretion of gonadotropins, as well as end

organs stimulation and clinical improvement (Besser, 1974; Mortimer
et al., 1974; Yoshimoto et al., 1975). In continuation of previous
studies (Borreman et al., 1975; Van Campenhout et al., 1974) we had
initiated somewhat similar studies to explore this possibility of
overcoming the negative response and of obtaining testicular or
ovarian stimulation in patients. The data obtained to discontinuation of these studies is presented herein as well as preliminary
results on the chronic administration of LH-RH to a series of
female patients with secondary amenorrhea.

The studies were done according to methods previously published (Antaki et al., 1974; Van Campenhout, 1975; Tolis et al.,
1974). In all cases, LH-RH (Ayerst) was administered subcutaneously
or intramuscularly. The plasma hormone assays were carried out
by the individual hospital's laboratory, which accounts for the
difference in reporting units. Since the studies were considered
exploratory and were discontinued, no attempt was made to equate
the data between clinics.

In Table I are presented the results of administrating
large doses of LH-RH to four hypogonadal patients. The patients,
selected as representative of four clinical conditions, each
received a course of 1 mg of LH-RH subcutaneously, every twelve
hours, for a period of seven days. In all four patients, noteworthy is the improvement in the level of circulating testosterone.
This was particularly striking in patient F.D. whose testosterone
levels rose from 185 ng/dl at beginning of treatment, to 580 ng/dl
prior to the last dose of LH-RH on day 7 of administration. Noted
also, except in patient G.P., were increases in plasma testosterone
within six hours following LH-RH administration, concomittant to
the rises in circulating gonadotropins.

In normal males, the intramuscular administration of 1 mg of
LH-RH induced an increase in plasma LH and FSH, as well as in plasma
testosterone, as shown in Table II. Similar results had been obtained previously with the subcutaneous administration of 1 mg of
LH-RH (Bremner et al., 1972). Two modalities of LH-RH administration were attempted in two patients with hypogonadotropic hypogonadism. One patient received a single daily injection of 1 mg LH-RH
for seven days; the other received twice daily injections of LH-RH
for seven days. The results are presented in Table III. Both
patients responded to treatment; the stronger results were seen in
patient R.S. who received LH-RH twice daily. On day 7 of treatment,
this patient had plasma testosterone levels within the normal range
for adult males.

Because these two sets of data generally indicated that the
parenteral administration of large doses of LH-RH produced in male
hypogonad patients an improved primary and secondary response

TABLE I: PLASMA HORMONAL RESPONSES TO SUBCUTANEOUS LH–RH IN
           MALE HYPOGONAD PATIENTS

PATIENT	TIME (min)	LH mIU/ml**	FSH	T* ng/dl	LH mIU/ml**	FSH	T* ng/dl
M.B. (Age 17) Delayed Puberty		(100µg s.c., Day 0)			(1000µg s.c., Day 7)		
	0	17.2	3.9		8.7	3.6	81
	30	34.5	5.6		17.0	4.0	
	45	39.7	5.9		17.0	4.3	
	60	43.5	5.9		18.0	4.2	
	120	43.5	6.3		12.0	3.4	78
	180						155
	240						192
G.P. (Age 19) Leydig Cell Defic- iency		(100µg s.c., Day 0)			(1000µg s.c., Day 7)		
	0	13.6	2.9	45	26.2	7.8	103
	30	19.9	2.8		31.0	7.6	
	45	15.1	3.3		24.0	6.8	
	60	15.8	3.3		29.0	9.6	
	90	15.0	3.0		30.0	7.8	
	120	22.6	3.3		24.0	7.8	120
R.B. (Age 39) 2° Hypogo- nadism		(100µg s.c., Day 1)			(1000µg s.c., Day 7)		
	0	10.7	1.8	83	7.0	2.6	103
	30	12.7	2.1		12.0	3.6	
	60	13.7	2.2		31.5	3.6	
	120	11.3	2.1		56.0	4.2	162
	180	10.5	2.7	160	56.0	4.2	
	240	9.7	2.6		65.0	4.4	151
F.D. (Age 20) 1° Hypogo- nadism		(500µg s.c., Day 0)			(1000µg s.c., Day 7)		
	0	3.1	3.8	185	9.2	6.2	580
	30	5.6	6.0		17.5	7.3	
	60	9.0	5.0		18.0	9.6	
	120	9.3	5.0	170	17.5	18.8	
	180	15.8	4.9	175	26.2	10.4	4600
	240						1010

* T = testosterone ** mIU/ml, 2nd I.R.P. - HMG.

in general agreement with the data of Mortimer et al., (1974),
further studies were discontinued.

TABLE II: PLASMA HORMONAL RESPONSES TO 1 MG INTRAMUSCULAR LH–RH IN NORMAL MALE SUBJECTS.

TIME	LH μg/ml*	FSH μg/ml*	Testosterone ng/dl
0 min	7.5±2.0	14.2±1.9	662±68
30 min	50.4±6.4	27.9±6.8	
60 min	43.8±5.9	26.2±5.3	
120 min	33.6±3.4	26.8±4.6	842±55
240 min	19.1±2.8	21.6±3.4	
360 min	14.6±1.6	23.9±3.6	759±65
24 hrs	5.9±1.2	14.9±2.9	670±36

* mean ± standard error of the mean, for 8 subjects, in μg/ml equivalents of LER 907 standard.

TABLE III: PLASMA HORMONAL RESPONSES TO INTRAMUSCULAR LH–RH IN TWO MALE HYPOGONADOTROPIC HYPOGONAD PATIENTS.

PATIENT Dosing	TIME after dose (min)	DAY 1 LH	FSH μg/ml**	T* μg/dl	DAY 7 LH	FSH μg/ml**	T* ng/dl
P.L.	0	4.2	10.5	75	7.5	14.0	103
Age 24	30	13.0	18.0		17.0	23.0	
1000 μg,	60	13.0	22.0		19.0	19.0	
i.m.	120	13.0	26.0	41	10.0	18.0	155
once	240	9.6	27.0		11.0	15.0	
daily	360	8.8	21.0	38	5.8	18.0	108
R.S.	0	<1	13.0	76	<1	50	760
Age 26	30	20.0	17.0		15.0	50	
1000 μg,	60	17.0	27.0		12.0	21	
i.m.	120	14.0	42.0	95	11.0	46	670
twice	240	9.8	33.0		3.7	46	
daily	360	2.0	42.0	148	<1	50	610

* T = testosterone   ** ng/ml, equivalents of LER 907 standard.

We investigated also whether the administration of LH–RH to secondary amenorrheic patients could stimulate ovarian steroido-genesis. In a series of four secondary amenorrheic patients, all

TABLE IV: PLASMA HORMONAL RESPONSES OF IDIOPATHIC SECONDARY
AMENORRHEIC PATIENTS TO NINE CONSECUTIVE 500 µg
DOSES OF SUBCUTANEOUS LH-RH

PATIENTS	TIME	DOSE NO. 1			DOSE NO. 9		
		LH mIU/ml	FSH mIU/ml	E$_2$* pg/ml	LH mIU/ml	FSH mIU/ml	E$_2$* pg/ml
D.D. (Age 22)	0	20.3	8.8	86	39.9	21.9	716
	30	176.3	19.0		143.2	24.5	
	60	70.3	27.5		83.8	47.5	
	120	73.2	33.5		100.4	53.2	
	240	71.5	28.0		155.9	49.0	
	360	51.3	23.6		107.8	50.7	
C.W. (Age 22)	0	11.0	6.3	60	11.0	5.6	64
	30	20.4	12.0		37.0	16.8	
	60	22.0	15.2		34.3	12.0	
	120	48.5	20.0		44.8	11.8	
	180	50.0	24.2		27.4	10.8	
	240	37.0	35.0		21.5	11.0	
	360	21.5	22.8	96	19.6	12.0	81
C.R. (Age 19)	0	16.9	11.2	155	18.9	7.4	71
	30	41.6	13.6		42.1	11.2	
	60	117.9	42.9		42.8	12.5	
	90	122.9	46.1		37.9	12.3	
	120	74.1	41.7	47	26.2	10.4	33
	240	54.2	24.1		19.2	4.3	
	360	40.4	25.9		-	-	
M.T. (Age 23)	0	11.9	7.9	43	27.2	9.3	72
	30	27.8	11.6		26.9	10.1	
	60	28.2	11.6		26.9	10.1	
	60	28.2	16.7		28.6	9.7	
	120	27.7	17.6	19	26.6	10.5	54
	240	24.0	22.9		18.8	8.6	
	360	19.0	17.3		15.5	7.9	

*E$_2$= Estradiol

of whom had demonstrated an adequate response to the standard 100
mcg diagnostic test, doses of 500 mcg of LH-RH were administered
every 12 hours for four days. The data are presented in Table IV.
Somewhat surprisingly, notwithstanding adequate responses in LH
and FSH, no increases in circulating estrogens were obtained except
in patient D.D., whose levels rose from 86 pg/ml to 716 pg/ml.
These data should be compared to the recent results of Nillius and
Wide,(1975) and Nillius et al., (1975), which established that the

administration of 500µg of LH-RH every 8 hours for twenty-eight days induced follicular development and steroidogenesis in secondary amenorrheic patients. It appears that large doses of LH-RH must be administered repeatedly to obtain sustained gonadotropins secretion and eventually, steroidogenesis with its physiological consequences. This hypothesis must be further evaluated and possible differences in responses between various types of male and female hypogonadism clearly delineated.

In summary, the use of LH-RH as a diagnostic test in adult hypogonadism is helpful not only to verify the presence of a gonadotropic reserve, but also, concurrently to other established clinical and laboratory procedures, to delineate pituitary from hypothalamic dysfunction. Ongoing studies in juvenile patients (Chaussain et al., 1974; Job et al., 1974 a,b; Reiter et al., 1975, a,b; Sato et al., 1974) are directed towards establishing the diagnostic and prognostic utility of the procedure in pediatric endocrinopathies. The possibilities of determining therapeutic modalities for the compound are suggested by our results and by those of Mortimer et al., (1975), Nillius and Wide (1975), and Nillius et al., (1975).

It is to be expected that at the next Symposium on Hypothalamus and Endocrine Functions, more definitive statements on these uses of LH-RH will be made.

REFERENCES

Antaki, A., Chapdelaine, A., Van Campenhout, J. and Rochefort, J.G., (1974), Union Med. Canada, 103, 1191-1200.

Besser, G.M., McNeilly, A.S., Anderson, D.C., Marshall, J.C., Harsoulis, P., Hall, R., Ormston, B.J., Alexander, L. and Collins, W.P., (1972), Brit. Med. J., 3, 267-271.

Besser, G.M., (1974), Brit. Med. J., 3, 613-615.

Borreman, E., Wyman, H., Rochefort, J.G. and Van Campenhout, J., (1975), Am. J. Obstet. Gynecol., 123, 580-589.

Bremner, W.A., Paulsen, C.A. and Rochefort, J.G. (1972), unpublished observations, Ayerst Research Laboratories.

Chaussain, J.L., Garnier, P.E., Binet, E. and Job, J.C. (1974), J. Clin. Endocrinol. Metab., 38, 58-63.

Ginsberg, J., Isaacs, A.J., Gore, M.B.R. and Havard, C.W.H., (1975), 3, 130-133.

Harsoulis, P., Marshall, J.C., Kuku, S.F., Burke, C.W., London, D.R. and Fraser, T.R., (1973), Brit. Med. J., 4, 326–329.

Job, J.C., Garnier, P.E., Chaussain, J.L., Scholler, R., Toublanc, J.E., and Canlorbe, P., (1974), 38, 1109–1114.

Job, J.C., Garnier, P.E., Chaussain, J.L., Toublanc, J.E. and Canlorbe, P., (1974), J. Pediatr., 84, 371–374.

Lunenfeld, B., Kohen, F., Eshkol, A., Beer, R., Zuckerman, Z., Birnbaum, N. and Glezerman, M., (1973), in: The Endocrine Function of the Human Testis (James, V.H.T., Serio, M., and L. Martini, eds.), Academic Press Inc., New York and London, pp. 561–584.

Mortimer, C.H., Besser, G.M., McNeilly, A.S., Marshall, J.C., Harsoulis, P., Turnbridge, W.M.G., Gomez-Pan, A. and Hall, R., (1973), Brit. Med. J., 4, 73–77.

Mortimer, C.H., McNeilly, A.S., Fisher, R.A., Murray, M.A.F., and Besser, G.M., (1974), Brit. Med. J., 4, 617–621.

Nillius, S.J. and Wide, L., (1975), Brit. Med. J., 3, 405–408.

Nillius, S.J., Fries, H. and Wide, L., (1975), Am. J. Obstet. Gynecol., 122, 921–928.

Reiter, E.O., Grumbach, M.M., Kaplan, S.L. and Conte, F.A., (1975a), J. Clin. Endocrinol. Metab., 40, 318–325.

Reiter, E.O., Kaplan, S.L., Conte, F.A. and Grumbach, M.M., (1975b), Pediatric Res., 9, 111–116.

Sato, T., Inoue, M., Masuyama, T., Suzuki, Y., and Izumisawa, A., (1974), J. Clin. Endocrinol. Metab., 39, 595–599.

Schally, A.V., Kastin, A.J. and Arimura, A., (1971), Fertil. Steril., 22, 703–721.

Taymor, M.L., (1974), Fertil. Steril., 25, 992–1005.

Tolis, G., Cruess, S., Goldstein, M., Friesen, H.G., and Rochefort, J.G., (1974), Can. Med. Assoc. J., 111, 553–556

Van Campenhout, J., Rochefort, J.G. and Chapdelaine, A., (1974), in "Rapport du 25e Congrès de la Fédération des Sociétés de Gynécologie et d'Obstètrique de Langue Française", (Vokaer, R., ed.), Desbergers Ltée, Montreal, pp 24–43.

Wentz, A.C., Jones, G.S., Rocco, L. and Matthews, R.R., (1975), Obstet. Gynecol., 45, 256-262.

Yen, S.S.C., (1975), Ann. Rev. Med., 26, 403-417.

Yoshimoto, Y., Moridera, K. and Imura, H., (1975), N. Engl. J. Med., 292, 242-245.

DIAGNOSTIC AND THERAPEUTIC USE OF LH-RH

IN THE INFERTILE MAN

Luis Schwarzstein

G.E.F.E.R. (Grupo de Estudios en Fertilidad y
Endocrinologia de Rosario)
Cordoba 1764, Rosario, Argentina

I would first like to acknowledge the organizers of this Symposium for their kind invitation. I am highly honoured by the opportunity given to me to join my efforts to those of colleagues working in the same field.

As an introduction, I should like to make a brief outline of the general knowledge which held the field of pathophysiologic interpretation and treatment of male infertility before the availability of LH-RH.

The cause of male infertility could be ascribed to a deficiency of gonadotrophic secretion (hypogonadotrophic hypogonadism) and urologic factors, as the most common etiology and also to specific testicular damage due to chromosomal, genetical, infectious and other causes, or several diseases or external factors, as well as clinical extragonadal diseases with alteration at the seminiferous tubular level.

However, it was not possible to find an explanation for several cases of oligospermia in the absence of evident modifications of the basal gonadotrophic levels. This last group, idiopathic normogonadotrophic oligospermia (I.N.O.) is still lacking a known etiology and its pathophysiology and treatment remain, up till now, as a gap in the knowledge of modern reproduction and endocrinology. I am not going to deal with immunological factors, since they form a vast and specific field in themselves.

Treatment of I.N.O. was based on the assumption that over-stimulation of the hypothalamo-hypophyseal-gonadal axis would lead to

73

an improvement of spermatogenesis. However, several patients treated with different treatment schemes, suitable for that purpose,
failed to reach success. An approach to the prognosis of therapeutical possibilities was based on histological findings of the testis (Meinhard et al., 1973; Schwarzstein, 1974; Schwarzstein et al.,
1975 a, b; Aafjes and Van Der Vijver, 1974). As a group, much better results are obtained in patients with less damage at the tubular level, as it can be seen in Figure 1 describing treatment of
patients treated with HMG. These data could have been predicted
since it is reasonable to expect a better therapeutical result
among patients with less damage.

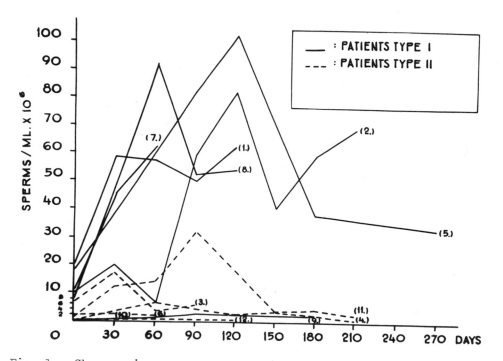

Fig. 1:   Changes in sperm concentration during treatment with HMG
          in 12 oligospermic subjects.
          Type 1 patients: Hypospermatogenesis or arrest up to the
                           spermatid stage.
          Type II patients:Arrest at spermatocyte I or spermatogo-
                           nial stages.

However, there are several patients, without a very severe damage,
in whom therapy is ineffective and on the other hand, in few pa-

tients having more severe damage, sometimes unexpected good results
are obtained.   All these facts face us with the necessity for a
better knowledge of the physiopathology of this disease.

The availability of LH-RH made the exploration of the hypophy-
seal-gonadal axis possible by means of a specific stimulus at the
pituitary level.   When we started investigations with LH-RH in male
infertility, we asked the following questions:

1. What was the dynamic response of LH, FSH and testosterone (T)
   in normal men?

2. Was there any difference between the responses of a normal population and patients with I.N.O.?

3. In case of a possible therapeutical application of LH-RH, what
   was the most proper dose to be used?

4. What would be the schemes of treatment to be used and what results to expect?

A few months ago, Dr. Andrew V. Schally gave us the opportunity
to use an analog of LH-RH, D-Leucine[6]-LH-RH-ethylamide and we could
then ask the above-mentioned questions with this new and more potent agent.

We will thus try to present our results following the order of
questions previously mentioned.

(1, 2) Dynamic response of normal subjects and oligospermic men to synthetic LH-RH

In a previous study (Schwarzstein et al., 1975 c), we demonstrated a circadian variation of the pituitary response to LH-RH.
Better responses were obtained during the morning hours, a fact
experimentally confirmed later by Debeljuk et al. (1975).   In that
study, we also showed that, in the presence of a normal LH rise
after LH-RH, significant increments of T occurred 16' to 30' after
the LH-RH injection.   Following this study, we performed a trial in
which we compared LH, FSH and T responses to a 50 µg I.V. LH-RH injection at 8 a.m. in normal and oligospermic men.

In figure 2, average responses in both groups can be seen.   Under these experimental conditions, the response in normal men is
characterized by increments of LH and FSH above 100% the basal values.

The minimal individual post-stimulatory levels of LH and FSH

were 15 and 12 mUI/ml, respectively T also showed increments of
generally more than 100% with post-stimulatory levels of no less
than 9 ng/ml.

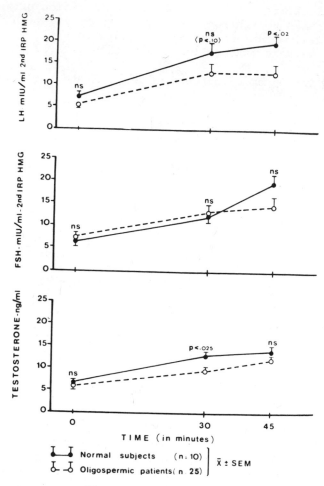

Fig. 2:   Serum levels ($\bar{x}$ ± S.E.M.) of LH, FSH and T basal (time 0)
          at 30 and 45 minutes after I.V. injection of 50 µg of LH-
          RH at 8 a.m. in 10 normal and 25 oligospermic men. The
          significance given on the graph corresponds to comparison
          between both groups (t tests for non-paired samples). Hor-
          monal levels at 30 and 45 minutes were significantly dif-
          ferent from those at time 0 in all cases (p < 0.001).

     Spontaneous variations of basal levels of LH and FSH are shown
in Figure 3. As it can be seen, neither the normal nor the oligospermic subjects have values above the mentioned figures. This
fact allows us to presume that post-stimulatory values found in

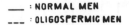

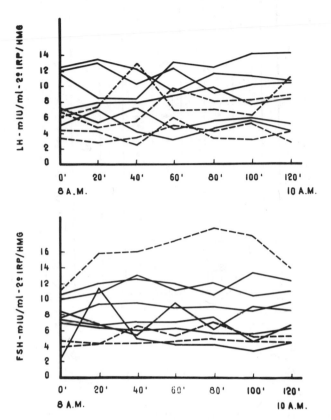

Fig. 3: Pulsatile secretion of LH and FSH in 9 normal and 4
         oligospermic subjects.

         Samples were taken every 20 minutes between 8 A.M. and
         10 A.M.

the patients studied can be attributed to the specific stimulus
used and not to spontaneous fluctuations.

    I.N.O. men had similar average basal values for the three hor-
mones, but post-stimulatory values showed significant differences
of LH and T between normal and oligospermic subjects.

    Figure 4 illustrates the individual values of LH. It seems
that the differences commented are due to a group of patients who
respond less than the normal group.

    In figure 5 T. individual values can be observed. Similarly,
a group of patients also responded with low T values. However,

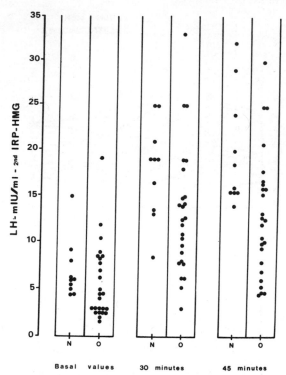

Fig. 4: Distribution of individual serum levels of LH, basal and 30 and 45 minutes after I.V. injection of 50 μg of LH-RH at 8 A.M. in 10 normal (N) and 25 oligospermic men (O).

these patients did not always correspond with those with low levels of LH, the correlation coefficient for both hormones being of 0.47.

These facts suggest that some of the so-called I.N.O. patients could have a latent impairment of their pituitary functional reserve and/or a latent alteration of the Leydig cell function. This last fact was previously suggested by Mecklemburg and Scherins (1974).

A correlation of these results with the testicular histology (both optical and ultrastructural) is now being performed.

In conclusion, the above findings show that, by means of an acute LH-RH test, it would be possible to separate different entities from the group of I.N.O. patients or, at least, to differentiate developmental stages of the disease.

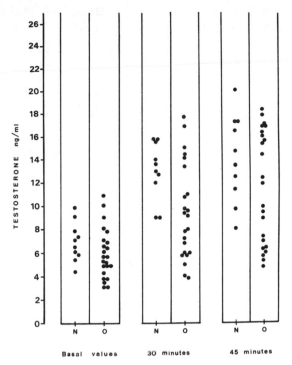

Fig. 5:   Distribution of individual serum levels of T under basal
          conditions and 30 and 45 minutes after I.V. injection of
          LH-RH at 8 a.m. in 10 normal (N) and 25 oligospermic (O)
          men.

(3) Dose of LH-RH and D-Leucine[6]-LH-RH-ethylamide to be used for
     treatment

     We can see in Fig. 6 the LH and FSH responses to I.M. LH-RH in-
jection at 4 doses of the neurohormone.

     As it can be seen, maximal responses are obtained by using 250
µg. With 500 µg, the responses were the same or even lower (Turner
et al., 1975).

     In Figure 7, the LH, FSH and T responses to the I.M. injection
of 2.5, 5, 10 or 20 µg of D-leucine[6]-LH-RH-ethylamide are shown.

     In this case, a dose-response relationship for both gonadotro-
pins was seen (r = 0.96 for LH and r = 0.99 for FSH). Maximal responses were obtained with 20 µg between the 4th and 6th hour after
the I.M. injection. T also showed a dose-response relationship
(r = 0.94). However, values obtained with 10 and 20 µg did not

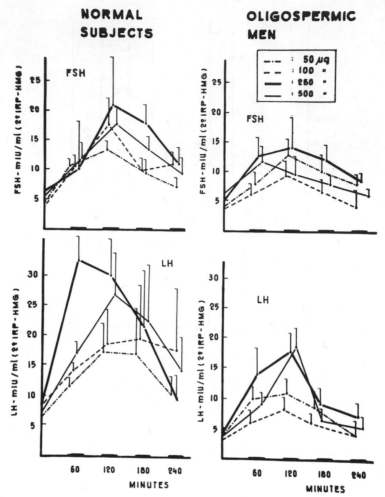

Fig. 6: Dose-response study to I.M. injection of LH-RH in normal and oligospermic men

differ significantly. The response of T showed a trend to stabilization at higher doses.

Another interesting observation emerging from these results is that maximal post-stimulatory values did not correlate significantly with the respective basal values. Although maximal values of FSH and LH obtained under the lowest (2.5 µg) and the highest (20 µg) dose of D-Leucine[6]-LH-RH-ethylamide correlated significantly, it did not occur for T. These results suggest that these patients have an individual pattern of pituitary response to the stimulus. The testicular response, on the contrary, seems to have a maximal threshold, in spite of very high gonadotropic stimulation.

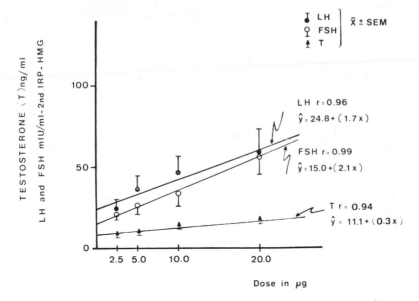

Fig. 7:   Response of LH, FSH and Testosterone to increasing doses of [D-leucine[6]] LH-RH-ethylamide

LH and FSH show increasing responses with maximal values after 20 µg. No significant difference exist between maximal and minimal average responses of LH, while for FSH the response after 20 µg differs significantly from those obtained with 2.5 and 5 µg.

Testosterone shows, however, a high correlation coefficient.

These facts seem to be confirmed when we correlate the LH, FSH and T maximal responses to LH-RH with those obtained with the analog. As it can be seen in Fig. 8, correlation between both responses are very significant for LH ($r = 0.72$) and for FSH ($r = 0.79$), but not for T ($r = -0.34$). These results seem to validate the hypothesis that it is possible to separate groups from the I.N.O. subjects by means of the dynamic bipolar exploration at the pituitary and gonadal levels although basal values do not differ.

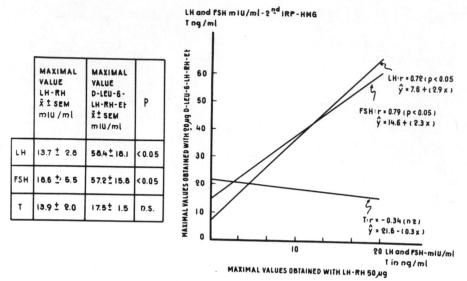

	MAXIMAL VALUE LH-RH $\bar{X} \pm$ SEM mIU/ml	MAXIMAL VALUE D-LEU-6- LH-RH-Et $\bar{X} \pm$ SEM mIU/ml	P
LH	13.7 ± 2.8	58.4 ± 18.1	< 0.05
FSH	18.6 ± 5.5	57.2 ± 15.8	< 0.05
T	13.9 ± 2.0	17.5 ± 1.5	n.s.

Fig. 8 :   Correlation between maximal responses of LH, FSH and
Testosterone obtained after injection of 20 µg of
[D-Leucine[6]]-LH-RH-ethylamide or 50 µg of LH-RH.

Average values and levels of significance are also
shown. Average results for LH and FSH were significantly higher after [D-leucine[6]] LH-RH-ethylamide,
while for testosterone, no significance was obtained.
Maximal values of LH and FSH correlated significantly
and positively, while for testosterone, the correlation
was not significant.

      As a final remark of diagnostic and prognostic implications
of LH-RH (and possibly of the analog), I should like to mention
that correlating therapeutical results with those of the acute
test in a trial that we are carrying on, high FSH responses and/
or low T responses in the presence of normal LH responses seem to
be associated with the worst therapeutical results. Further studies are however needed to confirm these first findings.

(4) Therapeutic use of LH-RH and of [D-Leucine[6]] -LH-RH ethylamide

According to the dose-response study already mentioned, we treated 21 patients with LH-RH according to two different schemes of treatment:

a) Long-term, that is at least 90 days of daily I. M. administration; and
b) Short-term, that is a 30- to 45-day course of treatment separated one from each other by intervals of one month.

Patients incorporated into the study were classified according to their testicular histology in two groups:

Group 1: presenting quantitative alterations of spermatogenesis or qualitative alterations up to the spermatid stage; and
Group 2: with more severe alterations of spermatogenesis up to spermatocyte I or spermatogonial stage.

Fourteen patients were included in Group 1 and seven in Group 2 (Table I). As it can be seen in Table 1, motility and vitality parameters did not differ between groups, but the number of sperms/ ml was significantly lower ($p < 0.05$) in Group 2 patients. Spermograms were performed monthly during and up to 150 days after cessation of treatment.

Results were assessed quantitatively by means of variance analysis involving the number of sperms/ml, the % of live and motile sperms and % of forward progressive sperms.

For qualitative assessment, frank improvement was arbitrarilly defined as the achievement of at least twice the initial values and over 30×10^6 sperms/ml, 50% of live and motile sperms or 30% of forward progressive sperms; improvement meant duplication without increase over previous levels and no change meant that duplication was not obtained. Finally, global assessment involved comparison of the results obtained in both biopsy groups under both therapeutic regimens Results obtained were classified as positive when all three parameters considered (number of sperms/ml; % of live and motile sperms and % of forward progressive sperms) showed frank improvement or when plain improvement was followed by impregnation; doubtful when improvement in the number of sperms/ml was obtained with improvement or frank improvement of the vitality and motility parameters; and negative when only slight improvement occurred only in the qualitative parameters or in none of the three parameters.

GROUP	SPERM /ml $\bar{X} \pm$ SEM x 10^6	RANGE OF SPERM/ml x 10^6	% OF LIVE AND MOTILE SPERM $\bar{X} \pm$ SEM	% OF FORWARD PROGRESSIVE SPERM $\bar{X} \pm$ SEM
1	7.9 ± 1.5	1.5 - 17	31.7 ± 4.3	12.5 ± 3.4
2	3.5 ± 0.9	0.5 - 7.5	34.4 ± 7.1	13.2 ± 4.1

Table I   Number of sperms/ml (x 10^6) and % of live and motile
            sperms and % of forward progressive sperms in Goups 1
            and 2, before the treatment ($\bar{x} \pm$ S.E.M. of at least 3
            sperm counts).

   In figure 9, we show the number of sperms/ml, the % of live
and motile sperm and the % of forward progressive sperms obtained
before treatment with LH-RH, and the maximal values during the
treatment.

   As it can be seen, a significant rise in all three parameters
but predominantly of the number of sperms/ml, occurred in Group 1.
Group 2 showed a rising trend but statistical significance was not
reached after the first course of treatment. The patients in Group
2 who received two courses of treatment experienced significant
qualitative and quantitative improvement.

   In Table II, qualitative assessment of the results in both
Groups are shown. The proportion of frank improvements was similar
in both groups as far as the parameters of vitality and motility
are concerned. This proportion, on the other hand, was significantly higher in Group 1 regarding sperm concentration.

   Of the 21 patients studied, six obtained the maximal sperm
concentration 30 or more days after treatment was discontinued. In
the same period, 10 subjects obtained the maximal percentage of live

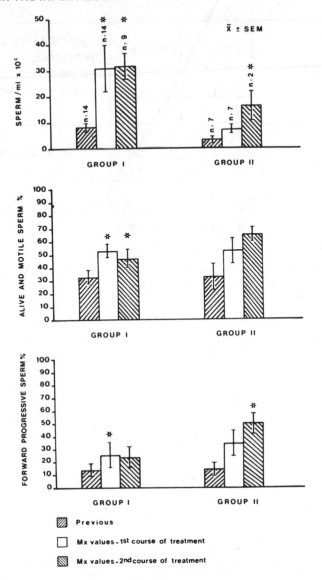

Fig. 9: Number of sperms/ml, % of live and motile sperms and % of
forward progressive sperms ($\bar{x}$ ± S.E.M.) before and after
treatment with synthetic LH—RH. The asterisks indicate
statistically significant differences (p < 0.05) with
treatment.

and motile sperm and 15 the maximal % of forward progressive
sperm.

PARAMETER		GROUP 1 n=14		GROUP 2 n=7		SIGNIFICANCE OF THE DIFFERENCE BETWEEN THE PROPORTIONS OF F.I. BETWEEN GROUPS
		n	%	n	%	
SPERM/ml	F.I.	7	50.0	0	0.0	2 α = 0.05
	I.	3	21.4	4	57.1	
	N.C.	4	28.6	3	42.8	
LIVE AND MOTILE SPERM	F.I.	7	50.0	4	57.1	2 α = n.s.
	I.	4	28.5	0	0.0	
	N.C.	3	21.4	3	42.8	
FORWARD PROGRESSIVE SPERM	F.I.	7	50.0	4	57.1	2 α = n.s.
	I.	4	28.5	0	0.0	
	N.C.	3	21.4	3	42.8	

Table II   Qualitative assessment of the results of number of sperm/
ml, % of live and motile sperm and % of forward progressive sperm, obtained in both groups and expressed in absolute and percentual terms.
FI means frank improvement; I means improvement and NC
means no change. The significance of the differences
between the proportions of FI between groups is also
shown.

Six out of seven patients in Group 1 who were followed up for
90 to 150 days after withdrawal of treatment retained sperm/ml values above the initial number, while this occurred in only 1 out
of 6 patients of Group 2 (differences between proportions $p < 0.02$).

In Table III, the overall results are shown classified according to the severity of testicular involvement and to the type of
treatment applied.

Four out of 5 patients receiving long-term treatment in Group
1 obtained positive results and three of them were able to impreg-
nate their wives. The same regimen resulted in one positive case,
with impregnation in Group 2.

	LONG-TERM TREATMENT			SHORT-TERM TREATMENT		
	POSITIVE	DOUBTFUL	NEGATIVE	POSITIVE	DOUBTFUL	NEGATIVE
GROUP 1	4	1	0	1	4	4
GROUP 2	1	3	1	0	1	1

Table III   Overall results of treatment with LH-RH classified according to the severity of testicular involvement and to the type of treatment applied.

With the "short-term" regimen, only 1 positive case occurred, with impregnation, belonging to Group 1. The significance of the difference between proportions, on comparing both treatment regimens was $p < 0.05$. No side effect was observed in any case.

In conclusion, it can be said that synthetic LH-RH was able to cause qualitative and quantitative improvements, chiefly in the post-treatment period, in patients with I.N.O. The cases with the best prognosis were those presenting hypospermatogenesis or alterations up to the spermatid stage, although improvement could also be achieved in some subjects with more severe disorders of spermatogenesis.

Treatment for at least 90 days at an average daily dose of 250 µg seems to offer the best therapeutic approach. Hypothetically, the therapeutic action of LH-RH might result from 2 mechanisms: one would be direct gonadotrophin release, the other would be restoration of normal pituitary gonadotrophin functional reserve (Mortimer et al., 1974; Yoshimoto et al., 1975).

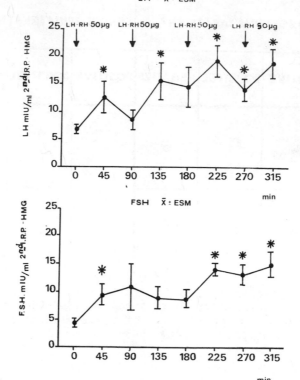

Fig. 10: LH and FSH levels after 4 successive I.V. injection of
LH-RH (50 µg each), every 90 minutes.

Taking into account all these considerations, it was thought
that a substance, analog to LH-RH, with more potency and long-lasting action, would combine a more intense and prolonged releasing
effect with the restoration of pituitary functional reserve, as
hypothetisized for LH-RH. A draw back for this idea could be that
a very strong and sustained stimulus could lead to pituitary and/
or testicular exhaustion.

On this basis, when Dr. Schally supplied us with [D-leucine[6]]-
LH-RH-ethylamide, a trial was initiated in which the analog was
administered I.M., during 90 days, to I.N.O. subjects.

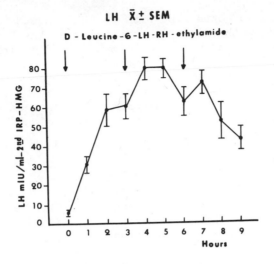

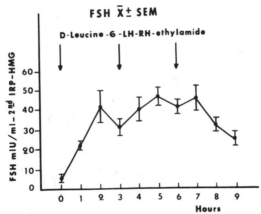

Fig. 11: LH and FSH levels after 3 successive I.V. injections of [D-leucine⁶]-LH-RH-ethylamide (20 µg each), every 3 hours.

By now, 4 patients have been treated with 5 µg of the analog per day, 5 with 10 µg per day and 5 with 20 µg per day; 50% of them having Type I testicular biopsy and the other 50% Type 2 biopsy.

No significant improvement has been seen, either in the concentration of spermatozoa or in the qualitative parameters, during treatment. We do not have a complete post-treatment control yet, so it is not possible to say if a rebound effect exists or not. We can say that results obtained so far and with the dose used do not seem very promising.

Finally, and in connection with the therapeutic results, I should like to show the findings obtained when LH-RH and [D-leucine[6]]-LH-RH ethylamide are administered several times during the day.

Figure 10 shows LH and FSH profiles after four 50 μg I.V. LH-RH injections given every 90 minutes. As it can be seen, the response of both hormones shows an increment after each successive injection, which is an evidence in favour of a potentiation of the pituitary response.

Figure 11 shows similar parameters, but after three I.V. injections of 20 μg of [D-leucine[6]]-LH-RH ethylamide, every 180 minutes. As it can be seen, the responses after the second injection are similar to or higher than those obtained after the first one. The third injection also elicited a response but levels felt quickly in comparison with the previous injections.

According to this, it would be of great interest to study the pituitary depletion of gonadotrophins after the analog application. We consider all the results described in this presentation as the beginning of a line of investigation. We think that, above all, research on physiopathological mechanisms should be emphasized. In fact, our experience with LH-RH and its analogs faces us with interesting results concerning the dynamic acute response and, specially, with some paradoxical therapeutical results.

ACKNOWLEDGEMENTS

Synthetic LH-RH has been kindly provided by Quimica Hoechst S. A. and antisera for LH, FSH and T determination by Serono-Immunochemical, Roma, Italy.

REFERENCES

- Aafjes, J.H. and Van Der Vijver, J.C.M. (1975) Fertil Steril 25, 809-812.

- Debeljuk, L.; Rozados, R; Daskal, H. and Villega Vélez, C. (1975) Neuroendocrinology 17, 48-53.

- Mecklemburg, R.S. and Sherins, R.J. (1974) J. Clin. Endocrinol. Metab. 38, 1005-1008.

- Meinhard, E.; McRae, C.U. and Chisholm, G.D. (1973) Brit. Med. J. 3, 577-579.

- Mortimer, C.H.; McNeilly, A.S.; Fisher, R.A., Murray, M.A. F. and Besser, G.M. (1974) Brit. Med. J. 4, 617-621.

- Schwarzstein, L. (1974) Fertil. Steril. <u>25</u>, 813-816.

- Schwarzstein, L.; Aparicio, N.J.; Turner, D.; Calamera, J.
  C.; Mancini, R. and Schally, A.V. (1975a) Fertil. Steril.
  <u>26</u>, 331-335.

- Schwarzstein, L.; Premoli, F. and Aparicio, N.J. (1975b)
  Int. J. Fertil., in press.

- Schwarzstein, L.; Laborde, N.P. de; Aparicio, N.J.; Turner,
  D.; Mirkin, A.; Rodriguez, A.; Rodrigue Lhullier, F. and
  Rosner, J.M. (1975c) J. Clin. Endocrinol. Metab. <u>40</u>, 313-
  317.

- Turner, D.; Turner, E.A. de; Schwarzstein, L. and Aparicio,
  N.J. (1975) Fertil. Steril. <u>26</u>, 337-339.

- Yoshimoto, Y.; Moridera, K. and Imora, A. (1975) New Engl.
  J. Med. <u>292</u>, 242-245.

THERAPEUTIC USE OF LUTEINIZING HORMONE-RELEASING HORMONE IN THE

HUMAN FEMALE

Sven Johan Nillius

Department of Obstetrics and Gynecology

University Hospital, Uppsala, Sweden

A gonadotropin-releasing hormone became available for clinical studies in 1971, when Schally and associates isolated, determined the structure and synthesized LH releasing hormone (LH-RH). It was hoped that this new hypothalamic hormone, among other things, would prove to be useful in the diagnosis and therapy of disorders of the hypothalamo-pituitary axis. The diagnostic value of the LH-RH test has recently been questioned by Mortimer et al. (1973) who reported that it was not possible to distinguish between hypothalamic and pituitary causes of hypogonadotrophic hypogonadism. However, the possibility of using LH-RH in the treatment of infertility in men and women is of great interest and the potential therapeutic role of LH-RH has to be thoroughly explored.

Anovulatory infertility is mostly caused by a dysfunction or failure at the hypothalamo-pituitary level with loss of the normal cyclic and sometimes also the tonic secretion of pituitary gonadotrophins. In the vast majority of anovulatory women, LH-RH has proved to be able to stimulate the release of both luteinizing hormone (LH) and follicle-stimulating hormone (FSH) from the pituitary. The LH-releasing effect of LH-RH has been utilized by many clinical investigators to induce LH surges in attempts to induce ovulation in women, where follicular maturation was either spontaneous or induced by agents stimulating gonadal function like clomiphene citrate or human menopausal gonadotrophins (HMG). In several clinical trials, investigators have also tried to utilize the FSH releasing effect of LRH to induce follicular growth and maturation in anovulatory women. This paper is a review of therapeutic studies with LH-RH in women.

TIMING OF OVULATION

There is need for a practical and reliable method for timing ovulation in women undergoing insemination therapy. Pinpointing of ovulation in normal women for standardisation of the rythm method of birth control was suggested by Schally et al. (1972) as one possible approach to the use of LH-RH for control of human fertility. Schally speculated that administration of LH-RH on a specific day of the cycle (e.g. days 12-14) might induce and pinpoint the exact time of ovulation.

Clinical trials with LH-RH for pinpointing ovulation in normal women have been performed in association with insemination therapy. Gigon et al. (1973) stressed the importance of ovulation timing in this situation. They analyzed 50 cases of successful artificial insemination and found that 11 pregnancies were obtained in 66 treatment courses without ovulation timing. When humen chorionic gonadotropin, HCG (5000 IU) or LH-RH (100 µg intramuscularly or intravenously over four hours on cycle days 13 and 14) was used for ovulation timing, 39 pregnancies were obtained after 72 treatment cycles. There were some indications which suggested that infusions of LH-RH may have been more effective than injections of HCG in timing ovulation accurately.

Intravenous infusions of LH-RH were also used bu Nakano et al. (1973, 1974) for timing of ovulation in ten normally ovulating women, who were treated with artificial insemination by donor (AID) in the pre-ovulatory phase of the menstrual cycle. Immediately after insemination, these women were given a 6-h infusion of 600 µg of LH-RH supplemented with a subcutaneous injection of 400 µg of LH-RH. The basal body temperature rose on the following day in seven of ten women. Two pregnancies occurred. The authors concluded that the triggering of ovulation by LH-RH is a convenient way of controlling the timing of ovulation, if follicular development of the ovary is sufficient.

A more practical route of LH-RH administration was chosen by Grimes et al. (1975), who used single injections of 100 µg of LH-RH via the subcutaneous, intravenous or intramuscular route in an attempt to trigger ovulation in 19 cycling women who were inseminated in the immediate pre-ovulatory period. In 20 of 37 treatment cycles, the hyperthermia response occurred one to three days after LH-RH administration suggesting that ovulation occurred as a direct consequence of administered LH-RH. Four pregnancies were obtained but two of them ended in spontaneous abortions. Poor corpus luteum function, which was observed in two patients, was suggested as a possible explanation for the discrepancy between apparent ovulation and pregnancy rates.

In normally ovulating women, it is not easy to prove a cause-and-effect relationship between the LH-RH treatment and ovulation. A double-blind study was therefore designed to compare the effect-iveness of LH-RH and placebo to trigger ovulation in 44 cycling women undergoing AID (Nillius et al. 1975b). Plasma levels of progesterone were used instead of basal body temperature recordings to assess the effect of treatment on ovulation. The women were randomized into two groups and received an intramuscular injection of either saline or 100 µg of LH-RH in association with insemina-tion. Nine of the 44 women had pretreatment progesterone levels of more than 2 ng/ml, indicating that ovulation already had occur-red. These patients were excluded from the study. The adminis-tration of LH-RH resulted in dramatic LH increases (Nillius et al. 1973a). Sixty minutes after the injection of LH-RH the mean LH level had increased to more than twice the average LH peak level observed during the normal menstrual cycle. A summary of some results from this study are shown in table I. It is evident from the table that

	LH-RH 100 µg I.M. n = 20	Saline I.M. n = 15
Ovulation	20/20	15/15
Plasma progesterone (>2 ng/ml)		
after 24 h	8/18	6/15
after 48 h	13/19	8/14
Pregnancies	3	2
Interval injection-menses		
mean, days	14.8	15.1
range	13-16	11-20

Table I. Results from a randomized double-blind study on ovulation timing in women undergoing insemination therapy, there were no significant difference between a single intramuscular injection of 100 µg of LH-RH and placebo in this study on ovulation timing in cycling women undergoing insemination therapy.

The practical intranasal route for LH-RH administration was then investigated in normal menstruating women. Pilot studies showed that small intranasal doses of LH-RH administered by a nasal spray (Hoechst) were effective in evoking great LH release in normal women. This is illustrated by Fig. 1, which shows levels of LH and FSH measured by the radioimmunosorbent technique of Wide et al. (1973), before and after multiple intranasal doses of LH-RH

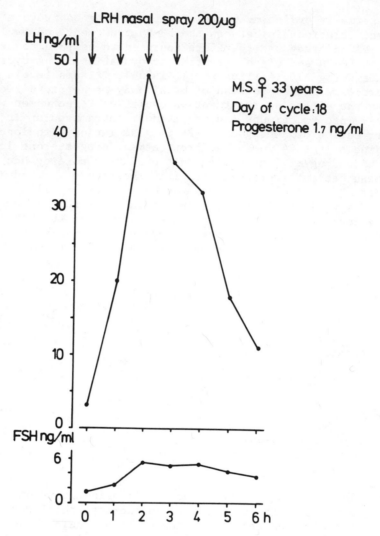

Fig. 1 Effects of intranasal administration of LH-RH on serum levels of LH and FSH in a woman in the pre-ovulatory phase of the menstrual cycle.

in a woman in the pre-ovulatory phase of the menstrual cycle. The pretreatment LH level was in the upper normal range of the folli-

cular phase of the menstrual cycle. After two spray applications
of 200 μg of LARH intranasally, the LH level had increased to 48 ng/
ml, i.e. to more than 5 times the average LH peak level of the normal menstrual cycle. LH levels of this magnitude are never observed in the normal menstrual cycle.

A new randomized double—blind study was then performed in 40
normally ovulating women undergoing AID (Nillius et al. 1976). LH-
RH (200 μg) or saline was administered by the nasaly spray twice at
an interval of one hour. This intranasal application was repeated
every eight hours for two days. Insemination was performed 8-12
hours after the first application. Preliminary results from this
study show that 50 per cent of the women treated with LH-RH had
plasma progesterone levels of more than 2 ng/ml 48 hours after the
first spray application as compared with 14 per cent in the group
treated with saline. The results suggest that multiple LH-RH administration by the intranasal route is effective in triggering ovulation in the pre-ovulatory phase of the menstrual cycle.

Thus, LH-RH might be of value for timing of ovulation in cycling
women undergoing insemination therapy. The optimal dose and therapeutic regimen remains to be established. It is possible that long-
acting depot preparations or potent analogues of LH-RH might be useful in this situation. In further studies, it seems essential to
investigate if the induction of an LH surge at a time when the follicle has not reached full maturity can have adverse effects on ovulation and corpus luteum function.

INDUCTION OF OVULATION

Induction of ovulation with LH-RH in an anovulatory woman was
first reported by Kastin and associates in 1971. In Kastin's study,
a 24-h intravenous infusion of porcine LH-RH was followed by ovulation, confirmed by pregnancy, in a clomiphene-responsive amenorrheic
woman, who was pretreated with 75 IU of human menopausal gonadotropins (HMG) for three days after a progestin-induced bleeding.

Clomiphene citrate was used by Keller (1972) to induce follicular maturation in 21 amenorrheic women, who were given an additional intravenous infusion of synthetic LH-RH to induce ovulation.
These women had previously not responded with ovulation to clomiphene alone. Twelve of the 21 women ovulated when infusion of 50
μg of LH-RH was given 6-7 days after administration of 100 mg of
clomiphene for five days. Two became pregnant. Ovulation could
not be induced in six of the patients who responded unfavourably
in a preliminary LH-RH test (12.5 μg I.V.). Nakano et al. (1974)
treated 18 previously clomiphene-unresponsive amenorrheic women
with 200 μg of LH-RH intravenously supplemented with 200 μg of

LH-RH subcutaneously 5-10 days after clomiphene administration (100 mg x 5). Nine patients ovulated but only one became pregnant. Figueroa Casas et al. (1975) attempted to induce ovulation by intravenous infusions and/or intramuscular injections of 50-500 µg of LH-RH during 25 treatment courses in patients where follicular maturation was either spontaneous or stimulated by LH-RH, clomiphene or HMG. Ten ovulations and two pregnancies were obtained during the treatment cycles.

HMG treatment until follicular maturation followed by LH-RH administration was used by Breckwoldt et al. (1974) in an attempt to induce ovulation in 13 patients with primary or secondary amenorrhea. LH-RH was infused intravenously at a rate of 50 µg/h over 2-8 hours. Eight of the 13 women had LH increases to preovulatory levels but only four of them showed signs of presumptive ovulation. One patient conceived. Pedersen et al. (1974) administered a single intravenous injection of 25 µg of LH-RH to five anovulatory women who were pretreated with HMG. Only one of the patients ovulated and this patient who had oligomenorrhea, developed symptoms of overstimulation: Two of three anovulatory women who were treated with HMG combined with a 4-h intravenous infusion of 50 µg of LH-RH showed signs of ovulation but no pregnancy occurred.

We have treated 21 amenorrheic women with LH-RH after pretreatment with HMG until follicular maturation (Nillius et al. 1973b,1974). The treatment was monitored by daily determinations of total urinary estrogens, measured according to the rapid method of Brown et al. (1968). When the total urinary estrogen excretion indicated follicular maturation, LH-RH was given instead of HCG in an attempt to induce ovulation.

An intravenous injection of 100 µg of LH-RH was given to fourteen women at the time of follicular maturation. Before the treatment, the same dose of LH-RH had been given to test the pituitary gonadotropic reserve capacity. The mean LH response to LH-RH in the group was unchanged after the induction of follicular maturation with increased estrogen secretion while the mean FSH response was markedly reduced. Some of the women responded with augmented LH responses to LH-RH after the pretreatment with HMG. However, ovulation did not occur in these women despite the fact that LH sometimes increased to preovulatory levels. One possible explanation for the failure to induce ovulation with a single intravenous injection of LH-RH may be the fact that the induced LH increase was a short duration. The raised LH level decreased within the first two hours after the LH-RH administration while the LH peak in the normal menstrual cycle has a duration of at least 24 h.

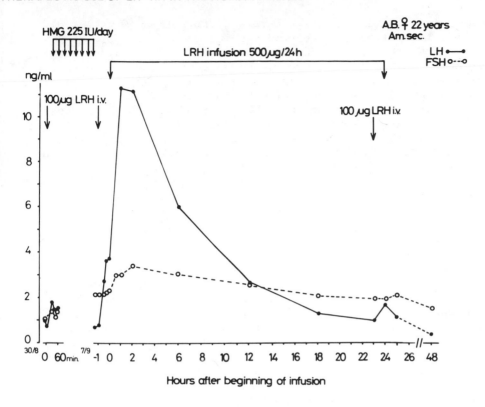

Fig. 2

Effects of intravenous LH-RH administration on serum levels of LH
and FSH before and after HMG induction of follicular maturation in
a woman with secondary amenorrhea.

A constant intravenous infusion of 500 µg of LH-RH over 24 h
was therefore administered into the other seven amenorrheic women,
who were pretreated with HMG until follicular maturation. LH and
FSH results from the LH-RH infusion in one of the seven women are
shown in Fig. 2. This 22-year-old amenorrheic woman had a very
small LH response to LH-RH before the treatment. On the ninth day
of treatment the LH response to LH-RH was augmented and when the
LH-RH infusion was started the LH level increased further and

reached normal mid-cycle peak levels of more than 10 ng per ml.
However, the raised LH level was not maintained for more than 4-6
hours. Then it fell back to the pretreatment level despite the
continuing infusion. Twenty-four hours later, a third LH-RH test
was performed. The result was a very small LH response. No signs
of ovulation were observed. Five of the seven women who were treated with 24 hour infusions of LH-RH after HMG treatment responded
in the same way. However, one woman had a pronounced LH increase
during 20 hours and she probably ovulated in association with the
LH-RH infusion. The results from the studies where we tried to
utilize the LH-releasing effect of LH-RH to induce ovulation in
amenorrheic women pretreated with HMG suggest that it is necessary
to have not only a mature follicle but also a sufficient pituitary
reserve capacity for LH secretion to be able to induce ovulation
with LH-RH.

During the pre-ovulatory phase of the normal menstrual cycle,
there is a greatly enhanced pituitary capacity to release LH in
response to LH-RH, presumably caused by the increased ovarian
secretion of estrogens during the late follicular phase of the
menstrual cycle (Nillius & Wide 1972, Yen et al. 1972). Such an
augmented pituitary reserve capacity for LH secretion may be a prerequisite for an ovulatory response to LH-RH treatment. Some
women with amenorrhea seem to be unable to respond to increasing
estrogen levels with these changes at the hypothalamic-pituitary
level. During LH-RH treatment, they may therefore respond with an
inadequate LH release at the time of full follicular maturation
with the result that ovulation fails to appear or alternatively
that a defective ovulation with insufficient corpus luteum function
occurs.

Thus, in amenorrheic women who require HMG treatment to stimulate follicular growth and maturation, LH-RH does not seem to be
suitable to replace HCG for induction of ovulation. In anovulatory
women who respond to clomiphene citrate with follicular maturation
but not ovulation, LH-RH might be useful for induction of ovulation.
However, if LH-RH has any advantages over HCG in this situation
remains to be proved.

INDUCTION OF FOLLICULAR GROWTH AND MATURATION

Human gonadotropin therapy is at present the treatment of
choice for induction of follicular growth and maturation in infertile amenorrheic women who have no evidence of endogenous ovarian
activity and do not respond to clomiphene citrate. Gonadotropin
treatment is very effective but unfortunately, it has considerable

disadvantages. A large individual variation in the ovarian sensitivity to gonadotropins necessitates the use of an individually
adjusted treatment scheme to achieve optimum results with a minimum
of adverse reactions. The therapeutic range is narrow. The difference between the effective dose and the dose producing hyperstimulation of the ovaries is very small. A careful monitoring
of human gonadotropin therapy is therefore necessary to avoid the
serious hyperstimulation syndrome. A high rate of multiple pregnancies is also an important drawback to gonadotropin therapy.
Furthermore, human gonadotropin preparations for treatment are
expensive. They are prepared by extraction from urine of postmenopausal women (HMG) or from human pituitary glands obtained at autopsy (human pituitary gonadotropins, HPG). When synthetic LH-RH
became available, it was therefore natural that clinical investigators displayed a keen interest in the possibility of replacing
human gonadotropins with synthetic LH-RH for induction of follicular growth and maturation.

    The first results from clinical trials where synthetic LH-RH
was used in an attempt to induce follicular growth and maturation
in anovulatory patients were reported by Zarate and associates in
1972. Ten women with "suspected hypothalamic anovulation" were
given daily intramuscular injections of 50 µg of LH-RH for 10 days
starting on day 5 after a progestin-induced bleeding. Four of
these women showed presumptive signs of ovulation and two became
pregnant. In a later study on 42 infertile women (18 with amenorrhea and 24 with oligomenorrhea), daily doses of 100-1000 µg of LH-RH
were administered intramuscularly over 5-20 days (Zarate et al. 1974).
When the total urinary estrogen excretion was around 60 µg/24 h,
10.000 IU of HCG were given on two consecutive days in an attempt
to induce ovulation. Signs of follicular growth were shown by 34
of the 42 patients but only ten women ovulated and seven of them
conceived. The best results were obtained in women with the Stein-
Leventhal syndrome. Patients who ovulated and became pregnant,
had previously proved to respond to clomiphene citrate. Seven
patients were given 500 µg of LH-RH intramuscularly three times
daily on days 5, 10, and 15 of the cycle but none of them ovulated.

    Keller (1973) reported one ovulation in two amenorrheic women
treated with two intramuscular injections of 25 µg of LH-RH per day
followed by two injections of 100 µg on the eleventh day. Both
these women had signs of estrogenic activity before treatment.
Nakano et al. (1974) treated five clomiphene-responsive amenorrheic
women with daily subcutaneous injections of 50 µg of LH-RH for 10
days after a progestin-induced bleeding. Two of these women experienced a uterine bleeding after the treatment but no signs of
ovulation were found. Zanartu et al. (1974) treated 15 women with
anovulatory sterility with various regimens of intramuscular and
intravenous LH-RH therapy. Six of these women had secondary ame-

norrhea while nine had irregular anovulatory cycles. Clinical
signs of ovulation were found in three of ten treatment cycles in
the amenorrheic patients and in ten of 18 cycles in the patients
with anovulatory cycles. Three pregnancies occurred. Figueroa
Casas et al. (1975) treated 15 women with idiopathic or functional
anovulation (8 with anovulatory or oligo-ovulatory cycles and 7
with amenorrhea) with daily intramuscular injections of 25-150 µg
of LH-RH over 6-14 days. Follicular maturation, assessed by cervical mucus reactions, was obtained in 6 of 12 treatment courses.
Clomiphene induced follicular maturation in 4 of the 6 patients
where LH-RH failed.

Although the studies referred to above suggested that it was
possible to induce follicular growth and maturation by LH-RH, the
results were rather disappointing. The ovulation and pregnancy
rates were not high. The percentage of ovulations was only 25 per
cent in the largest study (Zarate et al. 1974) where the LH-RH
treatment was monitored by daily urinary estrogen determinations
and repeated doses of HCG given to induce ovulation. The majority
of patients in these studies had evidence of endogenous estrogen
secretion or even irregular spontaneous bleedings, indicating that
they had at least some ovarian follicular activity before the
treatment. It is difficult to evaluate the effectiveness of LH-RH
to induce follicular growth and maturation in this group of
patients. In similar patients Evans et al. (1967) obtained an
ovulation rate of 39 per cent with placebo treatment alone.

In amenorrheic women with no evidence of endogenous estrogen
production before treatment, we were not able to induce follicular
maturation when daily doses of 80-240 µg of synthetic LH-RH were
administered for 7-21 days (Nillius et al. 1974). Similar results
were obtained by Breckwoldt et al. (1974). They treated three
amenorrheic patients, who had low pretreatment estrogen levels,
with daily subcutaneous injections of 100-200 µg of LH-RH over 18-
21 days without finding any signs of follicular activity.

Long-Term Treatment with High Doses of LH-RH

Prolonged treatment with higher doses of LH-RH (500 µg eight-
hourly) was successfully used by Mortimer et al. (1974) to induce
potency, puberty and spermatogenesis in hypogonadal men. With this
therapeutic regimen it proved to be possible to induce follicular
maturation in clomiphene-unresponsive amenorrheic women with no
signs of endogenous estrogen production (Mortimer et al. 1975,
Nillius et al. 1975a, Nillius & Wide 1975).

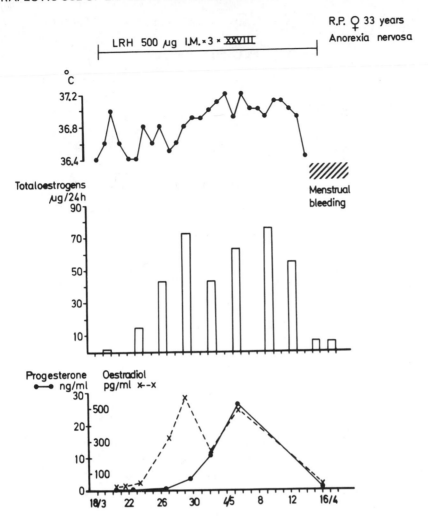

Fig. 3 Basal body temperature, total urinary estrogen excretion and blood levels of estradiol and progesterone during long-term treatment with 500 μg of LH-RH intramuscularly every eight hours in a woman with secondary amenorrhea (From Nillius et al. 1975a. Reproduced with permission of the publisher of Amer. J. Obstet. Gynec.).

Thirteen amenorrheic women have so far been treated by us with high doses of LH-RH in an attempt to induce follicular maturation and ovulation. Synthetic LH-RH, generously supplied by Farbwerke Hoechst AG, was administered subcutaneously or intramuscularly in a

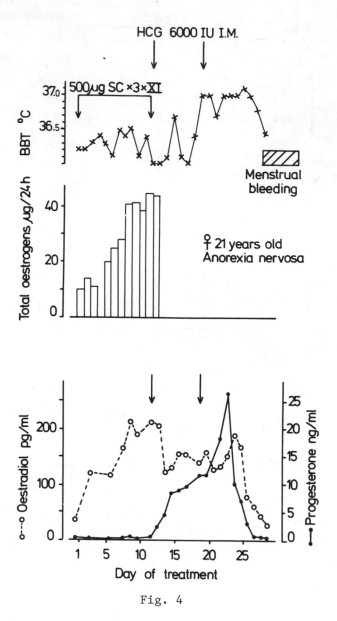

Fig. 4

Basal body temperature, total urinary estrogen excretion and blood levels of estradiol and progesterone during combined treatment with LH-RH and HCG in a woman with secondary amenorrhea.

dose of 500 µg every eight hours over 9-28 days. Follicular growth and maturation, as judged by increased estrogen levels in urine and blood, were induced in 14 of 16 treatment cycles after 9-23 days of therapy. One woman with hypogonadotrophic hypogonadism and another patient with normoprolactinemic post-partum amenorrhea did not show any evident increase in serum estradiol levels after four weeks of treatment.

Seven women were treated with LH-RH alone. Ovulation, as judged by increased serum progesterone levels, was induced in all these women. Hormone levels, during an ovulatory LH-RH treatment cycle are shown in Fig. 3. The estrogen patterns in urine and blood and the progesterone pattern in blood are similar to those seen during normal ovulatory menstrual cycles. In this patient, the progesterone level about one week after the basal body temperature shift was 26.4 ng/ml, i.e. a high normal luteal phase value. However, the maximum progesterone values during the luteal phases in four of the seven induced cycles were rather low, suggesting insufficient corpus luteum function.

LH-RH was therefore combined with HCG during seven treatment cycles. HCG was administered intramuscularly in a dose of 6000-9000 IU when the estrogen levels indicated follicular maturation or in the immediate postovulatory phase. During the luteal phase, one to three additional injections of 1500-6000 IU of HCG were given the support corpus luteum function. An example of this treatment scheme is given in Fig. 4. This amenorrheic woman with anorexia nervosa had previously been treated with 500 µg of LH-RH every eight hours over four weeks. During that first treatment with LH-RH alone, she responded with follicular maturation and ovulation as judged by the estradiol and progesterone patterns in blood. The luteal phase length was normal but the maximum progesterone value during the post-ovulatory phase was rather low, 7.7 ng/ml, which suggested a minor corpus luteum insufficiency. Menstruation occurred on treatment day 28. A new treatment (Fig. 4) was initiated three months later. On treatment day 12, when the estrogen levels in urine and blood indicated that follicular maturation had occurred, HCG was injected. The estrogen level in serum fell and the progesterone level increased, indicating that ovulation presumably occurred. The progesterone level rose to more function, and increased further when a second HCG injection was given during the mid-luteal phase. Six of the seven treatment cycles with LH-RH and HCG were presumptively ovulatory with normal luteal phase progesterone values.

Three involuntarily sterile amenorrheic women were treated with LH-RH combined with HCG. One of them conceived and thus proved that ovulation and normal corpus luteum function occurred during the LH-RH-HCG treatment. Results from the treatment which resulted in this pregnancy are shown in Fig. 5. The patient was a 28-year-old woman with 13 years of second amenorrhea and 4 hears of involuntary ste-

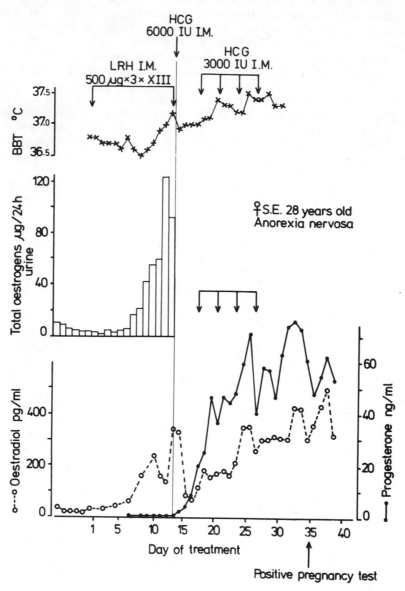

Fig. 5

Basal body temperature, total urinary estrogen excretion and blood
levels of estradiol and progesterone during combined treatment
with LH-RH and HGC in a woman with secondary amenorrhea (From Nillius & Wide 1975). Reproduced with permission of the publisher of
Brit. Med. J.).

rility. She had previously been treated with HMG which then was replaced with LH-RH during two treatment courses. The first treatment with LH-RH rapidly resulted in follicular growth. Full follicular maturation was obtained after only nine days of LH-RH therapy. This ovulatory treatment cycle did not result in conception. A second treatment course with LH-RH was started on cycle day 7. After thirteen days of treatment, the estrogen levels in urine and blood were increased to a level consistent with follicular maturation (Fig. 5). HCG was then administered and ovulation occurred as shown by the decrease of the estradiol level and increase of the progesterone level in blood. During the luteal phase of the induced cycle additional injections of HCG were given. The blood levels of estradiol and progesterone increased progressively. The pregnancy test was positive three weeks after ovulation, and she eventually delivered one healthy female child at term.

No side effects were observed during the prolonged LH-RH treatments. Three patients were given two treatment courses. There were no signs of secondary drug failure when therapy was reinstituted 1-3 months after the first treatment cycle.

To sum up, our study proves that LH-RH can be used alone or in combination with HCG to induce follicular growth and maturation, ovulation and pregnancy in amenorrheic women who have no evidence of endogenous ovarian activity. Thus, it seems possible to replace human gonadotropins with LH-RH for induction of follicular maturation and ovulation at least in some women with amenorrhea. The best results were obtained in patients with amenorrhea because of anorexia nervosa (Nillius et al. 1975a, Nillius & Wide, 1975). These patients had relative high FSH responses to LH-RH before treatment. Such prepubertal-like response patterns to LH-RH may be favourable for initiating follicular growth and maturation. It remains to be seen if LH-RH is equally effective in other women with amenorrhea.

Changes in the Pituitary Responsiveness to LH-RH during the Prolonged LH-RH Treatments

During the prolonged LH-RH treatments interesting qualitative and quantitative changes in the pituitary responsiveness to LH-RH were observed, especially in the patients with anorexia nervosa. This is illustrated by Fig. 6 which shows basal gonadotropin levels and LH and FSH responses to LH-RH before, during and after LH-RH treatment of the patient whose treatment cycle was shown in Fig. 3.

Before the treatment, the basal LH level was very low. There was a small but significan LH increase after intravenous LH-RH. The basal FSH level was higher and the FSH response to LH-RH was nearly two times higher than the LH response. This is a response pattern to LH-RH similar to what has been described in the prepubertal girl.

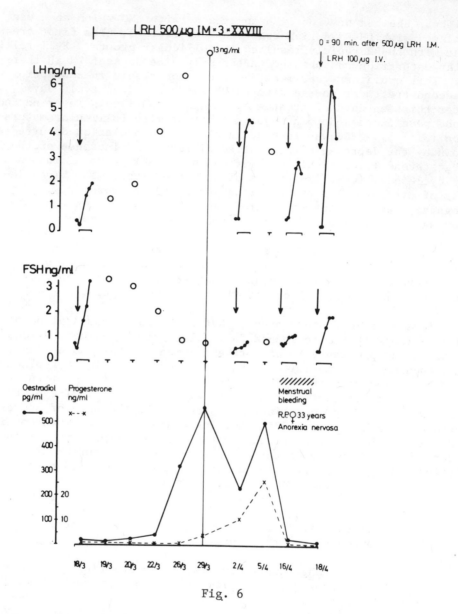

Fig. 6

Basal gonadotropin levels in serum and LH and FSH responses to LH-RH before, during and after prolonged LH-RH treatment of a woman with secondary amenorrhea.

During the first ten days of treatment, there was a progressive increase of the LH response to LH-RH parallel to the intreased estrogen secretion while the FSH response to LH-RH progressively de-

creased. On treatment day 11, the LH level was 13 ng/ml after LH–
RH administration, i.e. similar to the pre-ovulatory LH peak in the
normal menstrual cycle. The FSH level was only 0.7 ng/ml compared
with 3.3 on the second day of treatment. At the time of the maximum LH response the blood level of estradiol had increased from 20
to more than 500 pg/ml and there was also a small increase of the
progesterone level in blood. Influence of the gonadal steroids,
estradiol and possibly also progesterone, may be one possible explanation for these changes in the pituitary responsiveness to LH–
RH during the treatment.

These changes in the FSH response to LH–RH may give LH–RH
treatment an advantage over HMG treatment for induction of follicular growth and maturation. During HMG treatment, it is necessary
to monitor the treatment carefully by daily hormone determinations
to avoid complications such as the severe hyperstimulation syndrome.

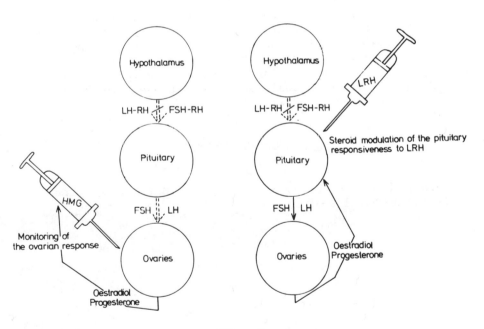

Fig. 7

Monitoring treatment with human gonadotropins and LH–RH.

The daily dose of HMG has to be adjusted according to the ovarian response (Fig. 7. Hyperstimulation of the ovaries might be easier to prevent during LH-RH treatments. The interrelationship between the pituitary and the ovaries which is present in patients treated with LH-RH, represents an internal control mechanism (Fig. 7). LH-RH induces synthesis and release of FSH and LH from the pituitary. The gonadotropins stimulate the ovaries to increased secretion of estradiol which then feeds back at the pituitary level to modulate the pituitary responsiveness of LH-RH (Fig. 7). The intact feedback system between the ovarian steroids and the pituitary may automatically prevent excessive FSH stimulation of the ovaries during prolonged treatments with high doses of LH-RH.

In summary, the results from therapeutic studies with LH-RH in the human female suggest that this hypothalamic hormone should find clinical application in the treatment of female infertility in the future. LH-RH might be useful for timing ovulation in association with insemination therapy, for inducing ovulation in anovulatory women pretreated with agents stimulating gonadal function, like clomiphene, and for replacing HMG for induction of follicular growth and maturation in some women with amenorrhea. It is possible that hyperstimulation of the ovaries, a serious complication to human gonadotropin therapy, might be easier to prevent during LH-RH treatments. Nevertheless, many more clinical studies with LH-RH must be performed before we can define the proper place for this hypothalamic hormone in the treatment of anovulatory infertility. The present therapeutic regimens are not very practical. Multiple injections of LH-RH have to be given each day over long periods to stimulate gonadal function. This problem might be solved by the use of long-acting superactive analogues of LH-RH. Clinical trials with such analogues are at present in progress and the results are awaited with interest.

ACKNOWLEDGEMENTS

This work was supported by the Swedish Medical Research Council (Grant No. 13x-3145).

REFERENCES

Breckwoldt, M., Czygan, P.-J., Lehmann, F. and
     Bettendorf, G. (1974) Acta endocr. (Kbh.), 75,
     209-220.
Brown, J.B., MacLeod, S.C., Macnaughtan, C., Smith, M.A.
     (1968) J. Endocr. 42, 5-15.
Evans, J.H., Taft, H.P., Brown, J.B., Adey, F.D. and
     Johnstone, J.W. (1967) J.Obstet. Gynaec. Brit. Cwl
     Cwlth. 74, 367-370.

Figueroa Casa, P.R., Badano, A.R., Aparicio, N.,
     Lencioni, L.J., Berli, R.R., Badano, H., Biccoca,
     C. and Schally, A.V. (1975) Fertil. and Steril.
     26, 549-553.
Gigon, U., Stamm, O. and Werder, H. (1973) Geburtsh. u.
     Frauenheilk. 33, 567-575.
Grimes, E.M., Taymor, M.L. and Thompson, I.E. (1975)
     Fertil. and Steril. 26, 277-282.
Kastin, A.J., Zarate, A., Midgley, A.R., Jr., Canales,
     E.S. and Schally, A.V. (1971) J. Clin. Endocr.
     33, 980-982.
Keller, P.J. (1972) Lancet 2, 570-572.
Keller, P.J. (1973) Amer. J. Obstet. Gynec. 116, 698-
     705.
Mortimer, C.H., Besser, G.M., McNeilly, A.S., Marshall,
     J.C., Harsoulis, P., Tunbridge, W.M.B., Gomez-Pau,
     A. and Hall, R. (1973) Brit. med. J. 4, 73-77.
Mortimer, C.H., McNeilly, A.S., Fisher, R.A., Murray,
     M.A.F. and Besser, G.M. (1974) Brit. med. J. 4,
     617-621.
Mortimer, C.H., Besser, G.M. and McNeilly, A.S.(1975)
     In: Proceedings of the Serono Symposium on Hypo-
     thalamic Hormones (Milan, 14-16 October, 1974)
     in press.
Nakano, R., Mizuno, T., Kotsuji, F., Katayama, K.,
     Washio, M. and Tojo, S. (1973) Acta obstet. gynec.
     scand. 52, 269-272.
Nakano, R., Katayama, K., Mizuno, T. and Tojo, S (1974)
     Fertil. and Steril. 25, 471-477.
Nillius, S.J. and Wide, L. (1972) J. Obstet. Gynaec.
     Cwlth. 79, 865-873.
Nillius, S.J. and Wide,L .(1975) Brit. med. J. 3,
Nillius, S.J., Friberg, J. and Wide, L. (1973a)Acta
     endocr. (Kbh.), Suppl. 177, 349.
Nillius, S.J., Gemzell, C. and Wide, L. (1973b)VII
     World Congress of Obstetrics and Gynaecology.
     Excerpta Medica International Congress Series
     No. 279, 184.

Nillius, S.J., Gemzell, C., Johansson, E.D.B. and Wide, L. (1974) In: Recent Progress in Reproductive Endocrinology (P.G. Crosignani and V.H.T. James, eds) Academic Press, London and New York, pp. 753-775.

Nillius, S.J., Fries, H. and Wide, L. (1975a) Amer. J. Obstet. Gynec. 122, 921-

Nillius, S.J., Friberg, J. and Wide, L. (1975b) Submitted for publication.

Nillius, S.J., Friberg, J. and Wide, L. (1976) In preparation

Pedersen, P.H., Falck Larsen, J., Micic, S. Roos, J. and Sele, V. (1974) Acta Obstet. Gynec. scand. 53, 89-95.

Schally, A.V., Arimura, A., Kastin, A.J., Matsuo, H., Baba, Y., Redding, T.W., Nair, R.M.G., Debeljuk, L., and White, W.F. (1971) Science 173, 1036-1038.

Schally, A.V., Kastin, A.J. and Arimura, A. (1972) Amer. J. Obstet. Gynec. 114, 423-442.

Wide, L., Nillius, S.J., Gemzell, C. and Roos, P. (1973) Acta endocr. (Kbh.) Suppl. 174, 1-58.

Yen, S.S.C., VandenBerg, G., Rebar, R. and Ehara, Y. (1972) J. Clin. Endocr. 35, 931-934.

Zanartu, J., Dabancens, A., Kastin, A.J. and Schally, A.V. (1974) Fertil. and Steril. 25, 160-169.

Zarate, A., Canales, E.S., Schally, A.V., Ayala-Valdes, L. and Kastin, A.J. (1972) Fertil. and Steril. 23, 672-674.

Zarate, A,, A., Canales, E.S., Soria, J., Gonzalez, A., Schally, A.V. and Kastin, A.J. (1974) Fertil. and Steril. 25, 3-10.

Somatostatin

CLINICAL IMPLICATIONS OF GROWTH HORMONE

RELEASE INHIBITING HORMONE (GH-RIH)

G.M. Besser

The Medical Professorial Unit

St. Bartholomew's Hospital, London, EC1A 7BE, England

GH-RIH (or somatostatin) was isolated as a cyclic tetradeca-peptide by Guillemin and his colleagues in 1973, and shown to inhibit growth hormone (GH) release in sheep in vivo and from isolated human acromegalic pituitary cells in vitro, Brazeau et al. (1973). Shortly afterwards, it was shown in in vivo studies in normal human subjects to suppress secretion of GH in response to all known stimuli, including insulin-induced hypoglycaemia, l-dopa, arginine, exercise and sleep (Hall 1973 ; Hansen et al., 1973; Mortimer et al., 1974; Siler et al., 1974). Surprisingly, even in normal subjects, the pituitary effects were not limited to actions on GH since TSH secretion after TRH was impaired although prolactin release after TRH was not reduced (Hall et al., 1973). This material did not affect pituitary LH, FSH or ACTH secretion. However, in addition to the actions on the pituitary, GH-RIH was shown to alter other hormonal secretions in normal subjects. Thus, pancreatic glucagon and insulin secretion were suppressed, as were gastrin, acid and pepsin secretion from the stomach (Mortimer et al., 1974; Alberti et al., 1974; Bloom et al., 1974; Gomez-Pan et al., 1975). There are preliminary studies suggesting that renin secretion can also be suppressed, but that parathyroid hormone secretion is not. These actions in normal subjects have also been investigated in states of abnormal hormonal secretion and these will now be reviewed.

ACROMEGALY

Infusions of GH-RIH have been shown to inhibit rapidly the secretion of GH in acromegalic subjects and the minimum effective dose rate appears to be of the order of 1.3 µg/min. (Besser et al.,

1974a). During short-term (1 hour) or prolonged (28 hours) infusions, not only are the basal blood levels reduced, but the frequently recurring spontaneous surges are obliterated as are the increases in response to food and the often seen paradoxical increments in response to glucose (Fig. 1) (Besser et al., 1974 a, b).

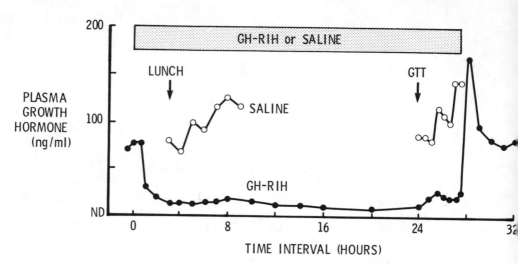

Fig. 1 Effect on circulating GH levels of 28-hr i.v. infusion of GH-RIH (1.3 µg/min) into a acromegalic patient compared with saline control in the same patient (GTT = 50 gm oral glucose tolerance test).

Urinary GH excretion rates are also greatly reduced. In so far unpublished studies, Drs. Lowry and Benker in our laboratories have shown that during such infusions, the nature of the circulating GH changes. Prior to the infusions, much of the circulating GH is present in the most biologically active monomeric form, but during the infusion, the monomeric and oligomeric GH are preferentially reduced so that the majority of any GH remaining in the plasma is in the less biologically active polymeric form.

During such 28-hour infusions, partial suppression of glucagon and insulin secretion has also been noted (Besser et al., 1974 b). In the acromegalic patients who were not diabetic, overall carbohydrate tolerance was not affected by suppression of GH, insulin and glucagon although the acute rise in blood sugar after food or oral

glucose was clearly increased (Fig. 2). The diabetic acromegalic
patients infused in the same way showed improved glucose tolerance
(Besser et al., 1974b).

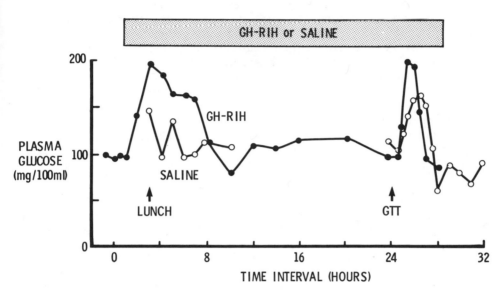

Fig. 2 Blood sugar levels in a non-diabetic acromegalic patient
infused with GH-RIH or saline as in Fig. 1.

        Great interest was therefore aroused concerning the possibili-
ty that GH-RIH could be used to treat acromegaly on a long-term basis. Unfortunately, the compound in both its linear and natural
cyclized forms is very short-acting, and has to be given parenterally by infusion. Useful suppression of GH is not obtained by subcutaneous, intramuscular or by bolus intravenous administration, and
the effects of the infusions pass off within a few minutes of stop-
ping the pump, often then showing a rebound secretion to much higher levels than before (Fig. 1). Attempts to lengthen the time course of action by administrating the tetradecapeptide with gelatin or
arachid oil were fruitless but adsorbing it onto protamine-zinc (by
the method used for making protamine-zinc insulin) resulted in a 4
to 5 hour duration of action after a subcutaneous injection (Besser
et al., 1974 a, b). Although long-acting analogues of GH-RIH have
been described (Brazeau et al., 1974), these have been shown not to
be long-acting in man (Evered et al., 1975). Finally, the original
interest in the use of this material for the treatment of acromega-

ly has been offset by the description of some side effects (see later), and still more by the description of the long-term efficacy in the treatment of acromegaly of the long-acting, orally administered dopaminergic agonist, bromocryptine (Thorner et al., 1975).

HORMONAL SECRETION FROM NON-PITUITARY TUMOURS

Patients with pancreatic tumours which secrete gastrin, glucagon, insulin or VIP (vasoactive intestinal polypeptide) have all been markedly reduced in each. Thus, in the Zollinger-Ellison syndrome, not only do circulating gastrin levels fall, but so does the excessive acid secretion and there may be relief of pain (Bloom et al., 1974). A patient with glucagon levels of between 800 and 950 pg/ml., in association with a presumed pancreatic tumour, became hypoglycaemic (blood glucose, 27 mg/100 ml) when the glucagon levels fell to 340 pg/ml, during an infusion of GH-RIH (Fig. 3), thus demonstrating that the glucagon was maintaining the blood sugar since in this case the low insulin levels were not altered (Mortimer et al., 1974).

We have studied 4 patients with pancreatic insulinoma in whom insulin levels have fallen during GH-RIH infusions. However, a recent report suggests that unlike the situation in normal subjects, tolbutamide-induced insulin secretion is not inhibited in patients with insulinomata (Lorenzi et al., 1975). Some patients with pancreatic tumours have profuse and lethal watery diarrhoea (the Verner-Morrison syndrome or "pancreatic cholera"). These tumours secrete large amounts of VIP into the circulation which seems to be responsible for the symptoms. We have studied 2 "vipoma" patients in conjunction with Dr. S.R. Bloom and Dr. M. Barraclough and shown that the VIP secretion can be inhibited by GH-RIH. We have also studied a patient with a malignant bronchial carcinoid tumour associated with elevated levels of GH and prolactin, and early clinical acromegaly but no evidence of a radiological pituitary lesion. The elevated GH levels have developed as the tumour disseminated, and it seems likely that the bronchial tumour is responsible. It is possible that the tumour could be producing catecholamines which are in turn releasing GH and prolactin from the pituitary, but it is more likely that these hormones are being produced by the tumour tissue ectopically although we have not yet been able to obtain the malignant tissue for hormone assay of extracts. Nevertheless, administration of GH-RIH intravenously resulted in a prompt lowering of the circulating GH levels (Fig. 4).

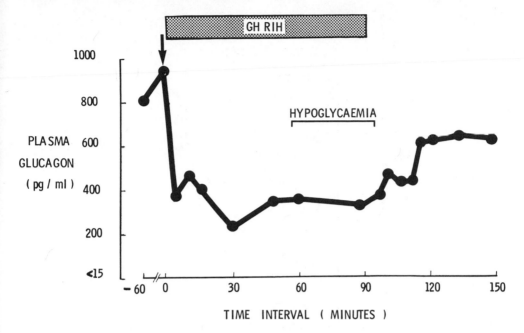

Fig. 3 Changes in plasma glucagon in a patient with a glucagon secreting tumour given an i.v. bolus (500 µg) followed by an infusion
of GH-RIH (6.7 µg/min).

PATHOLOGICAL SECRETION OF TSH, ACTH AND GASTRIC GASTRIN

It is difficult to demonstrate an action of GH-RIH on TSH in
normal subjects as the circulating levels are so low. However, we
have clearly shown that mildly elevated TSH levels are suppressed
during infusions of 6 hours or more of GH-RIH in a thyrotoxic patient rendered euthyroid with carbimazole (Besser et al., 1974 b),
and in a number of patients with myxoedema with markedly elevated
levels. Tyrrell et al. (1975) have recently reported that the very
elevated ACTH levels in patients with Nelson's syndrome are reduced
by GH-RIH although there are no other reports of alterations of ACTH
secretion by this peptide. Gastrin secretion from the stomach is
normally elevated in patients with pernicious anaemia in response
to the achlorhydria. These levels can be reduced by GH-RIH (Bloom
et al., 1974).

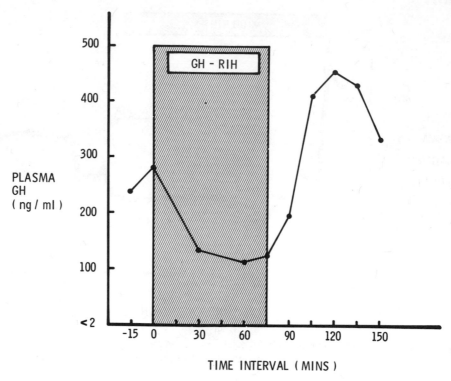

Fig. 4 Changes in circulating GH levels in a patient with a disseminated bronchial carcinoid tumour given an infusion of GH-RIH.

DIABETES MELLITUS

Many believe that increased GH secretion in diabetic patients
may be responsible for the angiopathic complications, and they hope
that treatment with GH-RIH would prevent these. However, as there
is currently no satisfactory form of the preparation for therapy,
there are no data to support this hope. Since there is good evidence that hyperglucagonaemia is involved in the development of diabetic ketoacidosis, it seems likely that GH-RIH would improve this
condition. Gerich et al. (1975) have shown that infusions of GH-RIH
may prevent development of ketoacidosis in diabetics on withdrawal
of insulin, but this topic is dealt with elsewhere in this symposium.
Inappropriately elevated glucagon and GH levels may be involved in
the instability of glucose control shown by some diabetics and it
has been suggested that GH-RIH might stabilize them. We have there-

fore infused one unstable diabetic patient with saline as a control
(24 hours) followed by GH-RIH (2 µg/min for 24 hours) under metabolic ward conditions. At home and during the control saline infusion, the blood sugar levels varied from above 300 mg/100 ml in the
morning to about 40 mg/100 ml in the afternoon when taking her usu-
al doses of insulin. When given GH-RIH but the same food and insulin, GH and glucagon levels were certainly reduced (Figs 5 and 6),
but the blood sugar levels felt dramatically and she required more
oral glucose for her hypoglycaemic attacks than before and indeed
was much more unstable (Fig. 7). Continuous GH-RIH delivery clearly did not help the control but it is possible that twice daily,
preprandial injections of protamine-zinc GH-RIH would be better
since this has a duration of action of 4 to 5 hours.

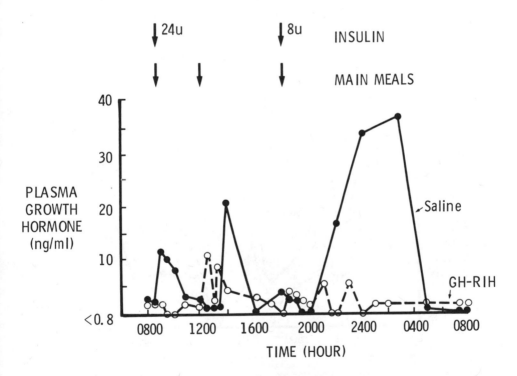

Fig. 5 Circulating GH levels in an unstable diabetic given a control saline infusion and a continuous infusion of GH-RIH.

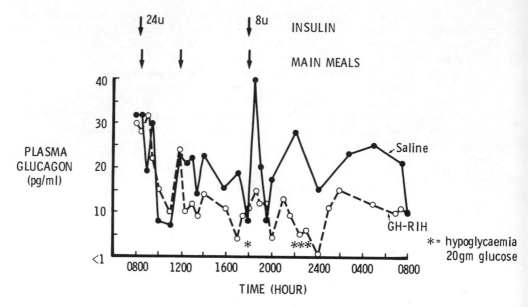

Fig. 6 Circulating glucagon levels in the same unstable diabetic patient shown in Fig. 5 given saline and GH-RIH infusions. The asterisks indicate symptomatic hypoglycaemia necessitating administration of oral glucose.

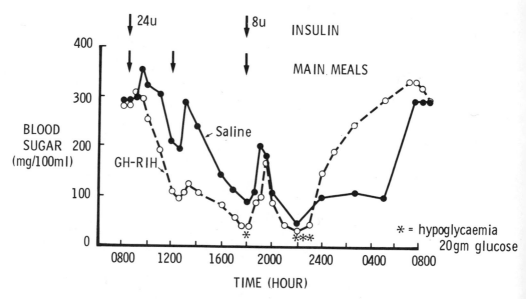

Fig. 7 Blood supar levels in the same unstable diabetic patient shown in Figs 5 and 6, given saline and GH-RIH infusions.

SIDE EFFECTS AND TOXICITY

Side effects of GH-RIH infusions have included abdominal pain
and diarrhoea usually when doses of more than 2 μg/min have been
given for more than 5 hours. Of greater concern are the reports
of alterations in platelet function. Studies in baboons showed
impairment of platelet agglutination, thrombocytopenia and death with
pulmonary haemorrhages in a high proportion of animals treated repeatedly, Koerker (1975), Koerker et al. (1975). Human studies have
shown rapid impairment of platelet agglutination to values of between 19 and 54% of control values after 6-hour infusions with doses of GH-RIH of between 3.4 and 6 μg/min of GH-RIH (Besser et al.,
1975). The effect was seen at 2 hours and continued to become more
marked after the end of the infusions. It may not reach a maximum
until 24 hours later but recovers after a few days. Thrombocytopenia was not seen but there was a marked increase in the immunoreactive fibrin degradation product, fragment FgE, suggesting significantly increased fibrinolysis. The full significance of these alterations is not clear since no workers have yet reported an increased bleeding tendency in patients given GH-RIH. However, it is e-
vident that further long-term infusions into human patients or volunteers would be unwise until these effects on the haemostatic mechanisms are fully elucidated. Our recent studies have shown similar but much shorter lived impairment of platelet agglutination after thyrotropin-releasing hormone infusions but not after the gona-
dotrophin-releasing hormone.

CONCLUSIONS

While GH-RIH is a highly active inhibitor of a specific spectrum of hormones, its potential place in therapy is uncertain. It
can be used to lower GH levels in acromegaly but as there is no satisfactory practical way of administering the peptide effectively
other than by infusion, it appears to have been superceded by bro-
mocriptine. It can reduce the excessive hormonal secretion from a
number of malignant tumours and temporarily aleviate the symptoms
and may therefore have a place in short-term management of such patients, particularly preoperatively. The place for GH-RIH in the
management of diabetes mellitus is also unclear. It cannot yet be
used to treat the angiopathy, and has yet to be shown to stabilize
unstable diabetic control. It does have an action preventing development of ketoacidosis but there is at this time no evidence that
this treatment is better than continuous administration of low doses of insulin. Unfortunately, further evaluation of the actions
of the synthetic tetradecapeptide as a therapeutic agent has been
delayed pending the investigation of the relevance of its potentially toxic side effects on the haemostatic mechanisms.

ACKNOWLEDGEMENTS

The work reported here has been done in collaboration with Professor R. Hall and his colleagues, Dr. A.V. Schally, Dr. A.J. Kastin, Dr. D.H. Coy, Dr. S.R. Bloom, and my colleagues at St. Bartholomew's Hospital. It has been supported by the Medical Research Council, the Joint Research Board of St. Bartholomew's Hospital, and the Peel Medical Research Trust. Figs 1 and 2 are reproduced with the permission of the Editor of the British Medical Journal.

REFERENCES

Alberti, K.G.M.M., Christensen, S.E., Iversen, J., Seyer-Hansen, K., Christensen, N.J., Hansen, Aa.P., Lundbaek, K. and Ørskov, H. (1973) Lancet, $\underline{i}$, 1299-1301.

Besser, G.M., Mortimer, C.H., McNeilly, A.S., Thorner,M.O., Bastistoni, G.A., Bloom, S.R., Kastrup, K.W., Hanssen, K.F., Hall, R., Coy, D.H., Kastin, A.J. and Schally, A.V. (1974a) Brit. Med. J. $\underline{4}$, 622-627.

Besser, G.M., Mortimer, C.H., Carr, D., Schally, A.V., Coy, D.H., Evered, D., Kastin, A.J., Tunbridge, W.M.G., Thorner, M.O. and Hall, R. (1974b) Brit. Med. J. $\underline{1}$, 352-355.

Besser, G.M., Paxton, A.M., Johnson, S.A.N., Moody, E.J., Mortimer, C.H., Hall, R., Gomez-Pan, A., Schally, A.V., Kastin, A.J. and Coy, D.H. (1975) Lancet, $\underline{i}$, 1166-1168.

Bloom, S.R., Mortimer, C.H., Thorner, M.O., Besser, G.M., Hall, R., Gomez-Pan, A., Roy, V.M., Russell, R.C.G., Coy, D.H., Kastin, A.J. and Schally, A.V. (1974) Lancet $\underline{ii}$, 1106-1109.

Brazeau, P., Vale, W., Burgus, R., Ling, N., Butcher, M., Rivier, J. and Guillemin, R. (1973) Science, $\underline{179}$, 77-79.

Brazeau, P., Vale, W., Rivier, J. and Guilemin, R. (1974) Biochem. Biophys. Res. Comm. $\underline{60}$, 1202-1207.

Evered, D.C., Gomez-Pan, A., Tunbridge, W.M.G., Hall, R., Lind, T., Besser, G.M., Mortimer, C.H., Thorner, M.O., Schally, A.V., Kastin, A.J. and Coy, D.H. (1975) Lancet $\underline{i}$, 1250.

Gerich, J.E., Lorenzi, M., Bier, D.M., Schneider, V., Tsalikian, E., Karam, J.H. and Forsham, P.H. (1975) New Eng. J. Med. $\underline{292}$, 985-989.

Gomez-Pan, A., Reed, J.D., Albinus, M., Shaw, R., Hall, R., Besser, G.M., Coy, D.H., Kastin, A.J. and Schally, A.V. (1975) Lancet, i, 888-890.

Hall, R., Besser, G.M., Schally, A.V., Coy, D.H., Evered, D., Goldie, D.J., Kastin, A.J., McNeilly, A.S., Mortimer, C.H., Phenekos, C., Tunbridge, W.M.G. and Weightman, D. (1973) Lancet, ii, 581-584.

Hansen, Aa.P., Ørskov, H., Seyer-Hansen, K. and Lundbaek, K. (1973) Brit. Med. J. 3, 523-524.

Koerker, D., cited by Ricketts, H.T. (1975) J. Amer. Med. Assn. 231, 391-392.

Koerker, D., Harker, L.A. and Goodner, C.J. (1975) New Eng. J. Med., in press.

Lorenzi, M., Gerich, G.E., Karam, J.H. and Forsham, P.H. (1975) J. Clin. Endocrinol. Metab. 40, 1121-1124.

Mortimer, C.H., Tunbridge, W.M.G., Carr, D., Yeomans, L., Lind, T., Coy, D.H., Bloom, S.R., Kastin, A.J., Mallinson, C.N., Besser, G.M., Schally, A.V. and Hall, R. (1974) Lancet, i, 692-701.

Siler, T.M., Yen, S.S.C., Vale, W. and Guillemin, R. (1974) J. Clin. Endocrinol. Metab. 38, 742-745.

Thorner, M.O., Chait, A., Aitken, M., Benker, G., Bloom, S.R., Mortimer, C.H., Sanders, P., Mason, A.S. and Besser, G.M. (1975) Brit. Med. J. 1, 299-303.

Tyrrell, J.B., Lorenzi, M., Gerich, J.E. and Forsham, P.H. (1975) J. Clin. Endocrinol. Metab. 40, 1125-1127.

SOMATOSTATIN AND THE ENDOCRINE PANCREAS

John E. Gerich

Metabolic Research Unit and
Department of Medicine
University of California
San Francisco, California 94143

Somatostatin is a 14-amino acid polypeptide originally isolated from the ovine hypothalamus by Guillemin and
his co-workers at The Salk Institute (Brazeau et al. 1973).
Because of its ability, at nanomolar concentrations, to
inhibit the secretion of growth hormone and its presence
in the hypothalamus of all species examined, it was believed to be a specific hypothalamic hormone (growth hormone release-inhibiting factor) analogous to prolactin
release-inhibiting factor (Guillemin & Vale, 1975).   Recent studies, however, indicate that somatostatin may have
more extensive biologic importance.   There is now considerable evidence that it exists outside the brain and hypo-
thalamus--most notably in the small intestine (Polak et
al. 1975, and Rufener et al. 1975b), stomach (Polak et al.
1975, Rufener et al. 1975b, and Arimura et al. 1975), and
D cells of the pancreatic islets of Langerhans (Polak et
al. 1975, Rufener et al. 1975b, Arimura et al. 1975, Luft
et al. 1974, Dubois 1975, Orci et al. 1975, Rufener et al.
1975a, Patel et al. 1975, and Goldsmith et al. 1975). Furthermore, somatostatin has now been shown to inhibit gastric (Barros D'Sa et al. 1975, Gomez-Pan et al. 1975, and
Arnold & Creutzfeldt, 1975) and pancreatic exocrine secretion (Creutzfeldt et al. 1975, and Boden et al. 1975) as
well as the release of numerous hormones other than growth
hormone (Guillemin & Vale, 1975).   The present report summarizes studies (particularly those performed in our laboratory) dealing with the effect of somatostatin on pancreatic endocrine function.

Koerker and her colleagues (Koerker et al. 1974) first

reported that, during infusion of somatostatin in the ba-
boon, both plasma insulin and glucagon levels declined.'
Subsequent studies from several laboratories performed in
vitro demonstrated that somatostatin acts directly at the
pancreatic level to inhibit insulin and glucagon secretion
(Curry et al. 1974, Efendic et al. 1974, Gerich et al.
1975f, Fujimoto et al. 1974, Turcot-Lemay et al. 1975,
Alberti et al. 1973, Iversen 1974, and Weir et al. 1974).
Several years previously, Hellman and Lernmark (Hellman
& Lernmark 1969) had reported that an extract of pancre-
atic alpha (D) cells inhibited insulin secretion in vitro.
With the demonstration that D cells contain somatostatin
(Polak et al. 1975, Rufener et al. 1975b, Arimura et al.
1975, Luft et al. 1974, Dubois 1975, Orci et al. 1975,
Rufener et al. 1975a, Patel et al. 1975, and Goldsmith et
al. 1975), it seems likely that this peptide may act as a

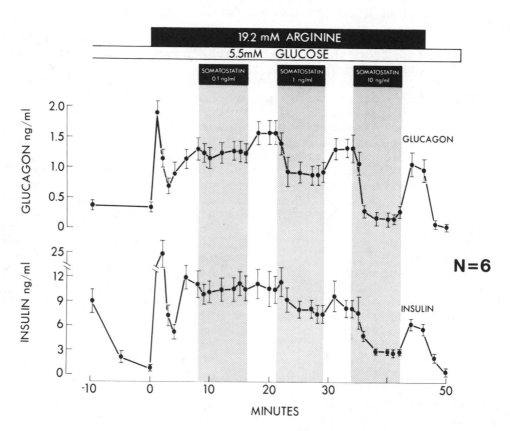

FIG. 1: Inhibition by somatostatin of glucagon and insulin
release from the rat pancreas perfused in vitro.

local regulator of insulin and glucagon secretion. As
shown in Fig. 1, release of these hormones from rat pan-
creases perfused in vitro during stimulation by glucose
(5.5 mM) and arginine (19.2 mM) is inhibited by somatostatin at concentrations as low as 10^{-9} M. Inhibition occurs
almost instantaneously and is rapidly reversible upon removal of somatostatin from the system. Dose-response results (Fig. 2), under the above experimental conditions,
suggest that glucagon secretion may be more readily inhibited than insulin secretion. Similar conclusions have
been drawn from other in vitro studies (Fujimoto et al.
1974), but these may be dependent on the experimental conditions (Johnson et al. 1975 and Bhathena et al. 1975).
Islets freshly prepared by the collagenase technique are
much less responsive to somatostatin than islets isolated
by the same procedure but subsequently cultured for

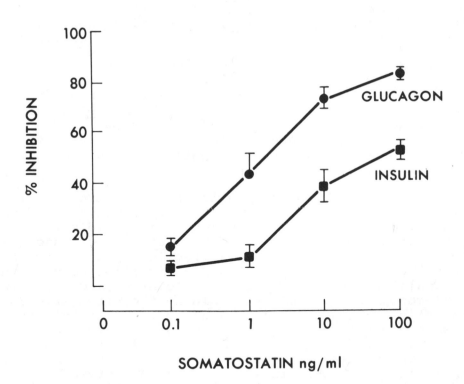

FIG. 2: Preferential, inhibitory effect of somatostatin on
glucagon and insulin release from the rat pancreas perfused
in vitro during stimulation by glucose (5.5 mM) and arginine (19.2 mM).

several days (Efendic et al. 1974, Fujimoto et al. 1974, Turcot-Lemay et al. 1975, and Johnson et al. 1975).

Virtually all known stimuli of insulin (i.e., glucose [Curry et al. 1974, Efendic et al. 1974, Gerich et al. 1975f, Fujimoto et al. 1974, Turcot-Lemay et al. 1975, Alberti et al. 1973, Chideckel et al. 1975, and Leblanc et al. 1975], glucagon [Gerich et al. 1974a and Chideckel et al. 1975], arginine [Koerker et al. 1974, Gerich et al. 1975f, Fujimoto et al. 1974, Iversen 1974, Johnson et al. 1975, Gerich et al. 1974c, Leblanc et al. 1975, and Mortimer et al. 1974], alanine [Sakurai et al. 1974], secretin [Chideckel et al. 1975], theophylline [Gerich et al. 1975f and Turcot-Lemay et al. 1975], tolbutamide [Gerich et al. 1974a and Chideckel et al. 1975], isoproterenol [Gerich et al. 1975f and Chideckel et al. 1975], calcium [Bhathena et al. 1975], and potassium [Turcot-Lemay et al. 1975]) and glucagon (arginine [Gerich et al. 1975f, Fujimoto et al. 1974, Iversen 1974, Johnson et al. 1975, Gerich et al. 1974c, Leblanc et al. 1975, and Mortimer et al. 1974], alanine [Sakurai et al. 1974], epinephrine [Weir et al. 1974 and Gerich et al. 1976], isoproterenol [Gerich et al. 1975f], theophylline [Gerich et al. 1975f], calcium [Bhathena et al. 1975], and hypoglycemia [Chideckel et al. 1975]) are blocked by somatostatin. Basal hormone secretion is also inhibited, even in patients with pancreatic islet-cell tumors secreting insulin (Curnow et al. 1975) or glucagon (Mortimer et al. 1974), as shown in Fig. 3. Curiously, however, insulin responses to tolbutamide are not blocked by somatostatin in patients with insulinomas (Lorenzi et al. 1975).

The exact mechanism by which somatostatin acts is unknown. Presumably, the initial step involves binding to a surface receptor. Because both the oxidized and reduced forms are equipotent (Efendic et al. 1974 and Leblanc & Yen 1975), receptor interaction does not appear to depend on integrity of the Cys-Cys disulfide bond. Since somatostatin has been reported to lower cyclic adenosine 3',5'-monophosphate (cAMP) levels in the pituitary (Borgeat et al. 1974), it has been suggested that this mechanism may cause inhibition of pancreatic hormone secretion. It seems doubtful, however, that a single action on cAMP metabolism can be the sole explanation because somatostatin inhibits not only insulin and glucagon responses to agents that elevate cAMP levels by activating adenylate cyclase (i.e., isoproterenol [Gerich et al. 1975f and Chideckel et al. 1975] and epinephrine [Weir et al. 1974 and Gerich et al. 1976]) but also responses to agents that elevate islet cAMP levels by inactivating cAMP phos-

phodiesterase (i.e., theophylline [Gerich et al. 1975f and
Turcot-Lemay et al. 1975] and tolbutamide [Gerich et al.
1974a and Chideckel et al. 1975]). Furthermore, inhibition by somatostatin is not augmented by an adrenergic receptor blockade (Efendic & Luft 1975). More likely, somatostatin acts later on in the secretory process, such
as by interfering with an action of cAMP or calcium
(Gerich et al. 1975f). Indeed, raising the perfusion calcium concentration has been reported to overcome partially
the inhibitory effects of somatostatin in vitro (Curry &
Bennett 1974 and Bhathena et al. 1975).

The ability to manipulate insulin and glucagon secretion with somatostatin has provided a useful tool for investigating the physiologic and pathologic interactions of
these hormones in man (Gerich et al. 1975c, Gerich et al.
1974b, Leblanc et al. 1975, Christensen et al. 1974,

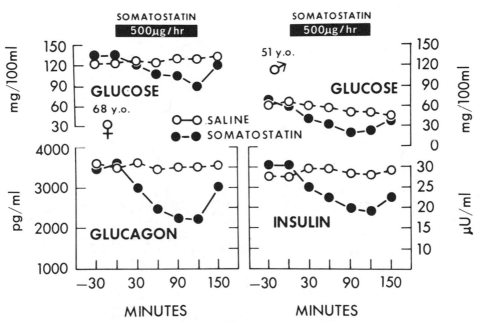

FIG. 3: Suppression of glucagon and insulin secretion in
patients with glucagon- and insulin-producing pancreatic
islet-cell tumors.

Alford et al. 1974, Gerich et al. 1975b, Gerich et al.
1975d, and Gerich et al. 1975e). Although the importance
of insulin in human substrate metabolism has been well established, before the discovery of somatostatin evidence
for the participation of glucagon was based largely on indirect observations and extrapolations from experiments
performed in other species (Unger & Lefebvre 1972). However, recent studies using somatostatin to inhibit human
glucagon secretion have provided direct evidence that the
pancreatic alpha cell is involved in several physiologic
and pathologic processes in man.

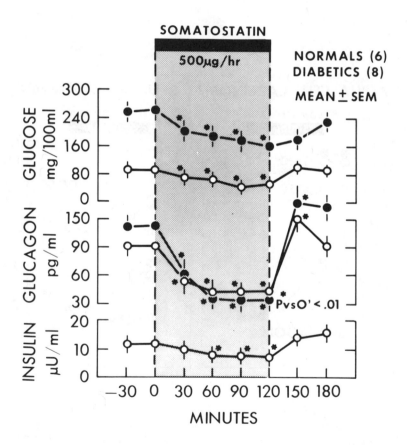

FIG. 4: Effect of somatostatin on fasting plasma glucose
levels in normal and insulin-dependent diabetic subjects.

When somatostatin is infused into normal human subjects after an overnight fast (Fig. 4), plasma glucose levels fall despite a decrease in circulating insulin levels. This cataglycemia appears to be a direct consequence of the somatostatin-induced inhibition of glucagon secretion, since somatostatin itself has no direct effect on either hepatic glucose production (Koerker et al. 1974, Chideckel et al. 1975, and Gerich et al. 1975a) or peripheral glucose utilization (Gerich et al. 1975c, Gerich et al. 1975a, Haas et al. 1975) and can lower plasma glucose levels in hypophysectomized individuals lacking growth hormone. Thus, in contradistinction to the previously widely held view that it was insulin predominantly that maintained euglycemia in man, studies with somatostatin indicate that glucagon may be at least as important as insulin by preventing hypoglycemia.

When somatostatin is infused into overnight-fasted, insulin-deficient diabetic subjects who have not received insulin for at least 24 hr (Fig. 4), plasma glucose levels decline during suppression of glucagon secretion. This decline is greater than that observed in the normal subjects and is positively correlated with the magnitude of fall in glucagon levels. Thus, in diabetics who are insulinopenic and have excessive glucagon secretion, fasting hyperglycemia does not result solely from insulin lack but is due to a large extent to excessive glucagon secretion. Thus, studies with somatostatin have delineated the interplay of pancreatic alpha- and beta-cell function regulating fasting plasma glucose levels in both normal and diabetic man.

To ascertain whether glucagon excess might also contribute to diabetic postprandial hyperglycemia, the effect of somatostatin on plasma glucose and glucagon responses to balanced meals was studied in insulin-dependent diabetic subjects (Fig. 5) (Gerich et al. 1975d). Somatostatin alone was more effective than insulin (15 U regular insulin administered subcutaneously 30 min before eating) in blunting glucagon responses and had approximately the same effect as insulin on plasma glucose rises. Since none of the patients experienced diarrhea or diminished plasma α-aminonitrogen responses, this diminution of postprandial hyperglycemia by somatostatin was attributable to the suppression of glucagon secretion. When insulin and somatostatin were given together, postprandial glucose levels fell instead of rising, despite no further suppression of glucagon secretion than that observed with somatostatin alone. These results thus demonstrate that inappropriate glucagon secretion contributes to excessive hyperglycemia

after meals in diabetic subjects and that suppression of
glucagon secretion renders exogenous insulin much more
effective. Similar results are observed when somatostatin
and insulin are given subcutaneously in the same syringe
(Fig. 6). Suppression of glucagon secretion lasts only
1.5 to 2 hr with this route of administration, even in
doses up to 8 mg (Gerich et al. 1974b)--a handicap current
ly necessitating intravenous infusion for prolonged studie
In contrast to the improvement in glucose tolerance seen
in insulin-dependent diabetics, plasma glucose responses
to meals or glucose are generally worsened by somatostatin
in normal and adult-onset diabetic subjects (Alberti et al
1973, Leblanc et al. 1975, and Mortimer et al. 1974)--not
an unexpected finding since both insulin and glucagon secretion are inhibited under these circumstances.

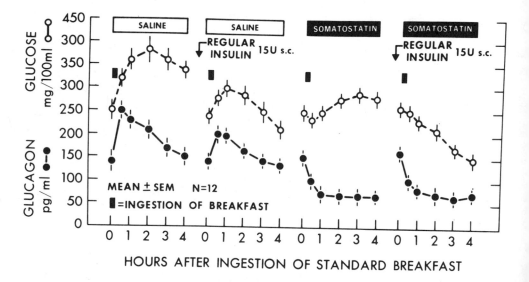

FIG. 5: Effect of somatostatin on postprandial hyperglycemia and hyperglucagonemia in insulin-dependent diabetic
subjects.

Another area in which somatostatin has proven useful as an experimental tool is the study of the hormonal basis for the development of diabetic ketoacidosis in man. Insulin lack has generally been considered the major factor. Nevertheless, plasma glucagon levels rise shortly after withdrawal of insulin from insulin-dependent diabetic subjects (Gerich et al. 1975g and Alberti et al. 1975), and extremely high levels are found in established ketoacidosis (Müller et al. 1973). Since glucagon has the potential to stimulate glycogenolysis, gluconeogenesis, lipoly-

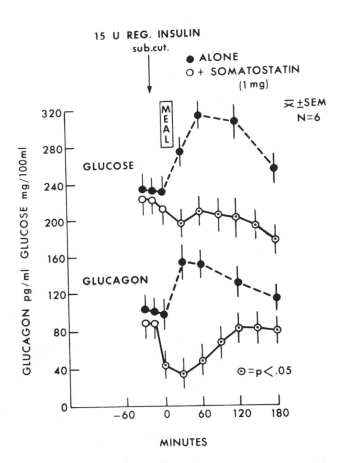

FIG. 6: Comparison of the effect of somatostatin and insulin administered subcutaneously in the same syringe and insulin alone on postprandial hyperglycemia and hyperglucagonemia in insulin-dependent diabetic subjects.

sis, and ketogenesis (Unger & Lefebvre 1972), it seemed
that it might play an important role in the development
of this condition. To investigate this (Gerich et al.
1975b and Gerich et al. 1975d), insulin was withheld from
ketosis-prone, insulin-dependent diabetics who had been

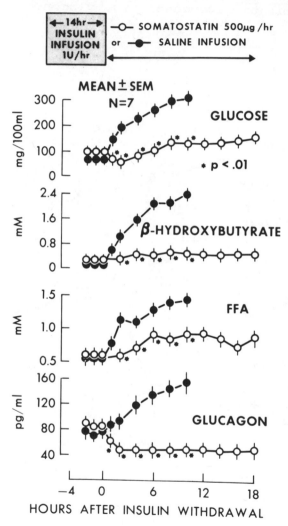

FIG. 7: Effect of somatostatin on plasma glucose, β-hydroxybutyrate, free fatty acid, and glucagon levels after
acute withdrawal of insulin from insulin-dependent diabetic subjects.

kept normoglycemic solely by prolonged intravenous regular insulin infusions; on one day saline was subsequently infused, and on another day somatostatin was infused. Figure 7 demonstrates that, when saline was infused (control

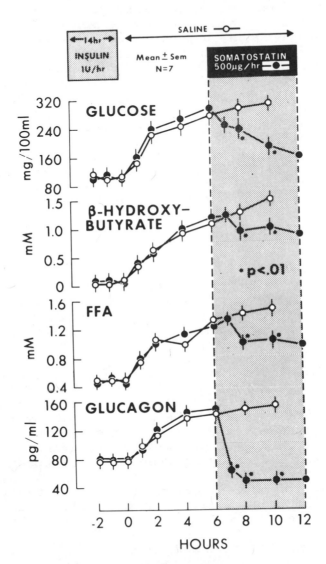

FIG. 8: Effect of glucagon suppression by somatostatin on plasma glucose, β-hydroxybutyrate, and free fatty acid levels 6 hr after withdrawal of insulin from insulin-dependent diabetic subjects.

studies), plasma glucagon, glucose, β-hydroxybutyrate, and
free fatty acid levels rise rapidly within 6 hr of insulin
deprivation; when somatostatin was infused to suppress
glucagon secretion, plasma glucose, β-hydroxybutyrate, and
free fatty acid levels rise minimally. This prevention of
diabetic ketoacidosis can be attributed predominantly to
suppression of glucagon secretion, since somatostatin itself has no direct effect on lipolysis or ketone body production (Gerich et al. 1976 and Gerich et al. 1975a) and
infusion of glucagon, but not growth hormone, completely
reverses the effects of somatostatin (reproducing values
observed during the control study [Gerich et al. 1975e]).
As shown in Fig. 8, when somatostatin is infused for 6 hr
to suppress glucagon secretion 6 hr after insulin withdrawal, plasma glucose levels fall toward normal and no
further rise in β-hydroxybutyrate and free fatty acid
levels occurs, despite the fact that subjects have now been
deprived of insulin for 12 hr. These studies thus demonstrate the important role of glucagon in diabetic ketoacidosis and indicate that insulin lack may be necessary, but
is not in itself sufficient, to initiate and maintain this
condition.

SUMMARY

Thus far, somatostatin has been used primarily as a
research tool to investigate pancreatic alpha- and beta-
cell function. On the basis of its ability to inhibit
insulin and glucagon secretion, several therapeutic applications have been suggested: e.g., as an adjunct in the
treatment of diabetes mellitus, or as a palliative agent
in inoperable islet tumors. Current experiments are underway to develop more specific analogs with longer durations of action to permit clinical evaluation of these
potential applications. The presence of somatostatin
within the pancreatic D cells raises the possibility that
it may function as a local regulator of insulin and glucagon release. Clearly, further work is needed to delineate the factors governing the secretion of somatostatin
and its mode of action. Such studies may uncover a new
class of syndromes resulting from D-cell dysfunction.

ACKNOWLEDGMENTS

These studies at the Metabolic Research Unit (Dr. P.
H. Forsham, Director) were performed in collaboration with
Drs. M. Lorenzi, V. Schneider, E. Tsalikian, J. H. Karam,
and D. M. Bier and Professor G. M. Grodsky. We thank Drs.

R. Guillemin and J. Rivier of The Salk Institute, San Diego, CA., for kindly providing somatostatin, and Gail Gustafson, Frances Sackerman, Ann Aldridge, Emily Gamble, Shiro Horita, and Dr. Satoshi Hane for technical assistance. These investigations were supported in part by the Levi J. and Mary Skaggs Foundation of Oakland, CA., the Susan Greenwall Foundation of New York City, and the National Institutes of Health (grants AM-12763-05 and HD 08340). Clinical studies performed at the General Clinical Research Center, University of California, were supported by the Division of Research Resources (RR-79), U. S. Public Health Service.

REFERENCES

Alberti, K.G.M.M., Christensen, N.J., Christensen, S.E., Hansen, Aa.P., Iversen, J., Lundbaek, K., Seyer-Hansen, K., and Orskov, H. (1973) Lancet 2, 1299-1301.

Alberti, K.G.M.M., Christensen, N.J., Iversen, J., and Orskov, H. (1975) Lancet 1, 1307-1311.

Alford, F.P., Bloom, S.R., Nabarro, J.D.N., Hall, R., Besser, G.M., Coy, D.H., Kastin, A.J., and Schally, A.V. (1974) Lancet 2, 974-976.

Arimura, A., Sato, H., DuPont, A., Nishi, N., and Schally, A.V. (1975) Fed. Proc. 34, 273 (Abstr.).

Arnold, R. and Creutzfeldt, W. (1975) Dtsch. Med. Wschr. 100, 1014-1016.

Barros D'Sa, A.A.J., Bloom, S.R., and Baron, J.H. (1975) Lancet 1, 886-887.

Bhathena, S., Perrino, P., Voyles, N., Smith S., Wilkins, S., Coy, D.H., Schally, A.V., and Recant, L. (1975) Diabetes 24 (Suppl. 2), 408 (Abstr.).

Boden, G., Sivitz, M., Owen, O., Essa-Koumar, N., and Londor, J. (1975) Science (in press).

Borgeat, P., Drouin, J., Belanger, A., and Labrie, F. (1974) Fed. Proc. 33, 263 (Abstr.).

Brazeau, P., Vale, W., Burgus, R., Ling, N., Butcher, M., Rivier, J., and Guillemin, R. (1973) Science 179, 77-79.

Chideckel, E.W., Palmer, J., Koerker, D.J., Ensinck, J., Davidson, M.B., and Goodner, C.J. (1975) J. Clin. Invest. 55, 754-762.

Christensen, S.E., Hansen, Aa.P., Iversen, J., Lundbaek, K., Orskov, H., and Seyer-Hansen, K. (1974) Scand. J. Clin. Lab. Invest. 34, 321-325.

Creutzfeldt, W., Lankisch, P.G., and Fölsch, U.R. (1975) Dtsch. Med. Wschr. 100, 1135-1138.

Curnow, R.T., Carey, R.M., Taylor, A., Johanson, A., and Murad, F. (1975) N. Engl. J. Med. 292, 1385-1386.

Curry, D.L. and Bennett, L.L. (1974) Biochem. Biophys. Res. Commun. 60, 1015-1019.

Curry, D.L., Bennett, L.L., and Li, C.H. (1974) Biochem. Biophys. Res. Commun. 58, 885-889.

Dubois, M. (1975) Proc. Natl. Acad. Sci. U.S.A. 72, 1340-1343.

Efendic, S. and Luft, R. (1975) Acta Endocrinol. 78, 516-523.

Efendic, S., Luft, R., and Grill, V. (1974) FEBS Lett. 42, 169-172.

Fujimoto, W.J., Ensinck, J.W., and Williams, R.H. (1974). Life Sci. 15, 1999-2004.

Gerich, J.E., Bier, D., Haas, R., Wood, C., Byrne, R., and Penhos, J.C. (1975a)Program of the 57th Annual Meeting of The Endocrine Society, New York, June 18-20, 1975, p. 128 (Abstr.).

Gerich, J.E., Lorenzi, M., Bier, D.M., Schneider, V., Tsalikian, E., Karam, J.H., and Forsham, P.H. (1975b). N. Engl. J. Med. 292, 985-989.

Gerich, J.E., Lorenzi, M., Hane, S., Gustafson, G., Guillemin, R., and Forsham, P.H. (1975c). Metab. (Clin. Exp.) 24, 175-182.

Gerich, J.E., Lorenzi, M., Karam, J.H., Schneider, V., and Forsham, P.H. (1975d) J.A.M.A. (in press).

Gerich, J.E., Lorenzi, M., Schneider, V., and Forsham, P. H. (1974a) J. Clin. Endocrinol. Metab. 39, 1057-1060.

Gerich, J.E., Lorenzi, M., Schneider, V., Karam, J.H., Rivier, J., Guillemin, R., and Forsham, P.H. (1974b) N. Engl. J. Med. 291, 544-547.

Gerich, J.E., Lorenzi, M., Schneider, V., Kwan, C.W., Karam, J.H., Guillemin, R., and Forsham, P.H. (1974c) Diabetes 23, 876-880.

Gerich, J.E., Lorenzi, M., Tsalikian, E., and Karam, J.H. (1976) Diabetes (in press).

Gerich, J.E., Lorenzi, M., Tsalikian, E., Schneider, V., Karam, J.H., Bier, D., and Forsham, P.H. (1975e) Clin. Res. 23, 421A (Abstr.).

Gerich, J.E., Lovinger, R., and Grodsky, G.M. (1975f) Endocrinology 96, 749-754.

Gerich, J.E., Tsalikian, E., Lorenzi, M., Karam, J.H., and Bier, D.M. (1975g) J. Clin. Endocrinol. Metab. 526-529.

Goldsmith, P., Rose, J., Arimura, A., Gerich, J., and Ganong, W. (1975) The Physiologist (in press).

Gomez-Pan, A., Reed, J.D., Albinus, M., Shaw, B., Hall, R., Besser, G.M., Coy, D.H., Kastin, A.J., and Schally, A.V. (1975) Lancet 1, 888-890.

Guillemin, R. and Vale, W. (1975) Rec. Prog. Horm. Res. (in press).

Haas, R., Clausen, E., Woods, C., Lorenzi, M., Bier, D., Hane, S., and Gerich, J.E. (1975) Clin. Res. 23, 110A (Abstr.)

Hellman, B. and Lernmark, A. (1969) Endocrinology 84, 1484-1488.

Iversen, J. (1974) Scand. J. Clin. Lab. Invest. 33, 125-129.

Johnson, D.G., Ensinck, J.W., Koerker, D., Palmer, J., and Goodner, C.J. (1975) Endocrinology 96, 370-374.

Koerker, D.J., Ruch, W., Chideckel, E., Palmer, J., Goodner, C.J., Ensinck, J., and Gale, C.C. (1974) Science
184, 482-484.

Leblanc, H., Anderson, J.R., Sigel, M.B., and Yen, S.S.C.
(1975) J. Clin. Endocrinol. Metab. 40, 568-572.

Leblanc, H. and Yen, S.S.C. (1975) J. Clin. Endocrinol.
Metab. 40, 906-908.

Lorenzi, M., Gerich, J.E., Karam, J.H., and Forsham, P.H.
(1975) J. Clin. Endocrinol. Metab. 40, 1121-1124.

Luft, R., Efendic, S., Hökfelt, T., Johansson, O., and
Arimura, A. (1974) Med. Biol. 52, 428-430.

Mortimer, C.H., Tunbridge, W.M.G., Carr, D., Yeomans, L.,
Lind, T., Coy, D.H., Bloom, S.R., Kastin, A., Mallinson,
C.N., Besser, G.M., Schally, A.V., and Hall, R. (1974)
Lancet 1, 697-701.

Müller, W.A., Faloona, G.R., and Unger, R.H. (1973) Am.
J. Med. 54, 52-57.

Orci, L., Baetens, D., and Rufener, C. (1975) Horm. Metab.
Res. (in press).

Patel, Y.C., Weir, G.C., and Reichlin, S. (1975) Program
of the 57th Annual Meeting of The Endocrine Society, New
York, June 18-20, 1975, p. 127. (Abstr.).

Polak, J.M., Pearse, A.G.E., Grimelius, L., Bloom, S.R.,
and Arimura, A. (1975) Lancet 1, 1220-1222.

Rufener, C., Amherdt, M., Dubois, M., and Orci, L. (1975a)
J. Histochem. Cytochem. (in press).

Rufener, C., Dubois, M., Malaisse-Lagae, F., and Orci, L.
(1975b) Diabetologia (in press).

Sakurai, H., Dobbs, R., and Unger, R.H. (1974) J. Clin.
Invest. 54, 1395-1402.

Turcot-Lemay, L., Lemay, A., and Lacy, P.E. (1975) Biochem.
Biophys. Res. Commun. 63, 1130-1138.

Unger, R. and Lefebvre, P. (eds.) (1972) Glucagon: Molecular Physiology, Clinical and Therapeutic Implications.
Pergammon Press, New York.

Weir, G.C., Knowlton, S.D., and Martin, D.B. (1974) Endocrinology <u>95</u>, 1744-1746.

Mechanism of Action of Hypothalamic Hormones and Steroid Feedback

NEW ASPECTS OF THE MECHANISM OF ACTION OF HYPOTHALAMIC REGULATORY HORMONES

F. LABRIE, A. DE LEAN, N. BARDEN, L. FERLAND,
J. DROUIN, P. BORGEAT, M. BEAULIEU and O. MORIN

Medical Research Council Group in Molecular
Endocrinology, Centre Hospitalier de l'Université Laval, Québec, G1V 4G2, Canada

Elucidation of the structure of the first hypophysiotropic hormone, TRH, from porcine (Bøler et al., 1969) and ovine (Burgus et al., 1969) hypothalami opened a new era in the field of neuro-endocrinology. This achievement was soon followed by the isolation of LH-RH, the neurohormone which stimulates the release of both LH and FSH (Matsuo et al., 1971; Burgus et al., 1971). More recently, the tetradecapeptide H-Ala-Gly-Cys-Lys-Asn-Phe-Phe-Trp-Lys-Thr-Phe-Thr-Ser-Cys-OH has been isolated from ovine and porcine hypotha-lami (Brazeau et al., 1973; Schally et al., 1975) on the basis of its ability to inhibit GH release and called somatostatin or GH-RIH.

Although important information on the role of hypothalamic hormones in the control of anterior pituitary function could be obtained using hypothalamic extracts at different stages of puri-fication, the relative ease of synthesis of these peptides and their analogs has opened new possibilities for studies of their mechanism of action. It has in fact led to a rapid expansion of our knowledge of the physiology of the hypothalamo-pituitary com-plex.

This presentation will first attempt to summarize the data describing the effect of three synthetic hormones, namely LH-RH, TRH and somatostatin, on cyclic AMP accumulation in anterior pi-tuitary gland. Since the characteristics of binding of TRH and properties of adenohypophyseal protein kinase and of some of its substrates have been described in recent reviews (Labrie et al.,

1975 a,b), these aspects will not be included in the present discussion. Emphasis will be given instead to the interactions between TRH and somatostatin on TSH and PRL secretion, the antagonism
between estrogens and thyroid hormone in the control of the number of TRH binding sites in adenohypophyseal tissue, the evidence
for an hypothalamic site of inhibitory action of thyroid hormone,
the evidence for a physiological role of somatostatin in the control of GH and TSH secretion, and the evidence for an hypothalamic
site of action of prostaglandins in the in vivo stimulation of LH,
TSH and PRL secretion.

Stimulatory effect of LH-RH and TRH on cyclic AMP accumulation in anterior pituitary gland

The action of many polypeptide hormones and of catecholamines
is at least partly mediated by changes of the levels of cyclic AMP
in target cells (Robison, Butcher and Sutherland, 1968). The first
suggestive evidence for a role of cyclic AMP as mediator of the
action of the hypothalamic releasing hormones in the anterior pituitary gland originated from the observations that cyclic AMP derivatives or theophylline, an inhibitor of cyclic nucleotide phosphodiesterase, stimulate the release of the six main anterior pituitary hormones. Stimulation or inhibition of adenylate cyclase
activity in specific pituitary cell types by the corresponding stimulatory and inhibitory hypothalamic regulatory hormones could thus
provide a mechanism of control of adenohypophyseal hormone secretion.

Much recent evidence indicates that cyclic AMP is involved as
mediator of the action of LH-RH in the anterior pituitary gland.
It is in fact well recognized that addition of LH-RH leads to a
stimulation of cyclic AMP accumulation in rat anterior pituitary
gland in vitro (Borgeat et al., 1972; Jutisz et al., 1972; Makino,
1973; Kaneko et al., 1973; Labrie et al., 1973; Borgeat et al.,
1974a). The concentration of LH-RH required for half-maximal stimulation of cyclic AMP accumulation is between 0.1 and 1.0 ng/ml
or between 1×10^{-10} and 1×10^{-9}M LH-RH (Borgeat et al., 1972).
A close correlation is always observed between rates of LH and FSH
release and changes of intracellular cyclic AMP concentrations, both
as a function of time of incubation and concentration of the neurohormone.

Moreover, when LH-RH analogs having a spectrum of biological
activity ranging from 0.001% to 500-1000% the activity of LH-RH
itself were used, the same close parallelism between stimulation
of cyclic AMP accumulation and both LH and FSH release was found
under all experimental conditions (Borgeat et al., 1974a). That
LH-RH exerts its action by activation of adenylate cyclase and
not inhibition of cyclic nucleotide phosphodiesterase is indi-

cated by the observation that a similar effect of the neurohormone
is observed in the presence or absence of theophylline (Borgeat
et al., 1972).

An even more striking correlation between changes of cyclic
AMP levels and rates of LH and FSH release was obtained with inhibitory analogs of LH-RH. In studies performed in collaboration
with Drs. Coy and Schally, we have recently found that peptide analogs in which the residues His and Leu at positions 2 and 6 are
replaced by D-Phe and a D-amino acid, respectively, have potent
anti-LH-RH activity both in vivo (Ferland et al., 1975) and in
vitro (Labrie et al., 1975c). When these analogs were studied in rat
hemipituitaries in vitro (Beaulieu et al., 1975), a striking correlation was found between the inhibition of adenohypophyseal cyclic AMP levels and rates of LH and FSH release. These observations add strong support to the already obtained evidence for a
mediator role of the adenylate cyclase system in the action of LH-
RH in anterior pituitary gland.

Although there was no doubt that theophylline and cyclic AMP
derivatives stimulate TSH release from anterior pituitary gland
in vitro (Wilber et al., 1969; Cehovic, 1969), more convincing
proof of the role of the adenylate cyclase system in the action of
TRH awaited the demonstration of a stimulation of cyclic AMP
accumulation in anterior pituitary gland by synthetic TRH.
Although the changes of cyclic AMP levels are of smaller magnitude
than those observed under stimulation by LH-RH, a significant increase (30% over control) is measured after 15 min of incubation
with 10^{-6}M TRH, while a maximal effect at 50% over control is found
after 2 h of incubation (Labrie et al., 1975a,b).

Inhibitory effect of somatostatin on cyclic AMP accumulation in anterior pituitary gland

Since we had previously found that a purified fraction of GH-
RH led to parallel stimulation of cyclic AMP accumulation and GH
release in rat hemipituitaries in vitro (Borgeat et al., 1973), it
was felt of interest to study the effect of somatostatin on the
same parameters.

Addition of somatostatin was found to lead to a rapid inhibition of adenohypophyseal levels of cyclic AMP accompanied by
decreased rates of secretion of both GH and TSH (Borgeat et al.,
1974b). A maximal inhibition of cyclic AMP levels (40-50% of
control) was in fact measured 10 min after addition of the tetradecapeptide. Since GH- and TSH-secreting cells account for 50
to 70% of the total cell population in the male rat adenohypophysis, the observed inhibition to 40 to 50% of control indicates
an almost complete inhibition of cyclic AMP levels in somatotrophs.

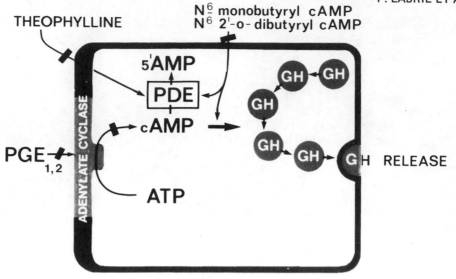

SOMATOTROPH
EFFECTS OF SOMATOSTATIN

Figure 1: Schematic representation of the inhibitory
effect of somatostatin on basal adenylate cyclase activity as well as on the basal and prostaglandin E_1- or
E_2-, theophylline-, N^6-monobutyryl cyclic AMP and N^6,
2'0-dibutyryl cyclic AMP-induced release of GH.

and thyrotrophs. As illustrated in Fig. 1, somatostatin not only
inhibits the basal GH release but also the release stimulated by
prostaglandins (Bélanger et al., 1974), theophylline (Borgeat et
al., 1974b) and derivatives of cyclic AMP (Vale et al., 1972; Bélanger
et al., 1974; Borgeat et al., 1974b). These data indicate that the
most likely mode of action of somatostatin is through inhibition
of adenylate cyclase activity at the plasma membrane level.

The data summarized so far clearly show that two synthetic
stimulatory hypothalamic hormones, TRH and LH-RH, as well as purified GH-RH, lead to parallel stimulation of cyclic AMP accumulation and specific hormone release while one inhibitory peptide,
somatostatin, leads to parallel inhibition of cyclic AMP accumulation and GH and TSH release. Such findings suggest strongly
that changes of adenylate cyclase activity are involved in the
mechanism of action of these peptides in the anterior pituitary
gland.

Characteristics of interaction between TRH and somatostatin

Since the possibility exists that the rate of secretion of both TSH and PRL may, up to an unknown extent, be dependent upon the relative concentrations of TRH (stimulatory) and somatostatin (inhibitory) in the portal hypothalamo-hypophyseal blood, we felt of interest to study in detail the characteristics of interaction of these two hypothalamic peptides on TSH and PRL secretion. These studies were performed with pituitary cells in culture.

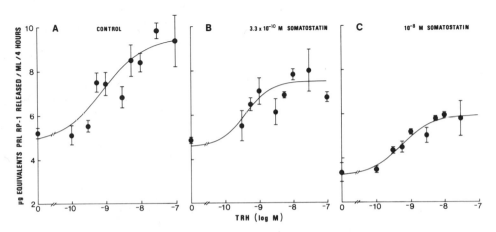

Figure 2: Effect of increasing concentrations of TRH on the release of PRL in female rat anterior pituitary cells in culture in the absence (A) or presence of 3.3 x 10^{-10}M (B) or 1 x 10^{-8}M (C) somatostatin, (from Drouin et al., 1976).

Fig. 2 shows that somatostatin (3.3 x 10^{-10} and 1 x 10^{-8}M) leads to a progressive inhibition of both basal and TRH-induced release of PRL in anterior pituitary cells in culture. It can be seen, however, that the TRH ED$_{50}$ for PRL release is not affected by the presence of somatostatin. Similar data were obtained on TSH release. These data showing no effect of somatostatin on the ED$_{50}$ value of stimulation of TSH (Drouin et al., 1976) or PRL (fig. 2) release by TRH indicate quite clearly that the two hypothalamic peptides act on different receptors in both TSH- and PRL-secreting cells. These data are supported by the findings that somatostatin does not affect the binding of [^{3}H] TRH to purified bovine adenohypophyseal plasma membranes (De Léan and Labrie, unpublished observations).

We have previously found that TRH stimulates while somatostatin inhibits cyclic AMP accumulation in anterior pituitary tissue. Since TRH receptors are associated, at least up to a major extent, with plasma membranes (Labrie et al., 1972; Poirier et al., 1972) which are also the site of adenylate cyclase (Poirier et al., 1974), it is likely that the first step in the action of these two peptides is binding to specific receptors localized on the external surface of the plasma membrane with resultant activation (for TRH) or inhibition (for somatostatin) of adenylate cyclase activity.

Antagonism between estrogens and thyroid hormone in the control of TRH binding sites

The data obtained so far on the characteristics of binding of [3H] TRH (Labrie et al., 1972; Grant et al., 1972) and its close association with adenylate cyclase activity (Poirier et al., 1972; Labrie et al., 1975a) indicate that the sequence of events in the action of TRH would presumably be: (1) binding of TRH to specific receptor sites on the external surface of the plasma membrane of thyrotrophs or mammotrophs, and (2) activation of adenylate cyclase with elevation of intracellular levels of cyclic AMP leading to activation of protein kinase, phosphorylation of protein substrates and altered rates of specific subcellular functions.

Since estrogens are well known to be potent stimulators of prolactin secretion (Nicoll and Meites, 1962) and TRH stimulates both TSH and PRL release in estrogen-treated rats (Vale et al., 1974), it became of interest to study a possible effect of estrogen treatment on TRH binding. As illustrated in Fig. 3, treatment of male rats with estradiol benzoate for 9 days (25 µg/day) leads to an approximately 2.5-fold increase of the total number of pituitary TRH binding sites without any detectable change of the affinity of the receptor for the neurohormone. Time-course experiments have shown that the increase of binding occurs between 2 and 4 days and that a plateau of stimulation is reached after one week of treatment (De Léan et al., 1976).

Since treatment with estrogens stimulates not only PRL but also TSH secretion in both intact and hypothyroid rats (Drouin et al., 1976) and thyroid hormone inhibits the secretion of both TSH (Bowers et al., 1967; Vale et al., 1968; Reichlin et al., 1970, 1974) and PRL (Yamahi, T., 1974; Drouin et al., 1976), it became of interest to study in more detail the characteristics of interaction between estrogens and thyroid hormones in the control of [3H] TRH binding sites and to attempt to correlate these changes of binding sites for TRH with the TSH and PRL responses to the neurohormone.

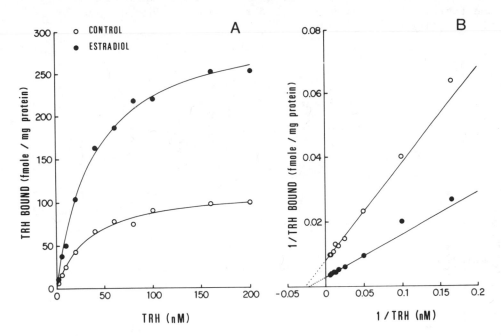

Figure 3: Effect of treatment with estradiol benzoate (25 μg/day x 9 days) on anterior pituitary [3H] TRH binding in male rats. [3H] binding was measured on adenohypophyseal homogenates as described (Labrie et al., 1972).

In rats made hypothyroid by chronic administration of propylthiou-racil, the number of pituitary TRH binding sites is increased approximately 2-fold while it is reduced after thyroid hormone treatment (Wilber and Seibel, 1973; De Léan et al., 1974).

Fig. 4 shows that although estrogen treatment has little ef-fect on the plasma TSH response to TRH in both intact (left panel) and hypothyroid (right panel) animals, it leads to 50% and com-plete reversal of the inhibitory effect of thyroid hormone in in-tact and hypothyroid animals, respectively. It can also be noti-ced that the basal levels of plasma TSH are increased in all groups after estradiol treatment.

The data indicating that binding to only a small fraction of the total population of cellular receptors is sufficient for full activation of adenylate cyclase activity (Birnbaumer and Pohl, 1973) suggest that the number of binding sites could be an important factor of control of cellular activity. An increase of the number of binding sites would permit a similar cellular response at a

lower concentration of the circulating hormone while a lowering of
the number of binding sites would require a higher concentration
of the circulating hormone.

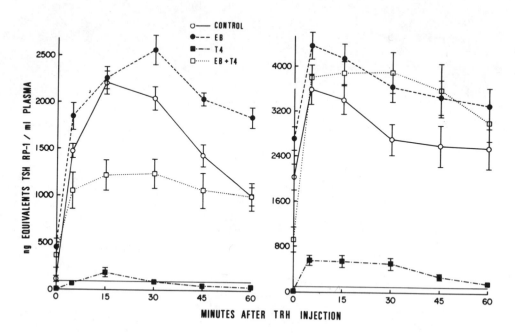

Figure 4: Effect of treatment for 9 days with estradiol benzoate (50 µg/day), L-thyroxine (10 µg/day) or
a combination of both on the plasma TSH response to
TRH (25 µg, i.v.) in intact (left panel) or hypothyroid
propylthiouracil-treated (right panel) male rats under
Surital anesthesia.

The present data indicate that the number of TRH binding sites
is under positive and negative control by estrogens and thyroid
hormone, respectively. It is also clear from Fig. 4 that this
antagonism exerted on the number of binding sites is reflected on
the plasma TSH response to TRH. Similar data are obtained on the
PRL response. Although it is tempting to suggest that changes of
the levels of TRH binding sites are responsible for the observed
changes of activity in both thyrotrophs and mammotrophs, the proof
of such a role remains to be obtained.

Evidence for an inhibitory effect of thyroid hormone at the hypotha-
lamic level

According to the classical model (Reichlin, 1966), the rate of

TSH secretion by the anterior pituitary gland is controlled by a stimulating factor, TRH, and an inhibitory influence, the level of circulating thyroid hormones (Bowers et al., 1967; Vale et al., 1968; Reichlin et al., 1970, 1974).

Our previous observation (Fig. 4, right panel) of a complete reversal of the inhibitory effect of thyroid hormone on the plasma TSH response to TRH in hypothyroid rats offered an ideal model for assessing a possible inhibitory effect of thyroid hormone at the hypothalamic level. In fact, the finding of decreased plasma TSH levels in the presence of a normal pituitary response to TRH would clearly indicate an inhibitory effect of thyroid hormone at the hypothalamic level. As illustrated in Fig. 5, the daily administration of 10 µg L-thyroxine inhibits plasma TSH to undetectable levels in control as well as hypothyroid rats (propylthiouracil-treated or thyroidectomized) and this inhibitory effect is not reversed by estrogen treatment.

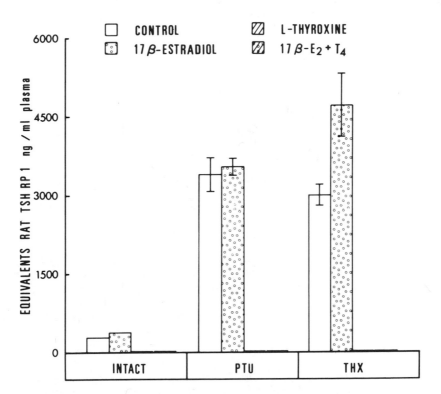

Figure 5: Effect of treatment for 9 days with estradiol-17β (10 µg/day), L-thyroxine (10 µg/day) or both on the basal levels of plasma TSH in intact, propylthiouracil-treated or thyroidectomized male rats.

Combination of these data and those of Fig. 4 indicate that
thyroid hormone exerts an inhibitory action at both the pituitary
and hypothalamic levels in the control of TSH secretion (Fig. 6).

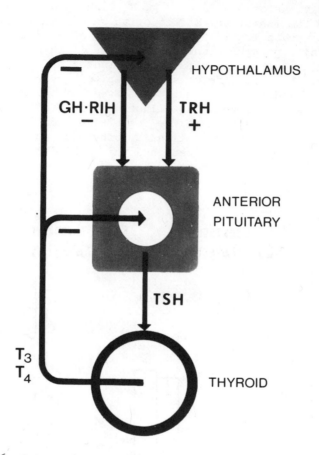

Figure 6: Schematic representation of the hypothalamic
pituitary thyroid axis. Thyroid hormone is shown to
exert an inhibitory action at both the hypothalamic
and pituitary levels. The inhibitory effect at the
hypothalamic level could be mediated by a decreased
release of TRH, an increased secretion of somatostatin
or an association of both.

Since, as shown later (Fig. 7), not only TRH but also somatostatin are involved in the physiological control of TSH secretion,
the inhibitory effect of thyroid hormone could be due to a decreased release of TRH or an increased secretion of somatostatin from
the hypothalamus or a combination of both.

Evidence for a physiological role of somatostatin in the control
of GH and TSH secretion

Although the presence of somatostatin in hypothalamic tissue
(Brazeau et al., 1973; Schally et al., 1975) and the demonstration
of its inhibitory effect on GH and TSH release (Brazeau et al.,
1974; Bélanger et al., 1974; Borgeat et al., 1974b; Vale et al.,
1974) after its exogenous administration both in vitro and in vivo
strongly suggested a role of the peptide in the control of GH
and TSH secretion, proof of its physiological role remained to be
obtained. It was thus felt of interest to study the effect of injection of a somatostatin antiserum on plasma levels of both GH
and TSH in the rat. In the event of a role of somatostatin in
the physiological control of GH and TSH secretion, the antiserum
should neutralize circulating somatostatin and lead to an increase of the plasma levels of these two hormones.

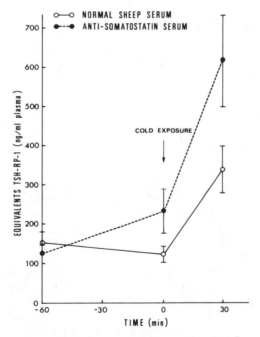

Figure 7: Effect of sheep anti-somatostatin serum on the
basal levels of plasma TSH and the response of the hormone to exposure to cold (5°C). 1.0 ml of sheep antiserum was injected through a catheter 1 h before exposure
to cold and plasma TSH measurements performed at the indicated time intervals.

Fig. 7 shows that administration of the somatostatin antiserum kindly provided by Dr. A. Arimura, New Orleans, not only leads to a 100% increase of basal plasma TSH levels measured 60 min after its injection but also potentiates (p<0.05) by about 80% the plasma TSH response measured 30 min after exposure to cold.

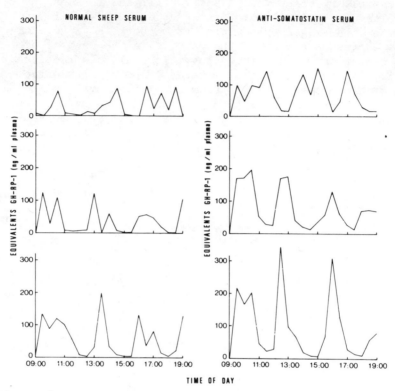

Figure 8: Representative patterns of plasma GH in freely-moving animals who received 1.0 ml of normal sheep serum (left panels) or the same amount of sheep anti-somatostatin serum (right panels). Blood samplings were performed every 30 min.

Since plasma GH levels in the rat show great variability (Schalch and Reichlin, 1968; Collu et al., 1973; Martin et al., 1975), plasma GH levels were measured every 30 min for a period of 10 h. Left panels of Fig. 8 show representative patterns of plasma GH levels in control rats injected with 1 ml of normal

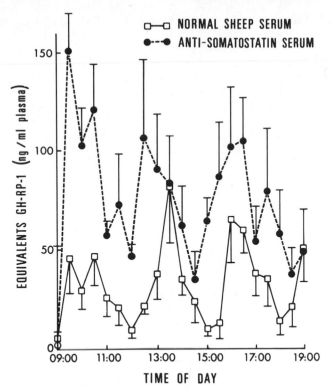

Figure 9: Effect of sheep anti-somatostatin serum on plasma GH levels. Data are presented as mean ± S.E.M. of 10 animals per group. Control rats received an equivalent volume of normal sheep serum.

sheep serum. Control animals show episodic bursts of plasma GH with levels ranging from 5 to above 200 ng/ml. In animals injected with somatostatin antiserum (right panels), the pulsatile release of GH is maintained but the amplitude of the peaks is increased 2- to 3-fold. Fig. 9 illustrates more precisely the effect of the somatostatin antiserum on plasma GH levels in a group of ten freely-moving animals. The area under the first plasma GH peak is increased 2 to 3-fold while the effect of the antibody, although still apparent, decreases progressively thereafter.

In the rat, cold exposure leads to a rapid increase of plasma TSH levels (Jobin and Fortier, 1965). The present findings that somatostatin antibody not only increases basal plasma TSH levels but also enhances its response to cold exposure suggest strongly that the tetradecapeptide plays a physiological role in the control of TSH secretion.

Data of Figs. 8 and 9 illustrate the pulsatile pattern of GH release in the control rat (Martin et al., 1975) with bursts of release occuring approximately every 3 h. It can also be clearly seen that neutralization of circulating somatostatin by the antibody leads to a general increase of plasma GH levels with maintenance of the pulsatile release of the hormone. These findings, beside indicating a physiological role of somatostatin in the control of basal GH secretion, suggest that the episodic bursts of GH release occuring in the freely-moving rat are not secondary to cyclic release of somatostatin but are likely to be due to intermittent release of GH-releasing hormone from the hypothalamus.

Evidence for a hypothalamic site of action of prostaglandins in the in vivo stimulation of LH, TSH and PRL release

Prostaglandins of the E type are well known to stimulate cyclic AMP accumulation in anterior pituitary gland (MacLeod and Lehmeyer, 1970; Zor et al., 1970; Borgeat et al., 1975). PGE_1 and E_2 are in fact the most potent activators of pituitary adenylate cyclase activity. They are in fact more potent than PGA_1 and A_2 while $PGF_{1\alpha}$ and $PGF_{2\alpha}$ exert a slight stimulatory effect only at high concentrations ($10^{-4}M$).

Since PGE-induced increases of pituitary cyclic AMP were measured in total anterior pituitaries, it was felt important to study the specificity of PG action by measuring changes of specific hormone release. In fact, cyclic AMP being a potent stimulator of the release of all six pituitary hormones, changes of specific hormone release should be a good indication of the cell types responsible for the increased cyclic AMP levels observed after addition of PGs.

As illustrated in studies performed with anterior pituitary cells in culture (Drouin and Labrie, 1976), PGE_1 has an important stimulatory effect on GH release only, a half-maximal (ED_{50}) stimulation of GH release being measured at 1 x $10^{-7}M$ PGE_1. Up to 3 x $10^{-4}M$, PGE_1 has no effect on LH, FSH and PRL release while TSH release is slightly but reproducibly stimulated (170% of control value) at concentrations higher than $10^{-6}M$.

Stimulation of GH release does not show an absolute specificity for PGEs since all eight primary prostaglandins are able to elicit GH release at high concentrations (Drouin and Labrie, 1976). PGEs are the most potent stimulators of GH release, a half-maximal stimulation by PGE_1 and E_2 being measured at 1-4 x $10^{-7}M$ while values of 3-10 x 10^{-6}, 1-3 x 10^{-5} and approximately 3 x $10^{-4}M$ are obtained for PGAs, PGBs and PGFs, respectively. The order of potency of the various PGs to stimulate GH release from anterior

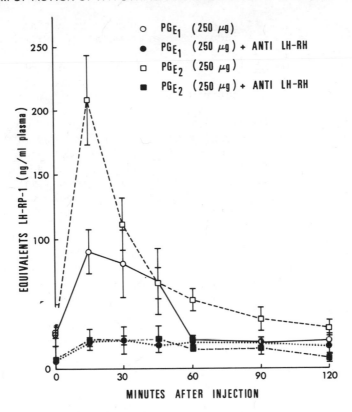

Figure 10: Effect of 1 ml anti-LH-RH serum on PGE₁- or
PGE₂-induced LH release in anesthesized female rats on
the afternoon of proestrus. The anti-serum was injected
1 h before PGEs through a canula inserted into the right
superior vena cava. Plasma LH concentrations are plotted
as mean ± S.E.M. of 6 to 8 rats.

pituitary cells in culture closely parallels the potency previously
observed on cyclic AMP accumulation. Such knowledge of the specificity of action of prostaglandins at the pituitary level should
then be of great help in the interpretation of _in vivo_ experiments.

It is well known that PGs of the E type stimulate LH release
after _in vivo_ administration. PGEs have in fact been found to
increase plasma LH levels in pentobarbital-blocked proestrus rats
(Tsafiri _et al._, 1973) as well as in steroid-primed ovariectomized

(Harms et al., 1974; Sato et al., 1974) and in intact male (Ratner et al., 1974) animals. Evidence for a stimulatory effect of $PGF_{2\alpha}$ on in vivo LH release has also been obtained in sheep (McCracken et al., 1973; Carlson et al., 1973).   These data do not however differentiate between an effect of PGs at the hypothalamic level on LH-RH release and a direct pituitary site of action on LH secretion.

Since the reports concerning the in vitro effects of PGs on LH release are conflicting (Ratner et al., 1974; Zor et al., 1970), it was felt important to examine the in vivo site of action of PGs using a LH-RH antiserum. In the event of an hypothalamic site of action of PGs, administration of the antiserum should neutralize the PG-induced LH-RH release and thus prevent the accompanying increase of plasma LH levels.

As clearly illustrated in Fig. 10, not only the basal plasma LH concentration was reduced by approximately 75% one h after injection of the antiserum but the treatment almost completely obliterated the plasma LH rise observed after injection of PGE_1 or PGE_2.   This observation of an almost complete inhibition of the PGE_1- or PGE_2-induced rise of plasma LH in animals treated one h previously with sheep anti-LH-RH serum leaves little doubt that the increased plasma LH levels observed in vivo after PGE administration are secondary to an effect of PGs on LH-RH release at the hypothalamic level.

Since PGE_1 and PGE_2 raise plasma LH levels in pentobarbital or thyamilal-treated animals, it is likely that parenterally administered PGs act directly on the nerve endings containing LH-RH (Pelletier et al., 1974) in the median eminence to induce release of the neurohormone.

Fig. 11 illustrates the stimulatory effect of PGE_2 on the plasma levels of both TSH and PRL in rats pretreated with estradiol benzoate. Since PGs do not affect PRL release in vitro and somatostatin does not affect basal or TRH-induced PRL release in vivo in the rat, it is likely that the observed stimulation of both PRL and TSH release after PGE_2 injection is secondary to increased TRH release from the hypothalamus. A decreased release of somatostatin could however be partly involved in the TSH response.

The previous data clearly show that at the pituitary level, PGs of the E type lead to parallel stimulation of cyclic AMP accumulation and GH release accompanied by a small but consistent stimulation of TSH release while the release of LH, FSH and PRL remains unchanged. As far as the hypothalamic site of action of PGs is concerned, data illustrated in Figs. 10 and 11 suggest that they might well be involved in the control of LH-RH and TRH secretion.

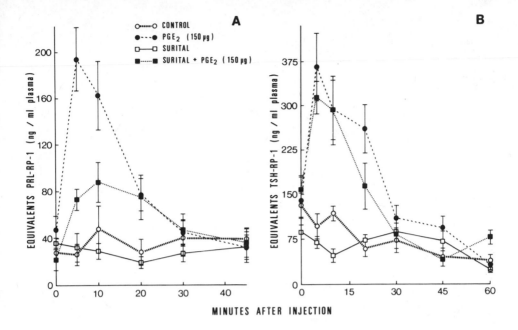

Figure 11:   Effect of 150 µg PGE₂ on plasma TSH and PRL
levels in male rats pretreated with estradiol benzoate
(25 µg/day) for 7 days.   Blood samples were collected
through a cannula in free-moving rats or under Surital
anesthesia.

Since PGs have been found to stimulate cyclic AMP accumulation in brain (Ramwell and Shaw, 1970; Wellman and Schwabe, 1973)
and there is much evidence for a role of cyclic AMP in neuronal
function (Bloom et al., 1975; Greengard, 1975), it was felt of
interest to study a possible stimulatory effect of systemically
administered PGs on cyclic AMP accumulation in the hypothalamus.
In order to prevent the important rise of cyclic AMP levels occuring at the hypothalamic level after decapitation, rats were
killed by microwave irradiation.   A significant stimulation of
cyclic AMP accumulation was apparent at a dose of 1 µg of PGE₁
while a maximal effect was seen at the dose of 100 µg.

Whilst the injection of 100 µg of PGE₁ was found to stimulate anterior pituitary cyclic AMP levels 100-fold, only a 2-fold
stimulation was seen in total hypothalamic tissue (Fig. 12).

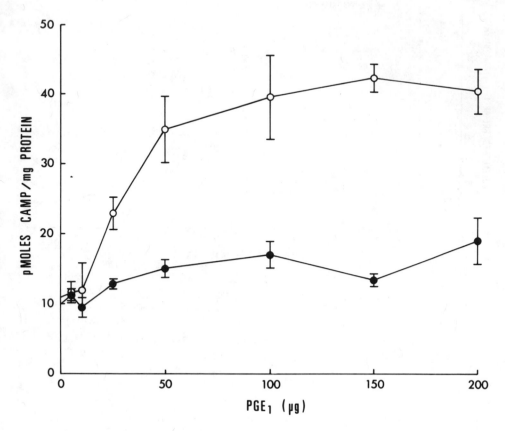

Figure 12: Effect of increasing doses of PGE$_1$ administered intravenously on the cyclic AMP levels in total hypothalamus (●——●) and median eminence (o——o) in rats
under Surital anesthesia killed by microwave irradiation
5 min after injection of PGE$_1$.

Measurements of cyclic AMP in the median eminence show that the
stimulation of cyclic AMP is restricted to this area and is about
4-fold at the highest dose of PGE$_1$ used. These changes of cyclic
AMP content in hypothalamic tissue after in vivo injection of PGs
may well be involved with the PG-induced release of LH-RH and TRH.

REFERENCES

Beaulieu, M., Labrie, F., Coy, D.H., Coy, E.J. and Schally, A.V. (1975) J. Cyclic Nucl. Res., in press.

Bélanger, A., Labrie, F., Borgeat, P., Savary, M., Côté, J., Drouin, J., Schally, A.V., Coy, D.H., Coy, E.J., Immer, H., Sestanj, K., Nelson, V., and Gotz, M. (1974) J. Mol. Cel. Endocrinol. 1, 329-339.

Birnbaumer, L. and Pohl, S.L. (1973) J. Biol. Chem. 248, 2056-

Bloom, F.E., Siggins, G.R., Hoffer, B.J., Segal, M. and Olivier, A.P. (1975) In "Advances in cyclic nucleotide research" (G.I. Drummond, P. Greengard and G.A. Robison, eds) Raven Press, pp. 603-618.

Bøler, J., Enzman, F., Folkers, K., Bowers, C.Y. and Schally, A.V. (1969) Biochem. Biophys. Res. Commun. 377, 705-

Borgeat, P., Chavancy, G., Dupont, A., Labrie, F., Arimura, A. and Schally, A.V. (1972) Proc. Nat. Acad. Sci. U.S.A. 69, 2677-2681.

Borgeat, P., Labrie, F., Poirier, G., Chavancy, G. and Schally, A.V. (1973) Trans. Ass. Am. Phys. 86, 284-299.

Borgeat, P., Labrie, F., Côté, J., Ruel, F., Schally, A.V., Coy, D.H., Coy, E.J. and Yanaihara, N. (1974a) J. Mol. Cel. Endocrinol. 1, 7-20.

Borgeat, P., Labrie, F., Drouin, J., Bélanger, A., Immer, H., Sestanj, K., Nelson, V., Gotz, M., Schally, A.V., Coy, D.H. and Coy, E.J. (1974b) Biochem. Biophys. Res. Commun. 56, 1052-1059.

Borgeat, P., Garneau, P., and Labrie, F. (1975) Can. J. Biochem. 53, 455-460.

Bowers, C.Y., Schally, A.V., Reynolds, G.A. and Hawley, W.D. (1967) Endocrinology 81, 741-747.

Brazeau, P., Vale, W., Burgus, R., Ling, N., Butcher, M., Rivier, J., and Guillemin, R. (1973) Science 179, 77-79.

Brazeau, P., Rivier, J., Vale, W., and Guillemin, R. (1974) Endocrinology 94, 184-187.

Burgus, R., Dunn, T.F., Desiderio, D. and Guillemin, R. (1969)
C.R. Acad. Sci. Paris 269, 1870-

Burgus, R., Butcher, M., Ling, N., Monahan, M., Rivier, J.,
Fellows, R., Amoss, M., Blackwell, R., Vale, W. and Guillemin, R.
(1971) C.R. Acad. Sci. (Paris) 273, 1611-1613.

Carlson, J.C., Barcikowski, B. and McCracken, J.A. (1973) J.
Reprod. Fertil. 34, 357-361.

Cehovic, G. (1969) C.R. Acad. Sci. Paris, 268, 2929-2931.

Collu, R., Jequier, J.C., Letarte, J. and Ducharme, J.R. (1973)
Neuroendocrinology, 11, 183-190.

De Léan, A., Beaulieu, D., and Labrie, F. (1974) Clin. Res.
22, 730A.

De Léan, A., Drouin, J. and Labrie, F. (1976) Manuscript in
preparation.

Drouin, J., De Léan, A., Rainville, D., Lachance, R. and Labrie,
F. (1976) Endocrinology, in press.

Drouin, J. and Labrie, F. (1976) Prostaglandins, submitted for
publication.

Ferland, L., Labrie, F., Coy, D.H., Coy, E.J. and Schally, A.V.
(1975) Fertil. Steril. 26, 889-893.

Grant, G., Vale, W. and Guillemin, R. (1972) Biochem. Biophys.
Res. Commun. 46, 28-34.

Greengard, P. (1975). In "Advances in cyclic nucleotide research"
(G.I. Drummond, P.Greengard, and G.A. Robison, eds) Raven Press
pp. 585-602.

Harms, P.G., Ojeda, S.R. and McCann, S.M. (1974) Endocrinology
94, 1459-1464.

Jobin, M. and Fortier, C. (1965) Fed. Proc. 24, 149-

Jutisz, M., Kerdelhue, G., Berauld, A. and Paloma de la Llosa,
M. (1972) In "Gonadotropins" (Saxena, B.B., Beling, C.G. and
Gandy, H.M., eds) Wiley Interscience pp. 64-71.

Kaneko, T., Saito, S., Oka, H., Oda, T. and Yanaihara, N. (1973)
Metabolism 22, 77-78.

Labrie, F., Barden, N., Poirier, G. and De Léan, A. (1972) Proc. Nat. Acad. Sci. U.S.A. 69, 283-287.

Labrie, F., Pelletier, G., Leamy, A., Borgeat, P., Barden, N., Dupont, A., Savary, M., Côté, J., and Boucher, R. (1973) In "Control of protein synthesis in anterior pituitary gland" Karolinska Symposium on Research Methods in Reproductive Endocrinology (E. Diczfalusy, ed.) Geneva, pp. 301-340.

Labrie, F., Borgeat, P., Lemay, A., Lemaire, S., Barden, N., Drouin, J., Lemaire, I., Jolicoeur, P. and Bélanger, A. (1975a) In "Advances in cyclic nucleotide Research" (Drummond, G.I., Greengard, P. and Robison, G.A., eds) vol. V, Raven Press, New York, pp. 787-801.

Labrie, F., Drouin, J., Ferland, L., Barden, N. and Bélanger, A. (1975b) In "Molecular Aspects of Hormone-Receptor Interaction" (G.S. Levey, ed.) Modern Pharmacology Series, Marcel Deker, New York, in press.

Labrie, F., Savary, M., Coy, D.H., Coy, E.J., and Schally, A.V. (1975c) Endocrinology, in press.

MacLeod, R.M. and Lehmeyer, J.E. (1970) Proc. Nat. Acad. Sci. 67, 1172-1179.

Makino, T. (1973) Am. J. Obst. Gynecol. 115, 606-614.

Martin, J.B., Tannenbaum, G., Willoughby, J.O., Renaud, L.P. and Brazeau, P. (1975) In "Hypothalamis Hormones chemistry, physiology, pharmacology and clinical uses" (M. Motta, P.G. Crosignani, and L. Martini, eds.) Academic Press, pp. 217-285.

Matsuo, H., Baba, Y., Nair, R.M.G., Arimura, A. and Schally, A.V. (1971) Biochem. Biophys. Res. Commun. 43, 1334-1339.

McCracken, J.A., Barcikowski, B., Carlson, J.C., Green, K., and Samuelsson, B. (1973) Adv. Biosciences 9, 599-624.

Nicoll, C.S. and Meites, J. (1962) Endocrinology 70, 272-277.

Pelletier, G., Labrie, F., Puviani, R., Arimura, A. and Schally, A.V. (1974) Endocrinology 95, 314-317.

Poirier, G., Labrie, F., Barden, N., and Lemaire, S. (1972) FEBS Letters 20, 283-286.

Poirier, G., De Léan, A., Pelletier, G., Lemay, A., and Labrie, F. (1974) J. Biol. Chem. 249, 316-322.

Ramwell, P.W. and Shaw, J.E. (1970) Rec. Progr. Horm. Res. 26, 139-173.

Ratner, A., Wilson, M.C., Srivastava, L. and Peake, G.T. (1974) Prostaglandins 5, 165-171.

Reichlin, S. (1966) In "Neuroendocrinology" (L. Martini and W.F. Ganong, eds) vol I, pp. 415-536, Academic Press, New York.

Reichlin, S., Martin, J.B., Boshans, R.L., Schalch, D.S., Pierce, J.G. and Bollinger, J. (1970) Endocrinology 87, 1022-1030.

Reichlin, S., Martin, J.B., Mitnick, M.A., Boshans, R.L., Grimm, Y., Bollinger, J., Gordon, J. and Malacara, J. (1974) Recent Progr. Horm. Res. 30, 229-286.

Robison, G.A., Butcher, R.W. and Sutherland, E.W. (1968) Ann. Rev. Biochem. 37, 149-174.

Sato, T., Taya, K., Jyuno, T., Hirono, M., and Igarashi, M. (1974) Am. J. Obst. Gynecol. 118, 875-876.

Schalch, D.S., and Reichlin, S. (1968) In "Growth Hormone" (A. Pecile and E.E. Müller, eds.) Excerpta Medica Amsterdam p. 211.

Schally, A.V., Dupont, A., Arimura, A., Redding, T.W. and Linthicom, G.L. (1975) Fed. Proc. 34, 584-586.

Tsafiri, A., Koch, Y. and Lindner, H.R. (1973) Prostaglandins 3, 461-467.

Vale, W., Burgus, R., and Guillemin, R. (1968) Neuroendocrinology 3, 34-46.

Vale, W., Brazeau, P., Grant, G., Nussey, A., Burgus, R., Rivier, J., Ling, N. and Guillemin, R. (1972) C.R. Acad. Sci. (Paris) 275, 2913-2916.

Vale, W., Rivier, C., Brazeau, P., and Guillemin, R. (1974) Endocrinology 95, 968-977.

Wellmann, W. and Schwabe, U. (1973) Brain Research 59, 371-378.

Wilber, J., Peake, G.T. and Utiger, R. (1969) Endocrinology, $\underline{84}$, 758-760.

Wilber, J.F. and Seibel, M.J. (1973) Endocrinology $\underline{92}$, 888-

Yamahi, T. (1974) Metabolism $\underline{23}$, 745-751.

Zor, U., Kaneko, T., Schneider, H.P.G., McCann, S.M. and Field, J.B. (1970) J. Biol. Chem. $\underline{245}$, 2883-2888.

STEROID BINDING IN THE HYPOTHALAMUS AND PITUITARY

Jean-Pierre RAYNAUD, Marie-Madeleine BOUTON,
Daniel PHILIBERT and Bernard VANNIER

Centre de Recherches Roussel-UCLAF
93230 Romainville, France

Over the last few years, biochemical studies have established
the existence of estrogen receptors in specific regions of the hypothalamus of adult male and female rats, presently indistinguisha-
ble from pituitary and uterine receptors, and of androgen receptors
in the hypothalamus of the adult male. As yet, the existence of
progesterone receptors is unproven (Kato, 1975).

The development of these receptors throughout foetal and neonatal life has been widely speculated upon, but so far, remains im-
precise. That steroid hormones exert an action on brain tissues is
indicated by countless observations on the effect of their neonatal
administration on the development of the hypothalamo-pituitary axis
and on sexual behaviour (Brown-Grant, 1974). As yet, however, their
specific action on the developing tissues of the very houng rat has
not been demonstrated and it has not been possible to assess whether
this action is via a receptor mechanism (Maurer, 1974; Barley et
al., 1974). This is to a large extent due to the lack of sensitivity of existing techniques.

Study of the ontogeny of steroid tissue hormone receptors is
further complicated by the presence of plasma proteins which specifically bind natural hormones. For instance, estradiol is bound
by EBP in the plasma of the pregnant mother, fetus and young animal
of several species (Raynaud et al., 1971; Raynaud, 1973; Swartz et
al, 1974). In the present studies, synthetic compounds were used
to measure hormone hypothalamic binding sites and to dissociate the
parts played by tissue and plasma binding in the activity of hormones in the young animal. Synthetic compounds, preferably with high
affinity for hormone receptors and not bound by plasma proteins,
were used (Raynaud et al., 1973a, b; Philibert and Raynaud, 1973;
Philibert and Raynaud, 1974a,b; Bonne and Raynaud, 1975).

EXPERIMENTAL RESULTS

ESTROGENS

Plasma binding : In the rat, estradiol binds to a specific binding protein in the plasma of pregnant animals, fetuses and
immature offspring of both sexes. As shown in Fig. 1, the concentration of this protein is very high in the fetus and decreases
linearly from birth with a half-life of 3.9 ± 0.3 days. It reaches
zero level at 29 days of age.

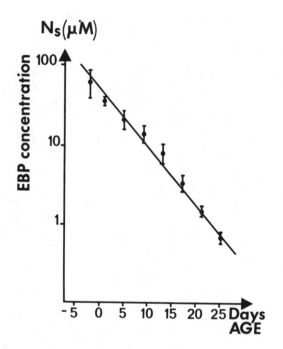

FIG. 1. Specific estradiol binding sites in rat plasma as a function
        of age

        1 ml of diluted plasma from Sprague-Dawley SPF rats of diffe-
rent ages (day 0 = birth) was placed in a Nojax dialysis bag and
dialyzed for 48 hr at 4°C against 15 ml of 0.1 M phosphate buffer
(pH 7.4) containing 0.1 nM 6,7[3H]-estradiol (56 Ci/mmole) and 0.2
to 1000 nM radioinert estradiol. The radioactivity of three 0.2 ml
aliquots from inside and outside the bag was counted. The number of
binding sites was evaluated from a proportion graph (Raynaud et al.,
1971).

The specificity of this binding protein was studied (Table 1). Among natural estrogens, estrone was more tightly bound and estriol much less tightly bound than estradiol. None of the non-estrogenic natural hormones studied (testosterone, androstanolone, progesterone and corticosterone) competed. Among synthetic estrogens, diethylstilbestrol, a non-steroidal compound, was slightly bound and 11β-methoxy-17α-ethynyl-estradiol (R 2858) was not bound at all. For this reason , R 2858 was considered an ideal tool, on the one hand, for the study of how a plasma protein, in this case EBP, can affect biological activity and, on the other hand, for the detection of target tissue estrogen binding sites in the presence of EBP.

TABLE 1. *Percentage decrease in plasma bound 6,7[^{3}H]-estradiol in the presence of radioinert steroid*

	10 nM	100 nM	1000 nM
ESTRADIOL	18	38	48
Estrone	33	48	59
Estriol	10	9	31
Testosterone	3	4	6
Androstanolone	0	0	9
Progesterone	4	2	1
Corticosterone	5	2	1
17α-ethynyl estradiol	4	6	33
17-deoxyestradiol	0	3	20
11β-methoxy-estradiol	10	4	8
11β-methoxy-17α-ethynyl estradiol	0	0	0
Diethylstilbestrol	0	9	30

1 ml of diluted plasma (1/100) from 20-day old female Wistar rats was placed in a Nojax dialysis bag and dialyzed for 48 hr at 4°C against 15 ml of 0.1 M phosphate buffer (pH 7.0) containing 0.15 nM 6,7[^{3}H]-estradiol (56 Ci/mmole) and various concentrations of radioinert steroid (10,100,1000nM). The percentage decrease in plasma bound 6,7[^{3}H]-estradiol was recorded.

Comparative activity of estradiol and R 2858 : Although R 2858 has a lower affinity than estradiol for the "8S" estradiol receptor in rat uterus cytosol, it is more uterotrophic than estradiol in the immature 3-week old rat. Its activity is directly related to its *in vivo* uptake and not to its *in vitro* affinity. The R 2858/estradiol uterotrophic activity ratio is even higher in the very young animal and decreases with age as EBP disappears (Table 2).

TABLE 2. *Uterine weight (mg) following a single subcutaneous injection of R 2858 or estradiol to rats of different ages*

Dose (µg)	5 DAYS R 2858	E	13 DAYS R 2858	E	21 DAYS R 2858	E	28 DAYS R 2858	E
0	7.81 ±0.25		19.01 ±0.79		23.62 ±0.86		38.97 ±1.48	
0.005	9.02 ±0.34 ***		33.47 ±0.99 ***		47.13 ±0.70 ***		39.66 ±1.83 ***	
0.05	10.20 ±0.26 ***	7.76 ±0.12	31.97 ±1.19 ***	19.93 ±0.42	49.37 ±2.29 ***	34.43 ±0.68 ***	61.59 ±2.97 ***	58.40 ±2.03 ***
0.5	8.94 ±0.43 ***	8.14 ±0.12	31.99 ±0.97 ***	20.77 ±0.81	61.62 ±2.01 ***	43.97 ±1.71 ***	69.89 ±2.04 ***	57.48 ±2.14 ***
5		7.97 ±0.13		22.97 ±1.58 ***		38.24 ±0.94 ***		79.92 ±3.63 ***

A single dose of R 2858 or estradiol (E) in 0.1 ml of a 10% solution of ethyl alcohol in saline was administered subcutaneously to 5,13, 21 and 28 day-old female Sprague-Dawley SPF rats. Control rats received solvent only. Since previous experiments had established that the compounds give rise to slightly different dynamic responses following a single injection and that the maximum response occurs between 24 and 40 hours, animal pairs were sacrificed at 24 hr and at 40 hr and the mean uterine weight for each pair was calculated. The overall mean responses for each dose were then evaluated and compared to control responses according to Dunnett's one-sided multiple comparison test (* $p < 0.5$, *** $p < 0.01$).

At 5 days of age, only R 2858 was able to induce a trophic response. The lowest dose was sufficient to induce the maximum response and must therefore have saturated the receptor. Estradiol was inactive whatever the dose. At 13 days of age, all R 2858 doses gave rise to a highly significant response and estradiol began to exhibit slight activity at the highest dose. R 2858 was at least 100 times as active as estradiol, since only 0.005 µg of R 2858

were necessary to induce a response greater than that given by 5 μg
of estradiol. At 21 days of age, all estradiol and R 2858 doses
gave rise to a highly significant response and roughly the same
uterine weight was obtained with 0.5 μg of estradiol as with 0.005μg
and 0.05 μg of R 2858. Statistical analysis (Duncan's test) established that the 0.005 μg dose of R 2858 was not significantly
different from 0.5 μg of estradiol. The R 2858/estradiol potency
ratio for 21 day-old rats was therefore between 10 and 100. At
28 days of age, the lowest R 2858 dose was no longer active and,
for the first time, estradiol induced the highest response. According to Duncan's test, the top estradiol and R 2858 doses are no
longer significantly different from each other, neither are the
remaining estradiol and middle R 2858 doses. The R 2858/estradiol
potency ratio was therefore between 1 and 10.

Administration of estrogens to pregnant rats is known to affect
the morphology of the fetal sexual organs. R 2858 gave rise to
exactly the same changes in the genital tract of the male rat fetus
as estradiol but at much lower doses (Fig.2). Following injection
of 50 μg and 250 μg of estradiol from day 16 to 20 of gestation,
one observe more or less total inhibition of the ventral and
dorsal prostatic buds, variable stimulation of the prostatic utricle, atrophy of the ejaculatory ducts and epithelial proliferation
of the urethral wall. These same effects were observed with as
little as 2 μg of R 2858. An approximate potency ratio was deduced
by comparing the effects of these marginally active doses. A dose
of 2 μg of R 2858 inhibited prostate formation more markedly than
50 μg of estradiol, yet not quite as markedly as 250 μg of estradiol giving an R 2858/estradiol potency ratio of 25 to 125. A comparison with younger control fetuses (21 days-old) established
that these effects were indeed due to perturbed sexual differentiation and not merely to differences in general development.

In a second study, the offspring of the treated mothers were
allowed to grow to adulthood and were then mated with normal part-
ners. Some pertinent results are given in Table 3. Bilateral testicular atrophy was observed only in those males from mothers
treated with the highest dose of both compounds. These rats were,
for the majority, unable to fertilize normal females, whereas at
lower doses, virtually all the males mated gave rise to a number
of implantations per pregnant female identical to control. The
female offspring were much more affected by the treatment. Fifty
percent developed persistent diestrus when the mothers had been
injected with a dose as low as 2 μg of R 2858. Moreover, at this
dose, only 58% of the females able to mate were still fertile
though they had only relatively few implantations. At the highest
dose of both compounds, all rats were in persistent diestrus.

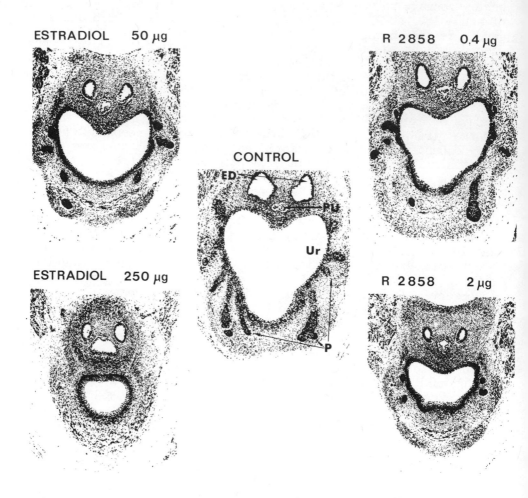

FIG.2. *Transversal sections of the sinus urogenitalis of male fetu-*
ses from treated and control mothers (ED = ejaculatory
ducts, PU = prostatic utricle, UR = urethra, P = prostate).

Pregnant Sprague-Dawley SPF rats were treated subcutaneously
with either R 2858 or estradiol in 0.5 ml of a 5% solution of benzyl
alcohol in sesame oil from day 16 to day 20 of gestation, day 1
being determined by the presence of spermatozoa in the vaginal
smears. At autopsy on day 22, the fetuses were excised. The abdominal region of male fetuses was embedded in paraffin, sectioned at
6 μ and every 5th section was stained with hematoxylin-eosin for
histological examination.

TABLE 3. *Some effects of treatment of pregnant rats with R 2858 or estradiol on 3 month old male and female offspring*

	MALES					FEMALES				
	Total no. of males	No. of mating males	No. of mated females	No. pregnant	Mean no. of implant-ations per rat	Incidences of crypt-orchidism & atrophy of testes (*= atrophy of one testis only)	Total no. of females	No. of mated females	No. of pregnant	Mean no. of implant-ations per rat	No. of females in persistent diestrus over 2 wks
0	*33*	*31*	*38*	*37*	*13*	*0/20*	*40*	*29*	*22*	*13*	*0/11*
R 2858										
0.4	23	22	32	27	13	0/23	24	19	16	9	0/5
2	35	30	35	31	13	1*/30	61	36	21	4	12/25
10	30	28	35	32	12	5*/30	33	4	1	1	28/29
50	27	6	12	1	9	16/24	24	0	0	0	24/24
ESTRADIOL										
50	20	18	22	22	13	0/20	30	21	18	11	0/9
250	19	17	22	19	13	1*/15	18	13	13	7	0/5
1250	6	0	0	0	0	6/6	10	0	0	0	10/10

Pregnant Sprague-Dawley SPF rats were treated subcutaneously with either R 2858 or estradiol in 0.5 ml of a 5% solution of benzyl alcohol in sesame oil from day 16 to day 20 of gestation, day 1 being determined by the presence of spermatozoa in the vaginal smears. The offspring, when adult, were mated with normal male and female rats. Male offspring were placed in a cage with 3 normal females for 8 nights. Each time a vaginal plug was detected, the female was removed and replaced. Female offspring were placed first with one set of 3 normal males proven fertile for 1 week and then with another set of 3 for a further week. The following criteria were used : male offspring were considered to have mated if a vaginal plug was detected in one or more of the normal females. Female offspring had mated if a vaginal plug was formed and was fertile if implanted.

Estrogen binding in the rat hypothalamus : Following administration of labelled estradiol to the 5-week old female rat, radioactivity was retained in the hypothalamus. This retention was preferential in the anterior and middle, but not posterior regions
as demonstrated by evaluating the ratio of the radioactivity levels
between presumed target and non-target tissues of similar cellular
structure (in this case the cerebral cortex). The ratio tissue/
cortex was markedly higher than 1 for the anterior hypothalamus
(5.6), somewhat higher for the middle hypothalamus (2.6), but
virtually equal to 1 for the posterior hypothalamus. This bound
radioactivity could be prevented in target tissues by the prior

TABLE 4 . *Preferential radioactivity uptake by the hypothalamus of
the 5-week old female rat following injection of 6,7[^{3}H]-
estradiol*

	*E			*E+E	*E+R2858
	dpm/mg or/µl	*t/c*	*t/p*	dpm/mg or/µl	dpm/mg or/µl
Anterior hypothalamus	162 ± 38	*5.6*	*1.1*	40 ± 4	27 ± 6
Middle hypothalamus	74 ± 4	*2.6*	*0.5*	33 ± 1	33 ± 7
Posterior hypothalamus	44 ± 8	*1.5*	*0.3*	25 ± 3	23 ± 5
Cerebral cortex	29 ± 3	*1.0*	*0.2*	28 ± 2	26 ± 4
Plasma	148 ± 9		*1.0*	138 ±25	182 ±31

5-week old female Wistar rats received an intravenous injection of
0.2 µg of 6,7[^{3}H]-estradiol (*E) (58 Ci/mmole) in 0.5 ml of saline
which, in certain cases, was preceeded by an injection of 2.5 µg
of radioinert steroid 30 min earlier. Two hours after tritiated
estradiol injection, the rats were decapitated. Their hypothalamus
was cut out as a block, limited anteriorly by a cut through the
center of the optic chiasma, laterally by the hypothalamic fissures,
and posteriorly by the anterior border of the mammillary bodies. The
depth from the basal surface of the hypothalamus was 2 to 3 mm. The
excised area was then divided into three parts : anterior, middle,
and posterior, which were homogenized in 1 ml of 0.32 M sucrose. The
radioactivity of plasma and of 0.2 ml aliquots of homogenate was
counted. Results are expressed as the mean uptake (±SEM) calculated
from measurements on 3 rats and as the ratio of the concentration
between tissue and cerebral cortex (t/c) or tissue and plasma (t/p).

administration of radioinert estradiol or R 2858. The most marked
inhibition   was obtained with R 2858 in the anterior hypothalamus ;
no inhibition   occurred in cerebral cortex.

    According to the sucrose density patterns in Fig.3, labelled
estradiol binds to a macromolecule present in cytosol from anterior
and middle hypothalamus. A "8S" peak, suppressible by the addition
of radioinert estradiol and more marked for anterior than middle
hypothalamus, was formed. This peak was absent on incubation of
labelled estradiol with cerebral cortex cytosol.

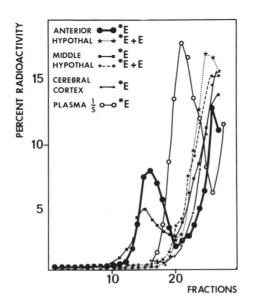

FIG.3. *Estradiol binding in the hypothalamus, cerebral cortex and
      plasma of the 5-week old female rat*

    Cortex and the anterior or middle hypothalamus of 5-week old
female rats were homogenized in 1 ml of 0.01 M Tris-HCl, 1.5 mM
EDTA, 12 mM thioglycerol buffer (pH 7.4) in an ice-cooled Teflon-
glass homogenizer ($\sim$660 mg tissue/ml buffer) and centrifuged at
105,000 x g for 1 hr at 4°C. The supernatant or 1 ml of 1/5-diluted
plasma was incubated for 30 min at 4°C with 0.2 nM 6,7[^{3}H]-estradiol
(*E) (58 Ci/mmole) either alone or in the presence of (20 nM) radioinert estradiol and then layered (0.3 ml) on a linear 6.5-20% (w/v)
sucrose gradient containing 10% glycerol (v/v). The gradients were
centrifuged at 47,000 rpm for 16 hr at 4°C in an SW 50.1 rotor
(Spinco L265B). The radioactivity of 2-drop fractions was counted
and expressed as a percentage of the radioactivity layered on the
gradient. Binding of estradiol to plasma ("4S") was taken as a
reference for the determination of the sedimentation coefficient.

Further experiments suggested that this hypothalamic cytosol estradiol-receptor complex may be translocated into the nucleus. Whereas the radioactivity in the crude nuclear fractions from anterior and middle hypothalamus increased during the 2 hours following injection of estradiol, that of the supernatant decreased correspondingly (Fig. 4). The radioactivity in all posterior hypothalamus fractions remained virtually constant.

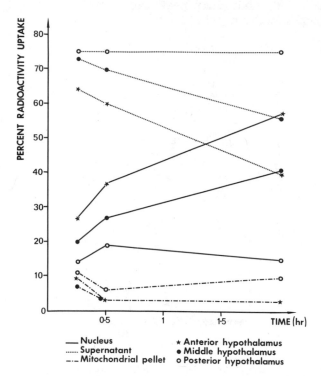

FIG. 4. Time-course of subcellular radioactivity uptake by the hypothalamus of the 5-week old female rat following injection of 6,7[^{3}H]-estradiol

5-week old female Wistar rats were decapitated at various times following an intravenous injection of 0.2 μg of 6,7[^{3}H]-estradiol (58 Ci/mmole) in 0.5 ml of saline. Tissue homogenates were prepared as described in the legend of Table 4 and were centrifuged for 15 mins at 800 g. The pellet constituted the crude nuclear fraction. The supernatant was further separated by centrifugation for 20 mins at 10,000 xg into a crude mitochondrial fraction(pellet) and a supernatant. The pellets were washed twice with 0.5 ml of 0.32 M sucrose and their radioactivity was extracted with 1 ml of ethanol. The radioactivity of each fraction was counted and expressed as a percentage of the total radioactivity taken up by each region of the hypothalamus.

Since estradiol has a higher affinity for the uterine cytosol receptor than R 2858, it was considered a more suitable compound for the detection of estrogen hypothalamic receptors in the 5-week old female rat.   In the young rat, however, it is retained in the vascular bed by EBP (Fig. 1) and R 2858, although less tightly bound by the uterine receptor, is more apt to detect any preferential radioactivity uptake since it is not bound by EBP (Table 1) and has easier access to all tissues (Raynaud, 1974). On injection of the same amount of radioactivity (10 µCi) to the two-week old female rat, more counts are recovered in the cortex and less in the plasma when R 2858 is injected than estradiol (estradiol : 86 ± 10 dpm/mg in cortex and 1522 ±.134 dpm/µl in plasma ; R 2858 : 191 ± 9 dpm/mg in cortex and 426 ± 40 dpm/µl in plasma).

Fig. 5 illustrates schematically the advantages in using R 2858 in the detection of preferential uptake in the young rat. Competition for radioactive estradiol (E*) binding by excess cold estradiol (E) gives the total binding to specific receptor and to EBP ; addition of diethylstilbestrol (DES), which as shown in Table 2 competes slightly for EBP binding, gives specific receptor binding and some EBP binding ; addition of excess R 2858 gives total specific receptor binding only. Competition for radioactive R 2858 binding by excess R 2858 also gives specific receptor binding only. Of these two methods of evaluating specific binding directly, the latter has a much higher sensitivity.

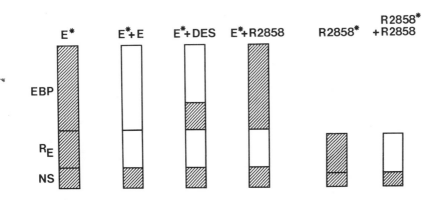

FIG. 5. Determination of receptor binding by displacement of radioactivity by addition of an excess of radioinert competitor.

The empty squares represent the type of binding which can be measured by the difference between the radioactivity recorded in the absence and presence of excess radioinert competitor (EBP = binding sites to EBP, RE = specific estrogen receptor sites, NS = non-specific binding).

This method was therefore used for the study of the ontogeny of estrogen receptors in several target tissues of the rat (Fig.6). Specific binding equivalent to or greater than 50% of plasma concentration could be significantly detected. Tissue responsiveness developed most spectacularly in the uterus. Preferential uptake was detected as early as 3 days after birth ; it increased markedly between days 3 and 8 and decreased slightly on day 15. On day 3, preferential uptake was also recorded for the pituitary but was lower than in the uterus ; the level remained constant until day 11 but increased on day 15. Much lower but significant values were observed for the hypothalamus from day 3.

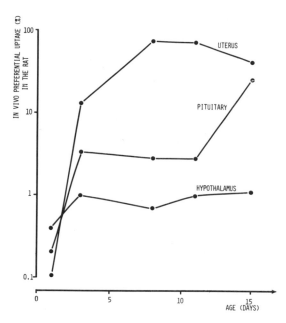

FIG.6. *In vivo preferential uptake by the hypothalamus, pituitary and uterus of female rats after injection of 6,7[3H]-R 2858*

Female Sprague-Dawley rats, 1 to 11 days old, received a subcutaneous injection of 0.2 nmoles of 6,7[3H]-R 2858 (48 Ci/mmole) in 0.1 ml of a 10% solution of ethanol in saline. The 15-day old rats received 0.4 nmoles. Another set of rats was injected with 2 µg of R 2858 30 min earlier. Two hours after tritiated R 2858 injection, the rats were decapitated and the uterus, pituitary and hypothalamus excised. Organ and plasma radioactivity was measured after combustion in an Oxymat auto-oxidizer. Results are expressed as specific uptake over plasma radioactivity (dpm/µl) as a function of age. The specific uptake (dpm/mg) was given by the difference in uptake when 6,7[3H]-R 2858 was injected alone or in the presence of excess radioinert R 2858.

PROGESTINS

<u>Influence of plasma binding on the detection of progesterone
receptors</u> : In the uterine cytosol of several species including the
rat, progesterone is bound by a "4S" CBG-like component which hin-
ders the detection of progestin-specific binding in the "8S"
region. To bring this latent binding to light, a highly potent progestin presumed to be active as a result of tight specific binding
to this receptor has been used as a tag. Fig.7 shows that whereas
progesterone is bound in the "4S" region only in uterine cytosol
from unprimed rats, R 5020 (17,21-dimethyl-19-nor-4,9-pregnadiene-
3,20-dione) is bound by a "7-8S" receptor.   This "8S" binding
is suppressible by radioinert progesterone.

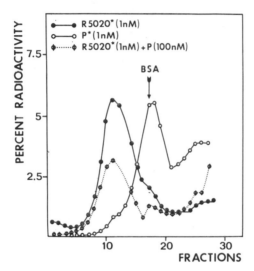

FIG.7. *Progestin-specific binding in the uterus of the unprimed*
     17-19 day old rat

The uteri of 17-19 day old Sprague-Dawley SPF rats were excised, weighed, minced, pooled, homogenized in 0.01 M Tris-HCl, 1.5 mM
EDTA buffer (pH 7.4) in an ice-cooled Teflon-glass homogenizer and
centrifuged at 105,000 x g for 90 min at 4°C. The supernatant was
incubated for 1 hr at 4°C with 2 nM 1-[^{3}H]-progesterone (27 Ci/
mmole) or 6,7[^{3}H]-R 5020 (51 Ci/mmole) either alone or in the presence of 100 nM radioinert progesterone and then layered (0.3 ml)
on a linear 5-20% sucrose gradient. The gradients were centrifuged
at 41,000 rpm for 16 hr at 4°C in an SW 50.1 rotor (Spinco L265B).
The radioactivity of 2-drop fractions was counted and expressed as
a percentage of the radioactivity layered on the gradient. BSA
(bovine serum albumin) was used as a marker.

Measurement of progestin binding sites by an in vitro exchange
method : Since R 5020 is not bound by CBG and since it forms a more
stable complex with the "8S" uterine cytosol receptor than proges-

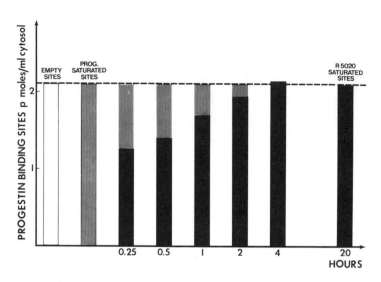

FIG. 8. Determination of optimal conditions for the measurement of
progestin binding sites by an in vitro exchange method

The uteri of immature Normandy rabbits (800 g) primed with
25 µg of estradiol administered percutaneously 5 days previously
were excised, weighed, minced, crushed in 0.01 M Tris-HCl, 0.25 M
sucrose (pH 7.4), homogenized (final dilution 1/25, w/v) in an
ice-cooled Teflon-glass homogenizer and centrifuged for 1 hr at
105,000 xg at 4°C. An aliquot of the supernatant (250 µl) was incubated with 25 nM 6,7 [^{3}H]-R 5020 (51 Ci/mmole) for 24 hr at 0°C,
alone or in the presence of 2500 nM radioinert R 5020. The remaining supernatant was preincubated with a saturating dose of radioinert progesterone and then incubated for the indicated time
intervals with 25 nM [^{3}H] 5020 in the presence or absence of 2500 nm
unlabeled R 5020. In each case, the concentration of bound tritiated R 5020 was measured on a 100 µl aliquot by adsorption of free
steroid by 100 µl dextran-coated charcoal (0.65-1.25%). The incubated supernatant was shaken in the presence of the charcoal for 10
min at 0°C in a microtiter plate, then centrifuged for 10 min at 800 x
Supernatant radioactivity corresponds to bound R 5020. The open
bar represents the number of total progestin binding sites in cytosol
non preincubated with progesterine. The shadowed bars indicate the
number of binding sites still covered by unlabeled progesterone
while the black bars represent the number of binding sites exchan-
ged by the labeled progestin after different time intervals.

terone, it is a highly suitable compound for the measurement of progestin binding sites.

As illustrated in Fig. 8, after 4 hours of incubation, binding sites, previously saturated with radioinert progesterone, are entirely occupied by labelled R 5020.

As illustrated in Fig. 9, the uterus contains by far the greatest number of progestin binding sites. Compared to a presumed non-target tissue such as the cortex, the hypothalamus has a similar number of sites, and the pituitary a significantly higher number of sites. No sites were detected in the plasma.

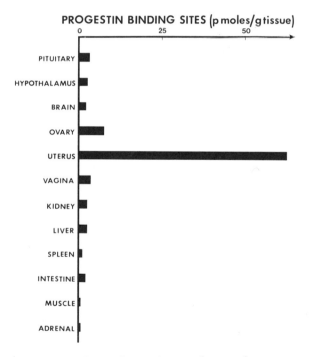

PROGESTIN BINDING SITES (p moles/g tissue)

FIG. 9. Progestin binding sites in various tissues of the estradiol-primed immature female rabbit

The number of progestin binding sites was determined in the cytosol fraction of various tissues by an *in vitro* exchange method using 6,7[³H]-R 5020 (incubation time 24 hours).

DISCUSSION

The study of the ontogeny of steroid hormone receptors in
very young rats is difficult owing to the lack of sensitive methods.   Autoradiography has enabled the detection of nuclear retention of estradiol in the hypothalamus as early as 2 days
after birth (Sheridan et al., 1974). However, this technique is
only qualitative.   Using sucrose gradient analysis, Kato et al.
(1974) have detected a rudimentary "8S" cytosol estradiol-receptor complex at 7 days of age.   It is difficult, however, to carry
out gradients in younger animals due to the small amount of tissue
available.   So far, *in vitro* competition studies have enabled the
detection of preferential estrogen uptake at 5 days of age (Kulin
and Reiter, 1972), but the high non-specific tissue binding affects the sensitivity of the method.

The present data suggest that a fruitful approach to the study of hormone mechanisms might be to use appropriate synthetic
compounds which enable the application of simple and sensitive
methods.   If the choice of synthetic compound is judicious, the
study of hormone mechanisms can be simplified both from a technical
and conceptual viewpoint. In the choice of these compounds, two
fundamental features have to be postulated and, if possible, proved : the compound should have the same activity as the natural
hormone in the tissue under study and this activity should be exerted via the same mechanism.   For instance, our results have shown
that, like estradiol, R 2858 (Moxestrol) is uterotrophic via binding to a cytosol uterine receptor (Raynaud et al., 1973). Furthermore, it has been observed that the estrogen R 2858, administered
to pregnant rats, manifests exactly the same kind of effects on the
genital tract of the fetus and on the fertility of offspring as
those induced by estradiol.   It has been postulated that these
effects might be through similar mechanisms and possibly due to
interference at the hypothalamo-pituitary level. In fact, it has
been demonstrated that the cytosol estradiol-receptor complex from
hypothalamus of the immature female rat is translocated to the nucleus (Raynaud, 1974; Clark et al., 1972) as has already been shown
for the uterine cytosol complex.

Three synthetic steroids which have been selected as hormone
receptor "detectors" will illustrate the technical advantages of
these compounds. Unlike estradiol and to a lesser extend DES,
R2858 is not bound at all by the estradiol binding protein present
in the plasma of the pregnant rat, fetus and immature rat of both
sexes (Raynaud et al., 1971; Swartz et al., 1974). Unlike progesterone, the progestin R 5020 is not bound by transcortin in any
species (Philibert and Raynaud, 1973; Philibert and Raynaud, 1974
a,b).   Moreover, it forms a more stable complex than progesterone
with the uterus cytosol "8S" receptor.   Unlike dihydrotestosterone,

R 1881 is not metabolized *in vitro* at 25ºC. Furthermore, it has a higher affinity for the cytosol prostatic androgen receptor and is not bound by sex steroid binding protein (Bonne and Raynaud, 1975). For these reasons, R 1881 and R 5020 may be considered as ideal compounds for the direct quantification of specific androgen and progestin binding sites respectively by a simple *in vitro* exchange method. To date, preliminary experiments using R 2858 for the direct measurement of preferential estrogen uptake and R 5020 for the measurement of specific progestin binding sites in the hypothalamus and pituitary have yielded interesting results. An estrogen receptor is probably present in the hypothalamus of the female rat 3 days after birth ; it is certainly already present in the pituitary at this time. No significant difference has been detected in the number of progestin binding sites in the cortex and hypothalamus of the immature female rabbit. The number of sites in the pituitary is however significantly higher than in the cortex.

The methods, however, still need perfecting. Apart from resolving difficulties such as the rapid excision of such a small and ill-delimited region of the brain as the hypothalamus in fetuses and very young animals without diluting the sample by neighbouring non-target tissue, it is still necessary to determine the optimum conditions for a preferably *in vitro* exchange technique. *In vivo*, the situation is further complicated by the difficulty in determining a dose which saturates the receptor. A tracer dose will establish whether the uptake is specific ; a saturating dose will enable the measurement of the number of binding sites.

As mentioned above, the use of synthetic compounds has not only technical, but also conceptual advantages. For instance, it may throw light on the influence of the balance of hormone levels on tissue binding. R 5020 is sensitive enough to detect progestin specific binding sites in an animal not primed with estrogen ; in particular, it has been used to demonstrate the induction of progestin-specific binding sites by estradiol in the immature rabbit uterus (Raynaud and Philibert, 1975). It is possible that with an appropriate estrogen priming dose and a suitable R 5020 dose for the exchange technique, it would be possible to reveal a similar induction mechanism in the pituitary and hypothalamus.

The use of R 2858 differentiates between activity due to a direct impact on the target tissues at the receptor level and activity due to the availability of the hormones at these target tissues. Owing to lack of plasma binding, administration of R 2858 to the rat has a far more marked effect than administration of estradiol on uterine weight, genital tract development (Vannier and Raynaud, 1975) and fertility. In view of these observations, it has been postulated that the estradiol binding protein might be present in low concentrations in maternal plasma in order to

modulate plasma estrogen levels, in high concentration in the fetal plasma in order to protect the developing sexual structures
whether at the genital tract or brain levels. In future studies
on sexual differentiation, however, other factors will have to be
taken into account, in particular the development of enzyme systems
which control gonadal and pituitary secretions.

Nevertheless, it is undeniable that these synthetic compounds
are useful tools in the study of the ontogeny of steroid hormone
receptors (McEwen et al., 1975) and a major step forward may be
made in the elucidation of hormonal mechanism in the young once
their use is coupled with radioimmunological determinations of
plasma steroid and gonadotrophin levels. In this way, it might
be possible to get a more precise understanding of the possible
role of steroid hormone receptor mechanism in sexual differentiation.

ACKNOWLEDGMENTS

The helpful collaboration of Mlle M. Orosco and the technical assistance of Mme D. Gofflo and Mme J. Humbert are gratefully acknowledged.

REFERENCES

Barley, J., Ginsburg, M., Greenstein, B.D., MacLusky, N.J. and
Thomas, P.J. (1974) Nature, 252, 259-260.

Bonne, C. and Raynaud, J.P. (1975) Steroids, in press.

Brown-Grant, K. (1974) International Symposium on Sexual Endocrinology of the Perinatal Period, INSERM, 32, 357-376.

Clark, J.H., Campbell, P.S. and Peck, E.J. Jr. (1972) Neuroendocrinology, 77, 218-228.

Kato, J., Atsumi, Y. and Inaba, M. (1974) Endocrinology, 94, 309-
317.

Kato, J. (1975) J. Steroid Biochemistry, 6, 979-987.

Kulin, H.E. and Reiter, E.O. (1972) Endocrinology 90, 1371-1374.

Maurer, R.A. (1974) Brain Research, 67, 175-177.

McEwen, B.S., Plapinger, L., Chaptal, C., Gerlach, J. and Wallach,
G. (1975) Brain Research, 96, 400-406.

Philibert, D. and Raynaud, J.P. (1973) Steroids, 22, 89-98.

Philibert, D. and Raynaud, J.P. (1974) Endocrinology, 94, 627-632.

Philibert, D. and Raynaud, J.P. (1974) Contraception, 10, 457-466.

Raynaud, J.P., Mercier-Bodard, C. and Baulieu, E.E. (1971) Steroids, 18, 767-788.

Raynaud, J.P. (1973) Steroids, 21, 249-258.

Raynaud, J.P., Bouton, M.M., Gallet-Bourquin, D., Philibert, D., Tournemine, C. and Azadian-Boulanger, G. (1973) Molecular Pharmacology, 9, 520-533.

Raynaud, J.P., Philibert, D. and Azadian-Boulanger, G. (1973) XIIIth International Symposium on Physiologic and Genetic Aspects of Reproduction, Bahia, pp. 143-160.

Raynaud, J.P. (1974) Drug Interactions, Ed. P.L. Morselli, S. Garattini and S.N. Cohen, Raven Press. pp. 151-162.

Raynaud, J.P. and Philibert, D. (1975) Fifth International Conference of Endocrinology, London, July 1975, Abstracts p. 35.

Sheridan, P.J., Sar, M. and Stumpf, W.E. (1974) Endocrinology, 94, 1386-1390.

Swartz, S.K., Soloff, M.S. and Suriano, J.R. (1974) Biochemica and Biophysica Acta, 338, 480-488.

Vannier, B. and Raynaud, J.P. (1975) Molecular and Cellular Endocrinology., in press.

ROLE OF SEX STEROIDS ON LH AND FSH SECRETION IN THE RAT

L. FERLAND, J. DROUIN and F. LABRIE

Medical Research Council Group in Molecular

Endocrinology, CHUL, Québec, G1V 4G2, Canada

Elucidation of the structure of LH-RH (Matsuo et al., 1971; Burgus et al., 1971) has opened new possibilities for studies of the factors involved in the control of LH and FSH secretion. This presentation will attempt to summarize the data describing the role of estrogens and androgens as specific and important modulators of gonadotropin secretion. Using the rat as model, evidence will be presented of a specific action of these steroids at the hypothalamic and pituitary levels.

The finding of increased plasma LH and FSH levels after castration in male and female rats (Ramirez and McCann, 1963; Legan et al., 1973) indicates that the global effect of both male and female gonadal steroids is inhibitory on both LH and FSH secretion. The inhibitory effect of estradiol and testosterone is further evidenced by decreased plasma levels of the two gonadotropins after administration of the steroids to castrated animals. Although the global effects of both androgens and estrogens are inhibitory on gonadotropin secretion, there are however good evidence for a stimulatory effect of estrogens at the pituitary level.

While the effects of estrogens and androgens on gonadotropin release are well recognized, data are still conflicting about their site of action. A widely used experimental approach to dissociate between hypothalamic and pituitary sites of action has been the implantation of small amounts of crystalline steroids in the pituitary and hypothalamus (Kingsley and Bogdanove, 1973; Smith and Davidson, 1974). In order to gain further evidence of the site of steroid action, a combination of in vivo and in vitro experiments will be presented.

<u>Role of estrogens in the control of gonadotropin secretion</u>
<u>Inhibitory effect of estrogens in vivo</u>

Since castration is well known to be followed by a rapid elevation of both plasma LH and FSH levels (Legan <u>et al</u>., 1973) which

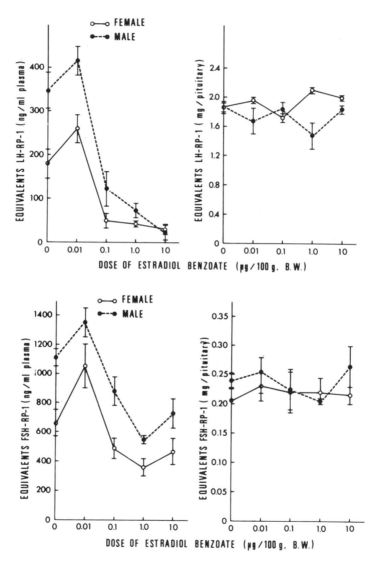

Figure 1: Effect of treatment of castrated male or female
rats with increasing doses of estradiol benzoate (0.01,
0.1, 1 or 10 µg/100 g, B.W.) twice a day for 7 days on
plasma LH and FSH levels and pituitary LH and FSH contents.

provides a sensitive model for studies of the inhibitory activity of steroids, castrated male and female rats were used in all following experiments.

Chronic treatment of castrated male or female rats with increasing doses of estradiol benzoate (0.01, 0.1, 1 or 10 µg/100 g, B.W.) twice a day for 7 days leads to an almost complete inhibition (10% of control) of plasma LH levels at doses equal to or higher than 0.1 µg. Such treatment does not affect significantly the pituitary LH and hypothalamic LH-RH contents. It should however be mentioned that the low dose of 0.01 µg estradiol benzoate induces a slight but consistent increase of plasma LH concentration in both male and female animals, thus indicating a positive feedback action of low doses of estradiol on the hypothalamic-pituitary axis (Swerdloff and Walsh, 1973).

In contrast with the almost complete inhibition of plasma LH level observed after estradiol treatment, a much smaller inhibition of plasma FSH is observed, the maximal inhibition being 50%. Such treatment with estradiol has no effect on pituitary FSH content. As observed for LH, the low dose of 0.01 µg estradiol benzoate leads to a slight increase of the plasma FSH concentration. These data are in agreement with previous studies (Legan et al., 1973) indicating that the global effect of estradiol, above a certain dose, is inhibitory on both LH and FSH secretion. These in vivo data obtained in castrated rats of both sexes indicate also some positive effect of the steroid on both LH and FSH secretion.

Stimulatory effect of estrogens in vivo

Although the effect of supraphysiological doses of estrogens is inhibitory on gonadotropin secretion, it is also clear that estrogens can have a positive effect on LH and FSH secretion. These data pertain to the induction of afternoon LH surges by injection of estradiol benzoate to ovariectomized animals (Baldwin et al., 1974), the induction of ovulatory LH surges by injection of estrogens at early stages of the estrous cycles (Everett, 1948) and the abolition of the ovulatory surge of LH at proestrus by administration of an estrogen antiserum (Jewelewicz et al., 1974). In order to investigate the positive action of estrogens at the pituitary level during the estrous cycle, the plasma LH response curve to LH-RH was studied in rats at different stages of the estrous cycle under conditions leading to blockage of endogenous LH-RH secretion (Surital or Pentobarbital anesthesia).

The subcutaneous injection of 200 ng of LH-RH leads to a much greater plasma LH response in the afternoon of proestrus than at any other stage of the estrous cycle. In fact, the response to LH-RH is approximately 7-fold higher on proestrus than diestrus I (Ferland et al., 1975). These data obtained in vivo could however

be influenced by some changes of endogenous LH-RH release occuring
even under Surital anesthesia, by changes of the transport or metabolism of exogenous LH-RH or by changes of the metabolism of LH
or to a combination of these factors.

In order to avoid these possible limitations of in vivo responses to LH-RH, a detailed study of the sensitivity to LH-RH
was performed in vitro using pituitaries collected at the different
stages of the estrous cycle. The data obtained after the first 45
min of incubation show a maximal pituitary sensitivity to LH-RH
on proestrus while the response is minimal on diestrus (Ferland
et al., 1975). That the changes of pituitary sensitivity to LH-RH
measured in vivo reflect changes of pituitary sensitivity is thus
ascertained by the similar changes of sensitivity to LH-RH measured in vitro. Since it is known that in the rat, estrogens levels
begin to rise on diestrus II with a peak occuring on the morning
of proestrus (Brown-Grant et al., 1970; Naftolin et al., 1972),
there is a good possibility that this estrogen surge is responsible
for the increased pituitary sensitivity to LH-RH during the afternoon of proestrus.

In agreement with this, we have found that administration of
ethinyl estradiol or 11β-methoxy ethinyl estradiol (R 2858) to
rats on diestrus I increases by 2- to 3-fold the plasma LH response to LH-RH measured on the following day. Further evidence of
the positive effect of estradiol on the pituitary LH response to
LH-RH is offered by the findings of a normal LH response to LH-RH
on the presumed day of proestrus in rats ovariectomized on the day
of estrus and treated with increasing doses of 11β-methoxy ethinyl
estradiol on the presumed day of diestrus II. All these studies
performed during the estrous cycle clearly show a positive role
of estrogens on the pituitary sensitivity to LH-RH.

Similar evidence of an estrogen-induced increased LH response to LH-RH was obtained using castrated animals. As indicated
by the areas under the plasma LH response curves to LH-RH (Fig. 2),
pretreatment with increasing doses of estradiol leads to 4- to 5-
fold higher LH responses at doses of 3 or 30 μg/day.

Such findings of an increased pituitary sensitivity to LH-RH
following estradiol treatment suggest a direct effect of estradiol
at the pituitary level. However, the recent observation of a potentiation of the LH and FSH responses to LH-RH by previous injection of this neurohormone clearly indicates that LH-RH itself
may be implicated in this increased pituitary sensitivity to the
neurohormone on proestrus (Ferland et al., 1975) and at midcycle
in women (Nillius and Wide, 1971; Yen et al., 1972).

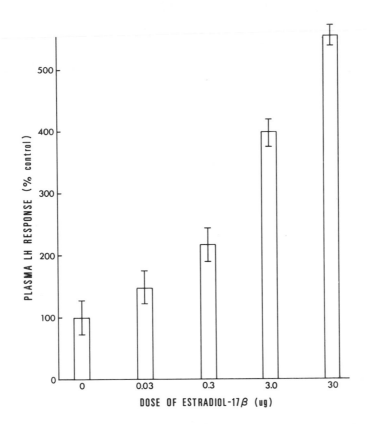

Figure 2: Effect of treatment of castrated (1 month previously) female rats with increasing daily doses of es-
tradiol-17β (0.03, 0.3, 3 or 30 μg) for 7 days on the
plasma LH response to LH-RH.   Animals were anesthesized
with Surital (50 mg/kg, i.p.) before subcutaneous injection of 200 ng LH-RH.   Results are expressed as
area under the plasma LH response curves (% of control).

        Fig. 3 shows the LH and FSH responses to three successive
injections of 50 ng LH-RH i.v.   A single dose of the neurohormone
injected in the afternoon of proestrus failed to increase significantly plasma levels of LH or FSH.   It can however be seen that
the response to LH-RH is 4- to 5-fold increased by a previous injection of the same dose of the neurohormone 60 min earlier. The
response to a third injection of LH-RH is even further increased
to approximately 20-times above control.

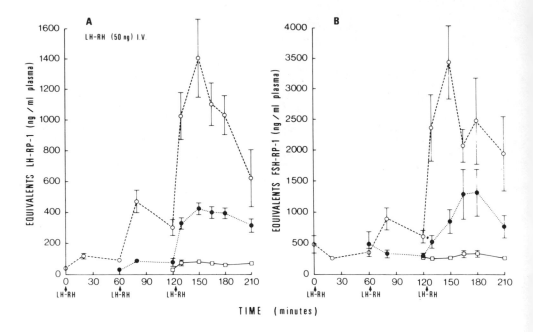

Figure 3: Effect of succesive injections of LH-RH on plasma LH and FSH release. Animals in the afternoon of proestrus were anesthesized with Surital (50 mg/kg, i.p.)
before intravenous injection of 50 ng of LH-RH at the
indicated times.

Taking into account the evidence already obtained of an essential role of estrogens in the increased pituitary sensitivity
to LH-RH, these data on the sensitization of the LH-RH response
by the neurohormone itself suggest that part of the increased
pituitary sensitivity may be due to an increased LH-RH secretion.

Stimulatory effect of estrogens in vitro

Although the in vivo experiments suggest that estrogens have
a positive effect directly at the pituitary level, confirmation of
these findings had to be obtained by in vitro experiments using
pituitary cells in culture.

In order to investigate the in vitro effect of estradiol, cells
were preincubated for different periods of time in the presence or
absence of 10^{-8}M estradiol before a short incubation of 5 h with
LH-RH (10^{-10}M). As illustrated in Fig. 4, pretreatment with the

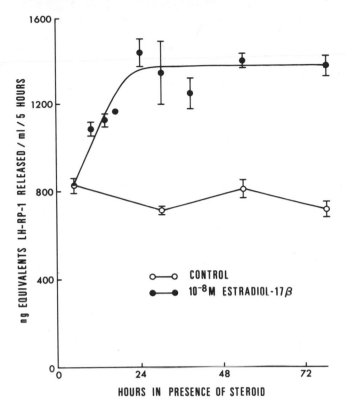

Figure 4: Time-course of the stimulatory effect of 10^{-8}M estradiol-17β on the LH response to 1×10^{-10}M LH-RH in anterior pituitary cells in primary culture.

estrogen leads to an approximately 70% increase of the LH response to LH-RH, the effect being maximal after 20 h of incubation with the steroid. These data indicate clearly that estrogens can have a positive action directly at the pituitary level on the LH response to LH-RH. This effect may, up to an unknown extent, be responsible for the increased LH responsiveness to LH-RH observed in vivo during the estrous or menstrual cycles (Ferland et al., 1975; Nillius and Wide, 1971; Yen et al., 1972) or after treatment with estrogens.

There is however one exception to these observations of a positive feedback effect of estrogens on the LH response to LH-RH.

In fact, when the time-course of pituitary sensitivity to LH-RH
is examined after a single injection of estradiol, the lowered
plasma levels of LH measured 4 h after injection of the steroid
are accompanied by a decreased pituitary sensitivity to LH-RH
(data not shown). A progressive return to normal of both plasma LH levels and its response to LH-RH are observed between 12
and 24 h after injection of the steroid. These data are in agreement with the observations (Negro-Vilar et al., 1973) that a small
dose of estradiol could inhibit LH release acutely (within 6 h)
in the ovariectomized rat, this inhibition being accompanied by a
reduced sensitivity of the pituitary response to LH-RH.

It should however be mentioned that the low level of plasma
LH observed 4 h after injection of estradiol-17β could well be
explained by an inhibition of LH-RH release thus resulting in a
decreased pituitary sensitivity to LH-RH without any direct inhibitory effect of the estrogen at the pituitary level. In fact,
the present data suggest that the effect of estradiol is exclusively positive at the pituitary level while the effect on LH-RH
secretion can be stimulatory or inhibitory depending upon the dosage used.

Role of androgens in the control of gonadotropin secretion

In vivo studies

Although it is well known that androgens administered systemically inhibit plasma levels of LH and FSH in both rat (Mahesh
et al., 1972; Beyer et al., 1972; Bodganove, 1967; Schally et al.,
1967; Swerdloff et al., 1972) and man (Peterson et al., 1968; Lee
et al., 1972), data are still conflicting about the site of androgen action. In fact, data derived largely from implantation experiments have suggested a direct action of androgens at the pituitary level (Kamberi and McCann, 1969; Kingsley and Bogdanove,
1973) while convincing evidence for an hypothalamic site of action has also been presented (Smith and Davidson, 1967).

In order to gain better knowledge of the site of feedback action of androgens, the relative potency of systemically administered androgens on the inhibition of plasma LH and FSH concentrations was compared with the effect of the steroids on the pituitary response to LH-RH.

As mentioned previously, the effect of androgens on plasma
levels of LH and FSH is exclusively inhibitory. In fact, chronic
treatment of castrated male or female rats with testosterone (T)
propionate (25 or 125 µg/100 g, B.W.) twice a day for 7 days leads
to an almost complete inhibition (83 to 99%) of plasma LH levels
in animals of both sexes. Pituitary LH and hypothalamic LH-RH

contents remain unchanged under such androgen treatments (Ferland et al., 1976). In contrast with the almost complete inhibition of plasma LH observed after T propionate treatment, a much smaller inhibitory effect is observed on FSH release, inhibitions of 36 and 50% being measured at the highest dose of T propionate in female and male animals respectively.

The same treatment has a stimulatory (30-40%) effect on pituitary FSH content. Similar effects of androgens on pituitary FSH content have already been reported (Bodganove, 1967; Kingsley and Bogdanove, 1973).

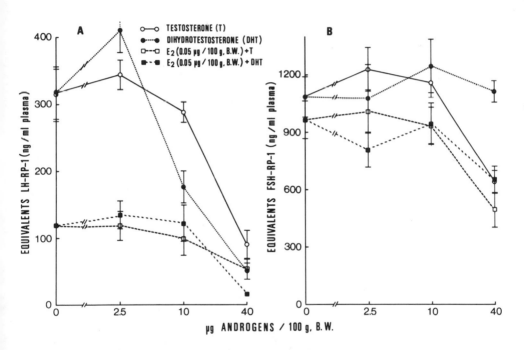

Figure 5: Effect of treatment with estradiol-17β (0.05 µg/100 g, B.W.) twice a day for 8 days alone or in combination with increasing doses of testosterone (T) or 5α-dihydrotestosterone (DHT) on plasma LH and FSH levels.

As illustrated in Fig. 5, T or DHT injected twice a day for 8 days at the dose of 2.5 µg/100 g, B.W., do not affect the plasma LH concentration. However, at the 10 µg dose, DHT inhibits plasma LH by 45% while T shows no significant effect. At the highest dose used (40 µg), both T and DHT treatments inhibit plasma LH to 15-25% of control. It can be clearly seen in Fig. 5 that T inhi-

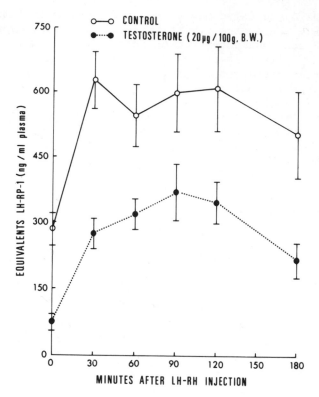

Figure 6: Effect of treatment of castrated female rats with testosterone (20 μg/100 g, B.W.) daily for 7 days on the plasma LH response to LH-RH. Animals were anesthesized with Surital (50 mg/kg, i.p.) before subcutaneous injection of 200 ng   LH-RH and measurements of plasma LH at the indicated time intervals.

bits plasma FSH concentration by approximately 40% only at the dose of 40 μg while DHT is without significant effect at any of the doses used. Since estradiol-17β (E_2) is known to inhibit plasma gonadotropin levels, it was felt of interest to study a possible interaction between E_2 and T or DHT on plasma LH and FSH levels. As shown in Fig. 5, E_2 (0.05 μg) leads by itself to a 60% inhibition of the plasma LH concentration while the slight inhibition of plasma FSH is not significant. When associated with E_2, T and DHT further decrease plasma LH already inhibited by treatment with the estrogen alone. This effect on LH is however observed only at the dose of 40 μg, DHT being somewhat more potent than T. In combination with E_2, both T and DHT (40 μg) depress the plasma FSH concentration by only 25-30%.

These data show clearly that treatment of male or female rats with T propionate leads to an almost complete inhibition of plasma LH and only to a partial inhibition (40%) of plasma FSH levels. These data are in agreement with the previous reports (Bogdanove, 1967; Swerdloff and Odell, 1968; Eldridge and Mahesh, 1974) of a greater sensitivity of LH than FSH release to the inhibitory action of androgens. The finding of an increased pituitary FSH content following T treatment has also been demonstrated by local implants of androgens (Kingsley and Bogdanove, 1973) and could thus be partly explained by a direct effect of androgens at the pituitary level. In agreement with previous reports (Swedloff and Odell, 1968; Beyer et al., 1972; Swerdloff et al., 1972; Beyer et al., 1974; Zanizi et al., 1973), the present experiments show that DHT is somewhat more potent than T to inhibit plasma LH levels in castrated rats. Data on plasma FSH are more conflicting, DHT having been found more potent (Beyer et al., 1972) or of equal potency (Kingsley and Bogdanove, 1973; Mahesh et al., 1972). Although no satisfactory explanation is available, changes of the levels of 5α-reductase activity (Denef et al., 1973) or androgen receptors under different endocrine states may well lead to apparent changes of the relative potencies of T and DHT.

The next experiments were aimed at dissociating the inhibitory effect of T and DHT at the hypothalamic and/or pituitary levels. As clearly illustrated in Fig. 6, while the basal plasma level of LH is decreased to about 40% of control after treatment for 7 days with 20 μg of T/100 g, B.W., the plasma LH response to LH-RH remains unchanged after such androgen treatment. This finding of a decreased rate of LH secretion in the presence of a normal pituitary response to LH-RH indicates strongly that at the dose used, T exerts its inhibitory action at the hypothalamic level.

As illustrated in Fig. 7, treatment of castrated male rats with increasing doses of DHT leads to parallel inhibition of basal plasma LH and of its response to exogenous LH-RH, an almost complete inhibition being observed after treatment with 125 μg/ 100 g, B.W. twice a day for 7 days. While Fig. 6 clearly suggests the hypothalamus as a site of inhibitory action of T, Fig. 7 shows that DHT treatment can lead to a decreased plasma LH response to LH-RH, thus indicating a pituitary site of action. Treatment of male rats with T has also been found to suppress the pituitary LH response to LH-RH (Debeljuk et al., 1972). Although it can be argued that the observed inhibition of the LH response to LH-RH after androgen treatment could well be secondary to a decreased LH-RH secretion, a pituitary site of action of androgens will be confirmed in the following series of experiments.

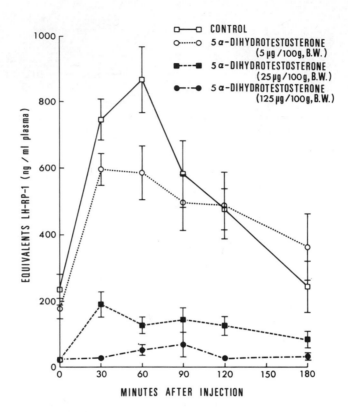

Figure 7: Effect of treatment of castrated male rats
with increasing doses of 5α-dihydrotestosterone (5,
25 or 125 µg/100 g, B.W.) twice a day for 7 days on
the plasma LH response to LH-RH.   Animals were anesthesized with Surital (50 mg/kg, i.p.) before subcutaneous injection of 200 ng   LH-RH and measurements
of plasma LH at the indicated time intervals.

In vitro studies

Since LH-RH stimulates both LH and FSH release (Schally et al.
1971; Borgeat et al., 1972), the divergence between LH and FSH secretion occurring under various physiological conditions (Bogdanove, 1967) could be best explained by differential effects of
steroids at the pituitary level on the secretion of these two hormones.

Our findings of a lowered LH response to LH-RH after DHT
treatment (Fig. 7) and the suggestions derived from implantation
studies (Kamberi and McCann, 1969; Kingsley and Bogdanove, 1973)
of a direct pituitary site of action of androgens indicated the interest of in vitro studies of the direct effect of androgens at the
pituitary level on LH and FSH secretion.

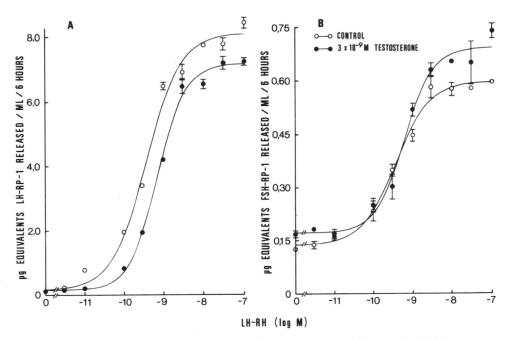

Figure 8: Effect of increasing concentrations of LH-RH
on LH (A) and FSH (B) release by anterior pituitary cells
in primary culture. Cells were pre-incubated for about
40 h in Dulbecco's modified Eagle medium containing dextran-coated charcoal-adsorbed sera in the presence (●) or
absence (o) of 3 x 10^{-9}M testosterone. Results are presented as mean ± S.E.M. of triplicate determinations.

As illustrated in Fig. 8A, pretreatment with 3×10^{-9}M T leads to a marked inhibition of the LH responsiveness to LH-RH, the LH-RH ED_{50} being increased from 3×10^{-10} to 1×10^{-9}M upon addition of the androgen. It can also be seen in Fig. 8A that incubation with T for 40 h does not affect spontaneous LH release and only slightly inhibits the maximal LH response to high LH-RH concentrations. In contrast with the LH data, it can be seen that in the same experiment (Fig. 8B), T does not significantly affect the LH-RH ED_{50} (3×10^{-10}M) of FSH release. Both the spontaneous and the maximal release of FSH are however slightly (15-20%) but consistently increased after androgen pretreatment. Maximal inhibition of the LH response to 3×10^{-10}M LH-RH is observed after about 48 h of preincubation with 10^{-8}M T. A very similar time course is obtained with 10^{-8}M 3α-androstanediol.

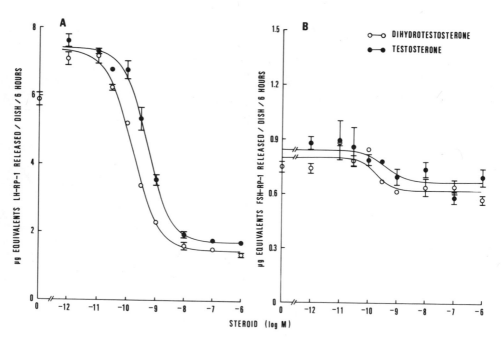

Figure 9: Effect of increasing concentrations of 5α-dihydrotestosterone (o) or testosterone ($\bullet$) on LH (A) and FSH (B) response to 1×10^{-10}M LH-RH.

Since the inhibitory effect of T on the LH response to LH-RH is more pronounced at low concentrations of the neurohormone, dose-response curves of T or DHT on LH and FSH release were studied at 1×10^{-10}M LH-RH. As illustrated in Fig. 9A, T and DHT exert the same maximal inhibitory effect (15-

20% of control) on the LH response to LH-RH. DHT is however approximately 3 times more potent than T, their ED_{50} values being of 1.6 x 10^{-10}M and 5 x 10^{-10}M, respectively. Both androgens show a slight tendency to inhibit the FSH response to 1 x 10^{-10}M LH-RH. It should be noticed that this small effect on FSH release is detected at the same concentrations of T and DHT which were found to lead to almost complete inhibition of LH release. Under similar conditions, dehydroepiandrosterone is without effect on the LH responsiveness to LH-RH while Δ^4-androstenedione inhibits LH-RH-induced LH release at an ED_{50} value of about 1 x 10^{-8}M (data not shown).

Since the observed changes of acute LH and FSH responses to LH-RH could be secondary to alterations of hormone cell content, it was felt important to investigate a possible effect of T on these parameters. As clearly indicated in Fig. 10A, the decreased LH

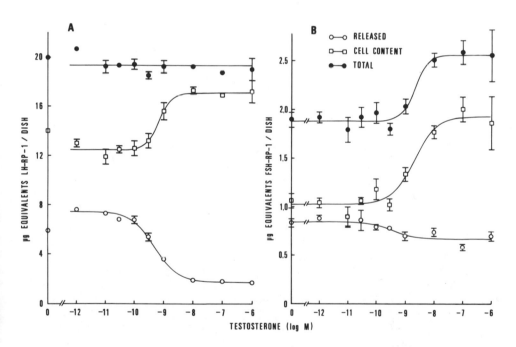

Figure 10: Effect of increasing concentrations of testosterone on LH (A) or FSH (B) response to 1 x 10^{-10}M LH-RH (o—o), cell content at the end of incubation (□—□) and total hormone (release + cell content), (●—●). Cells were preincubated for 40 h with the indicated concentrations of testosterone before a 5 h incubation with 1 x 10^{-10}M LH-RH. Similar results were obtained with 5α-dihydrotestosterone.

responsiveness to LH-RH observed with T (lower curve) is strictly
paralleled by an increased LH cell content (middle curve), total
LH (medium + cell content) remaining constant (upper curve) even
after 48 h of incubation in the presence of increasing concentrations of T.   In contrast with LH data, it can be seen in Fig. 10B
that preincubation with T leads to a significant increase (approximately 30%) of total FSH.   Similar results were obtained with
DHT and Δ^4-androstenedione.   The slight but reproducible inhibitory effect of T on 10^{-10}M LH-RH-induced FSH release can again be
noticed (lower curve).

The present data show clearly that the androgens T, DHT and
5α-androstane 3α, 17β-diol have not only specific but also opposite effects at the pituitary level on the control of LH and FSH
secretion.   In fact, pretreatment of pituitary cells in culture
with T markedly inhibits the LH response to LH-RH, while its effect on FSH is slightly stimulatory on the maximal response to
LH-RH.

While the inhibitory effect of androgens on LH release is
exerted at both the hypothalamic and pituitary levels (Ferland
et al., 1976; Drouin and Labrie, 1976), their inhibitory effect
on FSH release appears to be restricted to the hypothalamus.
Such findings can offer an explanation for the much reported observations in rat (Swerdloff et al., 1972; Eldridge and Mahesh,
1974; Ferland et al., 1976) and man (Swerdloff and Odell, 1968)
of a greater sensitivity of LH than FSH release to androgen administration.

In summary (Figure 11), the present studies performed in vivo
and in vitro indicate than androgens exert their inhibitory effect
of LH release at both the hypothalamic and pituitary levels while
their inhibitory effect on FSH release appears to be restricted
to the hypothalamus.   These data offer an explanation for the differences observed in vivo between LH and FSH sensitivity to the
negative feedback of androgens.   The physiological significance
of the slight stimulatory effect of androgens on the cell content
of FSH remains to be investigated.   Relatively high doses of estrogens on the other hand, seem to have an inhibitory effect on gonadotropin secretion this action being restricted to the hypothalamic level.   Estrogens can however have a stimulatory effect at
the hypothalamic level while their effect at the pituitary level
appear to be exclusively stimulatory.   Indeed, estrogens have
been shown to increase the sensitivity of the LH response to LH-
RH both in vivo and in vitro.

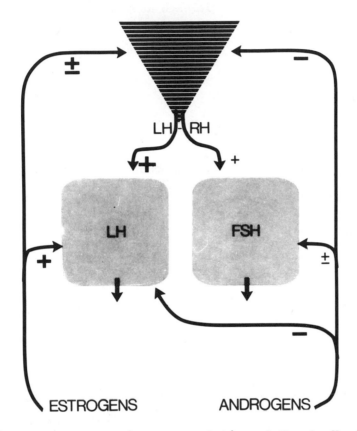

Figure 11: Schematic representation of the feedback effect of estrogens and androgens at the hypothalamic level on LH-RH release and at the pituitary level on LH and FSH secretion.

REFERENCES

Baldwin, D.M., Ramirez, V.D. and Sawyer, C.H. (1974) Fed. Proc. 33, 212.

Beyer, C., Jaffe, R.B. and Gay, V.L. (1972) Endocrinology 91, 1372-1375.

Beyer, C., Cruz, M.L., Gay, V.L. and Jaffe, R.B. (1974) Endocrinology, 95, 722-727.

Bogdanove, E.M. (1967) Anat. Rec., 157, 117-136.

Borgeat, P., Chavancy, G., Dupont, A., Labrie, F. Arimura, A. and Schally, A.V. (1972) Proc. Nat. Acad. Sci. 69, 2677-2681.

Brown-Grant, K., Exley, D. and Naftolin, F. (1970) J. Endocrinol. 48, 295-296.

Burgus, R., Butcher, M., Ling, N., Monahan, M., Rivier, J., Fellows, R., Amoss, M., Blackwell, R., Vale, W. and Guillemin, R. (1971) C.R. Acad. Sci. (Paris) 273, 1611-1613.

Debeljuk, L., Arimura, A. and Schally, A.V. (1972) Endocrinology, 90, 1578-1581.

Denef, C., Magnus, C. and McEwen, B.S. (1973) J. Endocrinol, 59, 605-621.

Drouin, J., and Labrie, F. (1976) Endocrinology, submitted for publication.

Eldridge, J.C. and Mahesh, B.V. (1974) Biol. Reprod. 11, 385-397.

Everett, J.W. (1948) Endocrinology 43, 389-392.

Ferland, L., Borgeat, P., Labrie, F., Bernard, J., De Léan, A. and Raynaud, J.P. (1975) Mol. Cell. Endocrinol. 2, 107-115.

Ferland, L., Kelly, P. and Labrie, F. (1976) Endocrinology, submitted for publication.

Jewelewicz, R., Ferin, M., Vande Wiele, R.L., Dyrenfurth, I. and Warren, M. (1974) Fertil. and Steril. 25, 290-291.

Kamberi, I.A. and McCann, S.M. (1969) Fed. Proc. 28, 382.

Kingsley, T.R. and Bogdanove, E.M. (1973) Endocrinology 93, 1398-1403.

Legan, S.J., Gay, V.L. and Midgley, A.R. Jr. (1973) Endocrinology 93, 781-785.

Lee, P.S., Jaffe, R.B., Midgley, A.R. Jr, Kohen, F. and Niswender, G.D. (1972) J. Clin. End. Metab. 35, 636-641.

Mahesh, V., Muldoon, T.G., Eldridge, J.C. and Korach, K.A. (1972) In "Saxena, B.B., Beling, C.G. and Gandy, H.M. (eds), Gonadotropins, Wiley-Interscience, N.Y.) p. 730-748.

Matsuo, H., Baba, Y., Nair, R.M.G., Arimura, A. and Schally, A.V. (1971) Biochem. Biophys. Res. Commun. 43, 1334-1339.

Naftolin, F., Brown-Grant, K. and Corker, S.C. (1972) J. Endocrinol., 53, 17-30.

Negro-Vilar, A., Ojeda, S.R. and McCann, S.M. (1973) Endocrinology 93, 729-735.

Nillius, S.J. and Wide, L. (1971) J. Obstet. Gynec. Brit. Common. 78, 922-927.

Peterson, N.T.Jr., Midgley, A.R.Jr. and Jaffe, R.B. (1968) J. Clin. End. Metab. 28, 1473-1478.

Ramirez, V.D. and McCann, S.M. (1963) Endocrinology 72: 452-455.

Schally, A.V., Carter, W.H., Arimura, A. and Bowers, C.Y. (1967) Endocrinology 81, 1173-1176.

Schally, A.V., Kastin, A.J. and Arimura, S. (1971) Fertil. Steril. 22, 703-721.

Smith, E.R. and Davidson, J.M. (1967) Am. J. Physiol. 212, 1385-1390.

Smith, E.R., and Davidson, J.M. (1974) Neuroendocrinology 14, 369-373.

Swerdloff, R.S. and Odell, W.D. (1968) Lancet 2, 683-687.

Swerdloff, R.S., Walsh, P.C. and Odell, W.D. (1972) Steroids 20, 13-22.

Swerdloff, R.S. and Walsh, P.C. (1973) Acta Endocrinologica 73, 11-21.

Yen, S.S.C., VanderBerg, C., Rebor, R. and Ehara, Y. (1972) J. Clin. Endocrinol. Metab. 35, 931-934.

Zanisi, M., Motta, M. and Martini, L. (1973) J. Endocrinol., 315-316.

THE ROLE OF ESTRADIOL IN MODULATING LH AND FSH RESPONSE TO

GONADOTROPIN RELEASING HORMONE

Robert B. Jaffe, William R. Keye, Jr.   and
John R. Young

Reproductive Endocrinology Center, Department of
Obstetrics and Gynecology, University of California
San Francisco, California 94143

In women, as well as in subhuman primates, it has been
suggested that estradiol may be involved in initiating the surge
of gonadotropins which occurs at midcycle. This suggestion is
based, in part, on the observations that estradiol reaches a peak
at or just prior to the midcycle gonadotropin surge (1), and that
the administration of estradiol to women and monkeys in the follicular phase of the menstrual cycle results in an increase in luteinizing hormone (LH) (2-5).

While the precise molecular mechanism by which estradiol may
act to initiate gonadotropin release has not been elucidated,
several mechanisms have been postulated. It has been suggested
that the midcycle surge of gonadotropins may be due to an increased
sensitivity of the pituitary to endogenous gonadotropin-releasing
hormone (GnRH or LRF) brought about by increasing levels of circulating estradiol (6). This suggestion was based on the observation
that the gonadotropin response to synthetic GnRH progressively increases as the time of ovulation is approached. It is also possible
that estradiol stimulates the release of endogenous GnRH or alters
its metabolism.

Initially, we performed studies designed to investigate the
effects of short-term (16 hr) constant infusions of 17β-estradiol
on 1) the responsiveness of the pituitary to GnRH, and 2) the
disappearance rate of GnRH (17).

In this study, fifteen healthy nulliparous women, ages 18-21
yr, with no history of gynecologic or endocrinologic disease or
previous use of oral contraceptives, were investigated. Each subject was studied on the second day of the menstrual cycle. An

211

intravenous infusion of normal saline was begun, and infused at
50 ml/hr.   Sixteen hours later, at 8 AM (t=0), a rapid intravenous
injection of normal saline was given.   Blood samples were obtained
through an indwelling venous catheter at t - 16 hr and at t - 30,
-15, 0, +5, +10, +15, +20, +25, +30, +45, +60, +90, +120, +180, and
+240 min.   Each sample was assayed for LH and follicle-stimulating
hormone (FSH).   In addition, the t = 0 sample was assayed for estradiol by radioimmunoassay.

    Each subject was studied again on the second day of one of the
subsequent three menstrual cycles.   In the second cycle studied,
each subject was assigned to one of three groups of five.   Group I,
the control group, received an intravenous infusion of normal saline.   Group II received an infusion of 17β-estradiol in normal saline, 0.05 μg/kg/hr. designed to achieve a circulating concentration
similar to that seen in the late follicular phase.   Group III received an infusion of 17β-estradiol, 0.10 μg/kg/hr, to achieve a
concentration similar to that at midcycle.   The infusions were
begun at t - 16 hr and discontinued at t + 240 min.   At 8 AM the
following day (t = 0), each subject received 50 μg GnRH in 5 ml of
normal saline as a rapid intravenous bolus.   The GnRH was kindly
supplied by Dr. S. Preston, Parke-Davis Research.

    Additional samples of blood were drawn from two subjects in
Group I and two in Group III at t + 2, +4, +8, +10, +15, +20, +25,
+30, +45, and +60 min., and assayed for GnRH.   The disappearance
rate of GnRH was determined as previously described (8).   The
gonadotropin responses to GnRH were determined by calculating the
mean increase in LH at t + 20 min and FSH at t + 45 min (average
times of maximal LH and FSH responses, respectively), and the mean
area subtended by the LH and FSH curves for each group of subjects.
Calculations were made after subtracting the mean baseline concentration (t - 30, -15, 0) from the subsequent values (t + 5 to t +
240).   Because of the disparate variances between groups, the
Kruskal-Waller test (9) was used to compare group responses.

    Daily oral basal body temperatures (BBT) or a luteal phase
blood sample for progesterone, or both, were obtained to provide
presumptive evidence for ovulation.

    The serum LH and FSH concentrations obtained throughout the
study period during the first (control) month (LH, 8.3 ± 0.3 mean
± se; FSH, 8.0 ± 0.3) were similar to those we have reported previously (10).   There was presumptive evidence of ovulation in
eleven of the subjects.   No basal body temperature record or progesterone concentration was available for the remaining 4 subjects.

    During the second month, serum estradiol concentrations at
t = 0 correlated with the rate of administration.   The control
group (no estradiol infused) had a mean serum estradiol

concentration of 61 $\pm$ 4 pg/ml (se); Group II, (0.05 µg/kg/hr) 151 $\pm$ 11; and Group III, (0.10 µg/kg/hr) 225 $\pm$ 54.

The infusion of 17β-estradiol was accompanied by a decrease in serum LH concentrations from 9.2 $\pm$ 1.5 (Group II) and 8.0 $\pm$ 1.8 (Group III) at t - 16 hr to mean baseline concentrations of 5.2 $\pm$ 0.5 (Group II) and 6.7 $\pm$ 1.8 (Group III). No significant change in LH concentrations occurred in response to the infusion of saline (Group I).

FSH concentrations decreased in response to the infusion of 17β-estradiol in 9 of 10 subjects in Groups II and III. The FSH concentrations fell from 11.4 $\pm$ 3.3 (t - 16 hr) to 5.7 $\pm$ 1.1 (mean baseline concentrations) in Group II, and 11.7 $\pm$ 3.7 to 7.3 $\pm$ 2.3 in Group III. No significant change in FSH concentrations occurred in response to the infusion of saline (Group I).

The mean ratio of FSH to LH (FSH/LH) at the time of admission, and prior to saline or 17β-estradiol administration, was 1.36 $\pm$ 0.53 for Group I, 1.2 $\pm$ 0.34 for Group II, and 1.51 $\pm$ 0.70 for Group III. Following the infusion of saline to subjects in Group I, or the low dose of 17β-estradiol to Group II, there was no significant change in FSH/LH. However, the higher rate of infusion of 17β-estradiol was associated with a greater decrease in FSH than LH in 4 of the 5 subjects in Group III. The average decrease in FSH/LH in these 4 subjects was 0.54 $\pm$ 0.03. The fifth subject had an increase in FSH/LH of 1.83.

The LH concentrations following GnRH administration during the second month of study are shown in Fig. 1.

LH values had begun to rise by t + 5 min in the control group. Peak response occurred at t + 20 min for 3 of the 5 subjects, and at t + 25 and 30 min in the other 2. LH concentrations then fell to near preinjection levels by 120 min. The rate of decline, as determined from a semilogarithmic plot of mean concentration vs. time, corresponded to a t$\frac{1}{2}$ of approximately 80 min. A greater increase in LH concentration was evident in the control group (I) than either of the estradiol treated groups (II and III). A definite but blunted response occurred in Group II, while there was no significant response in Group III.

A significantly greater increase in LH (ΔLH) occurred at t + 20 minutes in Group I than Group III ($p < 0.05$), as shown in Table 1. Similarly, there was a greater increase in LH secretion in Group I than III when the areas under the curves were compared ($p < 0.05$). While the differences between Groups I and II, and II and III were observed, they failed to reach statistical significance.

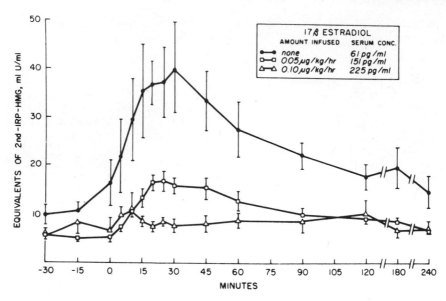

Fig. 1. Serum concentrations of LH (mean ± se) in response to
50 µg GnRH at t = 0 for Groups I (•–•), II (□–□), and III (Δ–Δ),
which received 17β-estradiol in amounts shown in inset. From: Keye,
W.R., Jr. and Jaffe, R.B. J Clin Endocrinol Metab <u>38</u>: 805, 1974.

Table 1. LH response to GnRH

Group	n	Mean baseline LH Concentration (±se) (mIU/ml)	Mean LH at t + 20 min (± se) (mIU/ml)	Mean area under curve (±se) (mIU/4hr)
I	5	12.2 ± 1.1	24.8 ± 4.3	2600 ± 806
II	5	5.2 ± 0.5	11.1 ± 2.0	1169 ± 297
III	5	6.7 ± 1.8	0.7 ± 1.8	292 ± 292

The FSH concentrations following the administration of GnRH
during the second month are shown in Fig. 2. The pattern of FSH
response was different from that of LH in the control group. FSH
levels began to rise by t + 15 min, with the mean peak value for
the group occurring at t + 45 min. However, no significant decline

in values had occurred by t + 240 min. It is apparent that the
infusion of 17β-estradiol also diminished the FSH response to GnRH.
While a significant increase in FSH occurred in Group I, there was
no significant response in either of the estradiol-treated groups.
The decrement in FSH concentration at t + 5 min for Group I (Fig.2)
is probably a statistical artifact, resulting from the absence of
a plasma sample from 1 subject whose pretreatment FSH concentrations
were higher than those of the other subjects.

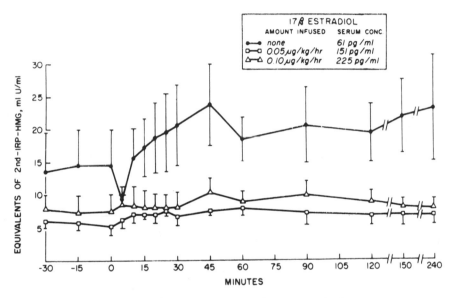

Fig. 2.   Serum concentrations of FSH (mean ±se) in response to
50 µg GnRH at t = 0 for Groups I (•–•), II (□–□), and III (Δ–Δ),
which received 17β-estradiol in amounts shown in inset.   From: Keye,
W.R., Jr. and Jaffe, R.B.   J Clin Endocrinol Metab <u>38</u>: 805, 1974.

The mean increase in FSH (ΔFSH) at 45 min for the control
group was significantly greater than in either of the estradiol-
treated groups (p<0.05) as seen in Table 2.   While an observable
difference in area under the FSH curves occurred between the control
and the estradiol-treated groups, these differences were not
significant.

Table 2.   FSH response to GnRH

Group	n	Mean baseline FSH concentration (±se) (mIU/ml)	Mean ΔFSH at t + 45 min (±se)	Mean area under curve (±se)
I	5	14.4 ± 5.6	8.0 ± 1.2	1395 ± 370
II	5	5.7 ± 1.1	1.5 ± 1.0	306 ± 202
III	5	7.3 ± 2.3	1.8 ± 0.9	274 ± 214

As seen in Table 3, the infusion of estradiol did not affect the maximal concentration of GnRH or its disappearance rate in the 4 subjects studied.

Table 3.   Maximal concentration and disappearance rate of GnRH

Subject	Group	Maximal GnRH concentration (ng/ml)	Disappearance rate of GnRH $(t_{\frac{1}{2}})$
1	I	5.0	4.09
2	I	5.7	4.52
3	III	4.4	4.30
4	III	6.6	3.30

Seven of the 8 subjects in whom serum progesterone values or BBT records were obtained had presumptive evidence of ovulation during the month in which GnRH or 17β-estradiol, or both, were administered.   No basal body temperature record or progesterone concentration were obtained from the other 7 subjects.

In the control group, GnRH induced a greater maximal increase in LH (max ΔLH) than FSH (max ΔFSH).   The ratio of the max ΔFSH/ max ΔLH was 0.40 ± 0.15.   The infusion of 17β-estradiol to subjects in Group II diminished the LH and FSH responses to a similar extent; the max ΔFSH/max ΔLH of 0.34 ± 0.05 is not significantly different from that of the control group.

The protocol used in this study was selected to mimic the conditions which exist in the midfollicular phase of the cycle and at the time of the midcycle gonadotropin surge.   By utilizing day two of the menstrual cycle to study the modulating effects of 17β–estradiol on the hypothalamic–pituitary axis, we chose a time when endogenous estradiol levels are relatively low and spontaneous release of gonadotropins is minimal (1). Progesterone concentrations at this time are similar to those seen at midcycle (1). Estradiol–17β was administered rather than synthetic estrogens (which do not increase the circulating concentrations of estradiol) to approximate more closely the estradiol milieu extant during several phases of the menstrual cycle. The dose of 50 μg GnRH was selected on the basis of previous data demonstrating a gonadotropin response similar to that seen at midcycle when this dose was employed (11).

While several other investigators have reported a decrease in gonadotropin concentrations during the administration of estradiol to women during the follicular phase of the menstrual cycle (2-4), the mechanism of this action has not been elucidated. The present study provides evidence that this suppressive action is due, at least in part, to a direct and inhibitory effect on pituitary responsiveness to GnRH.

The decrease in FSH/LH ratio following a high rate of estradiol infusion supports the previous contention that estradiol exerts a greater inhibitory action on the release of synthesis of FSH than LH (2). However, these data do not explain the greater suppression of FSH than LH, for following pretreatment with estradiol–17β, the response of FSH to GnRH was not inhibited to a greater degree than LH. It is possible that this greater suppression of FSH is the result of an estradiol induced decrease in the secretion of a separate FSH–releasing hormone (12-14).

Patterns of LH and FSH response following the administration of GnRH to women in the follicular phase of the menstrual cycle have been described previously (6). Our finding of an approximate rate of decline of LH, corresponding to a half–life of 56 min following its peak response to GnRH, is similar to that of 66.1 minutes reported by Yen et al. (6). In addition, we noted a more gradual decline in LH following pretreatment with estradiol. Yen et al. have reported a similar rate of decline in the late follicular phase (6). Whether this is due to a more sustained release of LH in response to GnRH or to a decreased rate of metabolism of GnRH is not clear. However, our finding that estradiol did not alter the maximal plasma concentration of GnRH or its rate of disappearance suggests that a decreased rate of metabolism of GnRH is not the causative factor.

The blunted gonadotropin response to GnRH in the presence of midcycle levels of estradiol is not consistent with the hypothesis that the preovulatory rise of estradiol increases the sensitivity

of the pituitary to GnRH. However, we postulated that the failure
of 17β-estradiol to increase pituitary responsiveness might have
been related to either the duration of the estradiol infusion or
the temporal relationship between the increasing estradiol concentration and the administration of GnRH. Studies utilizing the
rhesus monkey suggested that the positive feedback effect of estradiol may be both dose and time related (15,16).

Factors in addition to increased pituitary sensitivity to GnRH
may also be involved. It has been proposed that increased hypothalamic secretion of GnRH occurs at midcycle. It is also possible that
the metabolism of GnRH is altered at midcycle. However, our observation that estradiol does not affect the maximal plasma concentration or disappearance rate of GnRH suggests that estradiol does not
act in this way to initiate a gonadotropin surge.

Because of the study in the rhesus monkey that demonstrated
that estradiol effects upon gonadotropin release are dependent upon
the duration of administration as well as the circulating concentration which is achieved, we conducted a study in which estradiol
was administered for a more protracted period (6 days), beginning
on the first day of the menstrual cycle, a time when endogenous
estradiol is low (1). Utilizing this regimen, an augmentation of
both LH and FSH response to GnRH was demonstrated.

The study was conducted in the following manner: Twenty women
with regular menstrual cycles, and no history of gynecologic or
endocrinologic disease or previous use of oral contraceptives, were
divided into two groups. One group of 13 women served as the control (non estradiol-treated) group. Each subject received intravenous administration of 100 µg GnRH at t = 0 on 1 day during the
first week of the menstrual cycle. Blood samples (8 ml) were collected through an indwelling venous catheter at the following
times: t – 30, –15, 0, +5, +10, +15, +20, +25, +30, +45, +60, +90,
and +120 min. Responses in these subjects were combined for statistical analysis, as there was no difference in responses on these
days.

The other 7 women comprised the study (estradiol-treated)
group and were studied according to the following protocol: At
4 PM on the first day of the menstrual cycle, each subject received
an intramuscular injection of 5 µg/kg of estradiol benzoate (270–
330 µg) in sesame oil. Additional intramuscular injections of
2.5 µg/kg estradiol benzoate (135–165 µg) were administered at 8 AM
and 8 PM on days 2 through 6 of the menstrual cycle. At 8 AM (t =
0), on the 7th (7 subjects), 8th (4 subjects), and 9th (2 subjects)
days of the menstrual cycle, GnRH, 100 µg, was given as an intravenous bolus.

Blood samples were obtained by venipuncture at the time of each injection of estradiol benzoate; at t - 12, -10, -8, -6, -4, -2, -1 hr in 2 subjects; t - 30, -15, 0, +5, +10, +15, +20, +25, +30, +45, +60, +90, +120 minutes in all 7 subjects; and at t + 150, + 180, +210, +240 in 3 subjects on day 7 and 1 subject on day 9[1]. In addition, samples were obtained every 2 hr during the interval between the last estradiol injection and the administration of GnRH in 2 subjects.

The gonadotropin responses to GnRH were determined by calculating the mean maximal increase (Δ max LH and Δ max FSH) and the mean area subtended by the LH and FSH curves (integrated response) between t = 0 and t +120 min for each group of subjects. The area under each curve was calculated by connecting consecutive points by straight line segments and calculating the area under each segment by the method of triangulation. The total area under the curve was determined by the summation of the areas under the individual segments. Calculations were made after subtracting the mean base-line concentration (t - 30, -15, 0) from the subsequent values t + 5 to t + 120 min. Group responses were compared using the one-tailed Student's t test. The rate of decline of LH from the peak concentration was determined from a semilogarithmic plot of concentration vs. time, and is expressed as $t\frac{1}{2}$.

The composite patterns of LH responses to GnRH of subjects in the control and estradiol-treated (day 7) groups are shown in Fig. 3. In the control group, the increase in LH by t + 5 min, peak response at t + 25 min, and decline to near base line values at t + 120 is similar to that of a group of women in the early follicular phase which we reported in the previous study (17). Several differences between the mean responses in the control and estradiol-treated groups are apparent: 1) the mean LH response in the estradiol-treated group was greater than that of the control group; 2) as compared with the peak response of 37.4 $\pm$ 4.3 mIU/ml in the control group, which occurred at 25 min, the peak response (199.6 $\pm$ 44.1) in the estradiol-treated group was delayed, occuring at 120 min; and 3) the mean rate of decline ($t\frac{1}{2}$) of LH following the peak response was slower in the estradiol-treated than the control group (estradiol-treated group, 126.4 $\pm$ 29.1; control group 49.2 $\pm$ 5.6 min). As seen in Table 4, a significantly greater mean maximal increase in LH (Δ max LH) occurred in the group treated with estradiol on day 7 than the control group (p<0.01). Similarly, there was a significantly greater integrated LH response on day 7 when compared with that observed in the control group (Table 3) (p< 0.01). The average time of the Δ max LH of 98.6 $\pm$ 8.9 min in

---

[1] Samples from t + 150 to +240 min were collected in the last 3 subjects studied, as the analysis of the results from the first 3 subjects demonstrated a prolonged response to GnRH following estradiol pretreatment.

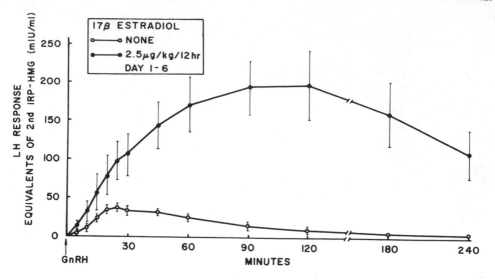

Fig. 3.   Net increase of serum LH (mean ± se) in response to gonadotropin releasing hormone (indicated as GnRH in this figure) (100
μg iv at t = 0 in women).   GnRH was administered on day 7 (•-•) of
the menstrual cycle following treatment with 5 μg/kg/day estradiol
benzoate on days 1-6.   Data from a control group of women (o-o)
who received GnRH on on occasion during the first week of the
menstrual cycle, but who did not receive exogeneous estradiol, also
are shown.   From: Jaffe, R.B. and Keye, W.R., Jr.   J Clin Endocrinol Metab 39: 850, 1974.

the study group was significantly later than 26.5 ± 0.9 min in the
control group.

     As seen in Fig. 4, and similar to the pattern of LH response,
the FSH response to GnRH in the estradiol-treated group was augmented and prolonged when compared to that of the control group.   The
peak response of 27.9 ± 6.8 mIU/ml, which occurred at 120 min in
the estradiol-treated group is significantly greater than that of
6.8 ± 1.9 which occurred at 45 min in the control group (p<0.01).
In addition, as seen in Table 4, the mean maximal increase (Δ max
FSH) and integrated response are significantly greater in the
estradiol-treated group on day 7 than in the control group (p<0.01

and p 0.01 in both cases). Whereas the average time of the Δ max
FSH was 58.8 ± 7.4 min in the control group, it did not occur until
107 ± 14.4 min in the estradiol-treated group.

Table 4. LH and FSH responses to LRF

	Mean maximal increase (from base line) mIU/ml		Integrated increase (area subtended by curve) IU/2 hr		
	LH	FSH	LH	FSH	Δ max FSH/Δ max LH
Control group	41.4 ± 4.7	9.3 ± 1.7	2.6 ± 0.3	0.8 ± 0.1	0.21 ± 0.03
Study group					
Day 7	216.9 ± 41.9	28.9 ± 6.4	18.2 ± 3.1	2.2 ± 0.5	0.24 ± 0.09
Day 8	168.8 ± 48.2	25.0 ± 5.4	14.9 ± 4.5	2.0 ± 0.4	0.18 ± 0.05
Day 9	104.5 ± 54.5	13.5 ± 0.5	9.2 ± 4.6	1.2 ± 0.1	0.18 ± 0.09

The augmentative effect of estradiol on LH and FSH responses
to GnRH which was seen 12 hr following the last injection of estradiol benzoate was still present at 36 and 60 hr.   Shown in Fig. 5
are the LH responses to GnRH in women who received estradiol benzoate on days 1-6 of the cycle, followed by LRF on days 7,8 and 9
(12,36 and 60 hr following the last injection of estradiol benzoate).
While the gonadotropin responses on days 8 and 9 were greater than
that of the control group, the augmentative effect of estradiol
appears to diminish as the interval between the last estradiol injection and the administration of LRF increases.   The augmented
mean maximal and integrated LH and FSH responses in the estradiol-
treated groups also decreased as this interval increased (Table 4).

Pretreatment with estradiol augmented the LH and FSH responses
to a similar extent, as the Δ max FSH/Δ max LH in the estradiol-
treated group on day 7 was similar to the control group.   Similarly, no significant differences in these ratios were noted on day 8
or day 9 when compared to the control group (Table 4).

Whereas in the mean baseline concentrations of LH on days 7
(14.7 ± 3.6), 8 (13.3 ± 4.4), and 9 (14.5 ± 1.5) were similar to
those in the control group (11.3 ± 0.7), the mean base line FSH
concentration on day 7 of 6.0 ± 0.9 was significantly less than
that of the control group of 11.9 ± 1.2.   The mean base line FSH
concentrations on day 8 (7.5 ± 2.5) and day 9 (10.0 ± 2.0) were
similar to the control group.   No significant change in serum LH
or FSH concentrations occurred during the administration of estradiol.   In addition, no spontaneous surge of gonadotropins occurred
in the 12-hr interval between the last injection of estradiol and
the administration of GnRH.

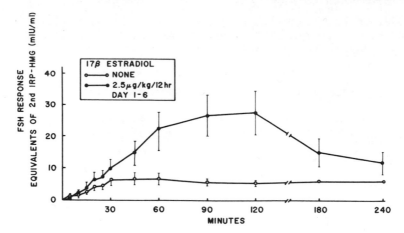

Fig. 4. Net increase of serum FSH (mean ± se) in response to gonadotropin-releasing hormone (GnRH) (100 μg iv at t = 0) in women.
LRF was administered on day 7 (•-•) of the menstrual cycle following
treatment with 5 μg/kg/day estradiol benzoate on days 1-6. Data
from a control group of women (o-o) who received GnRH on one occasion during the first week of the menstrual cycle, but who did not
receive exogenous estradiol, also are shown. From: Jaffe, R.B.
and Keye, W.R., Jr. J Clin Endocrinol Metab 39: 850, 1974.

The administration of this dose of estradiol during the first
6 days of the menstrual cycle delayed the onset of the next menstrual period. While there was no difference in the length of cycles
in subjects in the control and estradiol-treated groups prior to
participation in the study, the mean interval between menses during the month of study was 41.8 ± 1.5 days in the estradiol-treated
group and 30.2 ± 0.9 days in the control group. The longer interval in the estradiol-treated group was associated with a prolonged
follicular phase and normal luteal phase, as judged by basal body
temperatures.

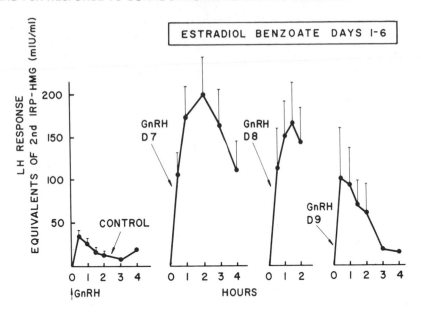

Fig. 5. Net increase of serum LH (mean ± se) in response to gonadotropin releasing hormone (GnRH, 100 μg iv at t = 0) in women. LRF
was administered on days 7, 8 and 9 of the menstrual cycle following treatment with 5 μg/kg/day estradiol benzoate on days 1-6. Data
from a control group of women who received GnRH on one occasion
during the first week of the menstrual cycle, but who did not receive exogenous estradiol, also are shown. From: Jaffe, R.B. and
Keye, W.R., Jr. J Clin Endocrinol Metab 39: 850, 1974.

This study demonstrated that exposure of the hypothalamic-pituitary axis to increased concentrations of estradiol for an appropriate length of time can significantly augment gonadotropin response
to GnRH in women. The amount of estradiol administered was similar
to the secretion rate of estradiol by the ovary during the late
follicular phase of the menstrual cycle (18). Thus, the data suggest that estradiol increases pituitary sensitivity to GnRH and
that this mechanism may be, at least in part, responsible for the
surge of gonadotropins at midcycle.

Among the several possible mechanisms by which estradiol may effect these changes are: 1) decreasing the metabolism of GnRH, 2) decreasing the metabolism of gonadotropins, 3) causing a spontaneous release of gonadotropins by positive feedback, 4) altering the secretion of endogenous GnRH, 5) increasing pituitary storage of gonadotropins, and/or 6) altering pituitary membrane permeability to gonadotropins, i.e., affecting gonadotropin release. That the biologic half-life of GnRH was not decreased is suggested by our finding that estradiol administration did not alter the immunologic half-life of exogenously administered GnRH in women (17). Nor does the metabolic clearance rate of LH appear to be altered by exogenous estrogen. Kohler et al. (19) administered a combination of ethinyl estradiol-3 methyl ether and norethynodrel to women of reproductive age and found no significant change in the metabolic clearance of LH. That the augmented response to GnRH is not dependent upon a surge of gonadotropins induced by the positive feedback effect of estradiol is suggested by our observation that no surge was present in sera obtained every 2 hr in the interval between the last estradiol injection and the administration of GnRH. The observation that LH and FSH concentrations did not decrease with this dose of estradiol suggests that the increased responses to GnRH are not simply a consequence of increased stores of LH and FSH resulting from an inhibition of LH release during the administration of estradiol.

The observation that gonadotropin responses can be augmented (present study) or blunted when exogenous GnRH has been administered following estradiol, suggests that one site of action of estradiol is the pituitary. However, it is possible that this effect also was brought about by stimulation of endogenous GnRH. For this latter possibility to obtain, though, this stimulation would have to have been achieved without a concomitant or subsequent increase in gonadotropins, as no such increase was seen in subjects prior to administration of exogenous GnRH.

The prolonged responses of LH and FSH following the administration of GnRH in the estradiol-treated women is similar to that seen in hypogonadal women (20). This prolonged response in our study may be related to the increased sensitivity of the pituitary, rendering it capable of continuing to respond to smaller amounts of GnRH than in untreated women. The question of whether the maximal concentration of estradiol reached results in the midcycle gonadotropin surge, or whether it is the decline from these peak levels with which the surge is associated, has been raised (20). Our finding that the augmentative effect of estradiol appeared to decrease as the interval between the last injection of estradiol

and the administration of GnRH increased points to the former possibility as being more likely. The observation by Korenman and
Sherman (18) that the midcycle surge of gonadotropins often begins
prior to the fall in circulating estradiol concentrations also supports this concept.

These findings suggest that the nature of the modulating effect
of estradiol (negative or positive) upon pituitary responsiveness
to GnRH is dependent upon the duration of exposure of the hypothalamic-pituitary axis to increased concentrations of estradiol.

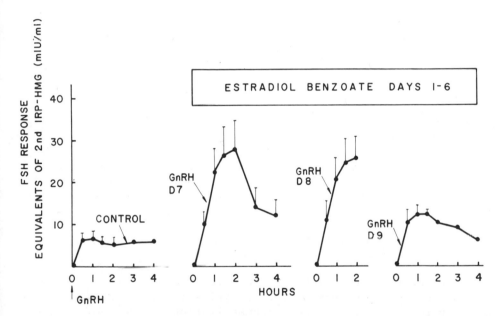

Fig 6. Net increase of serum FSH (mean ± se) in response to gonadotropin-releasing hormone (GnRH, 100 μg iv at t = 0) in women. GnRH
was administered on days 7, 8 and 9 of the menstrual cycle following
treatment with 5 μg/kg/day estradiol benzoate on days 1-6. Data
from a control group of women who received GnRH on one occasion during the first week of the menstrual cycle, but who did not receive
exogenous estradiol, also were shown. From: Jaffe, R.B. and Keye,
W.R., Jr. J Clin Endocrinol Metab 39: 850, 1974.

Therefore, we undertook studies to define the specific strength-duration characteristics of the relation between estradiol concentration and pituitary response to GnRH.

The following study was designed to elucidate the relation between the duration of elevated estradiol concentration and the modulation of pituitary response to GnRH.

Ten women with regular menstrual cycles and no history of physical findings of gynecologic or endocrinologic disease were studied. Studies were performed during two consecutive menstrual cycles.

During the first (control) cycle, each subject received 100 µg GnRH iv at t = 0 on day, 3,4,5,6, or 7 of the menstrual cycle. Blood samples were obtained through an indwelling catheter at t - 30, -15, 0, +5, +10, +15, +20, +25, +30, +45, +60, +90, and +120 min.

Each subject was studied again during the first week of the next menstrual cycle. At 8 PM on the first day of the menstrual cycle each subject received an i.m. injection of E_2B in sesame oil 5 µg/kg. Every 12 hr thereafter, additional injections of estradiol, 2.5 µg/kg, were administered for a total of 3,5,7,9, or 11 injections. GnRH, 100 µg iv at t = 0, was administered 12 hr following the last injection of E_2B, or after 36, 60, 48, 108, or 132 hr of estradiol administration (2 subjects at each time interval). Blood samples were drawn just prior to each E_2B injection, and at t - 14, -12, -10, -8, -6, -4, -2, -1 hr and t - 30, -15, 0, +5, +10, +20, +25, +30, +45, +60, +90, +120, +150, +180, +210, and 240 min. Each subject's gonadotropin response to GnRH during estradiol treatment (second or study month) was compared with her own response during the first or control cycle.

Each sample was assayed for LH and FSH. Selected samples were assayed for estradiol 17β.

The LH response during the study (estradiol pretreatment) and control (no estradiol pretreatment) cycles for individual subjects are compared in Fig. 7. The responses during the control months in 9 of the 10 subjects (Table 5) were similar to those which we previously reported for the early follicular phase. The response of the other subject (M.B.) was approximately three times greater.

Pretreatment of subjects with E_2B abolished the LH response in two subjects and augmented the responses in eight subjects. The nature of this modulating effect of estradiol was related to the duration of estradiol administration. When GnRH was infused after 36 hr of estradiol pretreatment the LH responses were abolished. In contrast, pretreatment with estradiol for 84, 108, or 132 hr

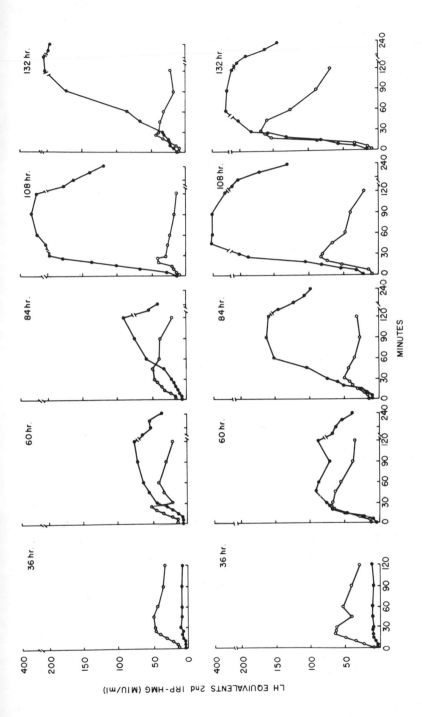

Fig. 7. LH responses to the iv injection of 100 μg gonadotropin releasing hormone to women in the early follicular phase of the menstrual cycle. The LH response for each subject studied during a control cycle (o-o) is compared to her response during a subsequent cycle in which she received estradiol benzoate (2.5 μg/kg i.m. every 12 hr after an initial injection of 5.0 μg/kg) for 36, 60, 84, 108, or 132 hrs (•-•). From: Keye, W.R., Jr. and Jaffe, R.B. J Clin Endocrinol Metab. In Press.

Table 5. LH and FSH responses to GnRh in the early follicular phase of the menstrual cycle

Subject	Serum estradiol concentration at t = 0 (pg/ml)	Maximal increase from baseline (mIU/ml)		Integrated response mIU/2hr	
		LH	FSH	LH	FSH
B.U.	42	54	9	4100	805
S.K.	33	36	2	2960	50
J.C.	66	58	6	4265	480
C.M.	55	38	5	1875	435
C.W.	N.D.*	34	6	2490	450
L.T.	44	36	14	1435	555
K.V.	48	74	13	4655	755
S.H.	25	33	6	1780	455
M.Z.	22	33	11	1340	420
M.B.	40	160	17	11405	1250

*N.D. = Not determined.

resulted in a marked augmentation of the LH response. Subjects who received 60 hr of estradiol also had responses that were augmented when compared to those seen during the control months, although the degree of augmentation was not as great.

In addition, the administration of estradiol for 60 to 132 hr prolonged, as well as augmented, the LH response. While peak responses occurred by t + 25 to t +45 min in the control cycle, they did not occur until t + 45 to t + 180 minutes in those women whose responses were augmented following E_2B pretreatment. In contrast to the rapid decline of LH following the peak response in the control cycle, a plateau of LH values at peak concentrations was seen for 30 to 150 minutes in most subjects during the study cycle.

The inhibitory effect of short term estradiol administration and augmentative effect of more prolonged estradiol treatment is also seen when the maximal LH responses (Δ max LH) and the integrated LH responses from the study cycle (Table 6) are compared with those during the control cycle (Table 5).

Pretreatment with estradiol also had an effect upon the FSH response to GnRH which varied with the duration of E_2 administration, as seen in Fig. 8 and Tables 5 and 6. Blunted responses occurred after short term estradiol administration, whereas augmented responses were seen following longer duration of estradiol pretreatment. No FSH response occurred when GnRH was given after 36 hr of E_2B administration (subjects S.K. and B.U.). While 60 hr of pretreatment with estradiol had no effect on FSH response to GnRH (subjects (J.C. and C.M.), augmented and prolonged responses were seen in five of six subjects who received estradiol for 84 or more hours prior to the administration of GnRH. A delayed and blunted response occurred in the other subject (M.Z.).

The mean serum estradiol concentration of 41.7 $\pm$ 4.7 pg/ml at t = 0 during the control month was similar to that previously reported during the early follicular phase and similar to but less than that at the time of the first estradiol injection during the study month.

Serum estradiol concentrations increased within two hours of an injection of E_2B, reached a maximum concentration by four hours, and were near preinjection concentrations by 12 hr (Fig. 9). The mean maximal increase in serum estradiol concentration following the injection of 2.5 µg/kg E_2B was 46.8 $\pm$ 11.81 pg/ml at 4 hr.

Shown in Fig. 10 are the serum estradiol concentrations determined at 12 hr intervals during the administration of E_2B. Since these determinations were performed on samples drawn just prior to each injection of E_2B, they represent the lowest estradiol concentration during each interval between injections. Estradiol

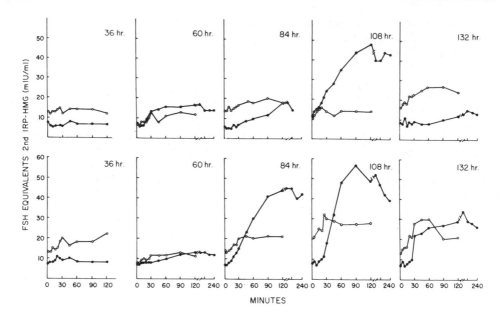

Fig. 8.   FSH responses to the iv injection of 100 µg gonadotropin releasing hormone to women in the early follicular phase of the menstrual cycle.   The FSH response for each subject studied during a control cycle (o-o) is compared to her response during a subsequent cycle in which she received estradiol benzoate (2.5 µg/kg i.m. every 12 hrs after an initial injection of 5.0 µg/kg) for 36, 60, 84, 108, or 132 hrs (•-•).   From: Keye, W.R. and Jaffe, R.B., J Clin Endocrinol Metab.   In Press.

concentrations rose progressively during the first 36 hr of E$_2$B injections.   Concentrations then remained relatively constant for the remainder of the study and ranged from 128 ± 43.0 to 186.2 ± 38.1 pg/ml from the 36th through the 132nd hr of study.   As seen in Table 5, the estradiol concentrations at the time of GnRH administration during the second month were in the mid- or late follicular phase range in all subjects (range: 85 to 183 pg/ml).   No significant change in LH or FSH concentrations occurred during the course of E$_2$B administration or during the interval between the last estradiol benzoate injection and the administration of GnRH.

Table 6. LH and FSH responses to GnRH in women pretreated with estradiol benzoate

Subject	Duration of estradiol benzoate administration (hrs)	Serum estradiol concentration at t = 0 pg/ml	Maximal increase (mIU/ml) from baseline		Integrated response (mIU/2hr)	
			LH	FSH	LH	FSH
B.U.	36	120	7	3	650	180
S.K.	36	N.D.*	6	0	515	-120
J.C.	60	126	86	10	8050	815
C.M.	60	85	70	6	5740	370
C.W.	84	146	84	12	5145	500
L.T.	84	228	154	38	12745	2485
K.V.	108	106	180	49	33855	3565
S.H.	108	114	306	36	26720	2505
M.Z.	132	85	217	7	11260	25
M.B.	132	141	284	27	34360	1190

*N.D. = Not determined.

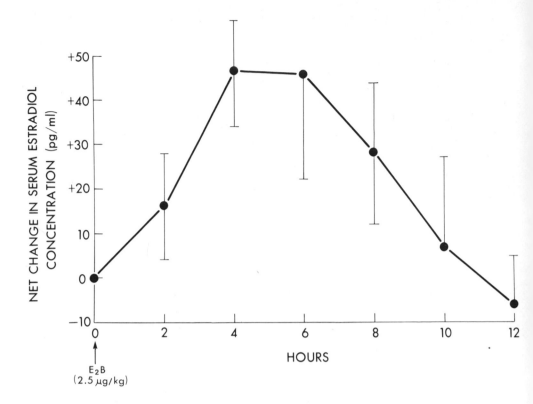

Fig. 9. Net change in serum estradiol (pg/ml) concentration following the administration of estradiol benzoate, 2.5 μg/kg i.m., to
10 normally menstruating women. From: Keye, W.R., Jr. and Jaffe,
R.B., J Clin Endocrinol Metab. In Press.

This study supports our earlier suggestion that the modulating
effect of estradiol (negative or positive) upon pituitary responsiveness to GnRH is dependent upon the duration of exposure of the
hypothalamic-pituitary system to increased concentrations of estradiol. The administration of estradiol in an amount approximating
the secretion rate of estradiol by the ovary during the late follicular phase of the menstrual cycle has 2 effects, depending upon the
duration of estradiol administration. The gonadotropin responses

to GnRH are abolished when GnRH is administered during the first 12 to 36 hr of estradiol administration. In contrast, gonadotropin responses are markedly augmented when the duration of estradiol administration was 84 to 132 hrs.

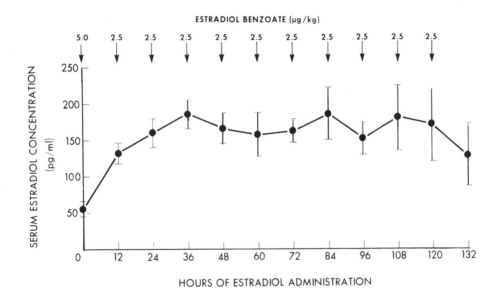

Fig. 10. Time course of serum estradiol concentrations following the administration of estradiol benzoate (2.5 µg/kg i.m. after an initial injection of 5.0 µg/kg i.m.) to 10 women in the early follicular phase of the menstrual cycle. From: Keye, W.R., Jr. and Jaffe, R.B., J Clin Endocrinol Metab. In Press.

This duration-dependent response to estradiol also has been reported in rats by Libertun et al (22). They found that the injection of 100 µg estradiol benzoate partially blocked the gonadotropin response to GnRH within one hr, and augmented the gonadotropin response after six to ten hrs.

Studies in women with abnormalities of menstrual function, utilizing synthetic estrogens, also have suggested duration-related responses. Yen et al (23) found that the administration of the synthetic estrogen, ethinyl estradiol, to four hypogonadal amenorrheic women resulted in an initial augmentative effect on pituitary response to GnRH during the first two weeks of estrogen administration. This was followed by a diminished response during the third and fourth weeks. Taymor (24) reported that the LH response to GnRH was blunted at 5 hr and augmented at 49 hr after the intramuscular injection of estradiol benzoate to a woman with "hypothalamic amenorrhea". On the basis of these studies, the authors concluded that gonadal steroids, estradiol in particular, have a modulating effect on the gonadotropin response to GnRH, and that this response is related to the duration of exposure of the hypothalamic-pituitary system to increased concentrations of estradiol. However, these results have questionable relevance in the study of the role of estradiol in the modulation of pituitary responsiveness to GnRH in the normal menstrual cycle, since the studies were performed on women with altered hypothalamic-pituitary function (23,24), in one study utilizing the pharmacologic preparation, ethinyl estradiol (23). The experimental design of our study differs from those mentioned above in three aspects: 1) to approximate more closely the estradiol milieu extant during the mid- and late follicular phase, we administered estradiol in an amount approximating the secretion rate of estradiol by the ovary during the late follicular phase of the menstrual cycle; 2) we studied women with regular menstrual cycles rather than women with altered hypothalamic-pituitary function; and 3) to reduce the influence of endogenous gonadal steroids or changing concentrations of estradiol, we studied subjects in the early follicular phase of the menstrual cycle.

Since serum estradiol concentrations at 36 hr (when gonadotropin responses were blunted) were similar to those at 60, 84, 108, and 132 hr (when gonadotropin responses were augmented) these results support the concept that the modulating effect of estradiol (i.e. the increased sensitivity to GnRH in the late follicular phase) is related to the duration of exposure of the hypothalamic-pituitary system to the increased concentrations of estradiol.

In this study the degree of augmentation of pituitary responsiveness to GnRH is seen to be dependent upon the _duration_ of exposure of the pituitary to a fixed increased concentration of E_2B. After the initial rise of circulating estradiol, essentially the same circulating concentration was achieved irrespective of the duration of pretreatment.

The final study was designed 1) to delineate further the strength-duration characteristics of estradiol modulation of pituitary response to GnRH by varying the _concentration_ of E_2B

administered while keeping the duration of exposure constant, and
2) to correlate the results obtained with reproductive hormone
events in the normal menstrual cycle.

Sixteen women with regular menstrual cycles and no history or
physical findings of significant gynecologic or endocrinologic disease were studied. Studies were performed during two or more menstrual cycles.

During the first (control) cycle, each subject received 100 µg
GnRH iv at t = 0 on day, 3, 4, 5, 6, or 7 of the menstrual cycle.
Blood samples were obtained through an indwelling catheter at
t - 30, -15, 0, +5, +10, +15, +20, +25, +30, +45, +60, +90, and +120
minutes in all subjects and additionally at +180 and +240 minutes
in 14 of the 16 subjects.

Each subject was studied again during the first week of a subsequent (study) menstrual cycle. Three subjects participated in
two study cycles. In these three subjects, each treatment cycle
was separated by four or five consecutive normal menstrual cycles.
Thus, the 16 subjects participated in a total of 19 study cycles.
Subjects were assigned to six study groups based upon the concentration of E2B administered. Six concentrations were studied: 0.3
µg/kg/12 hr (n = 3), 0.6 µg/kg/12 hr (n = 4), 1.25 µg/kg/12 hr (n =
3), 2.5 µg/kg/12 hr (n = 3), 3.75 µg/kg/12 hr (n = 3) and 5.0 µg/
kg/12 hr (n = 3).

At 4 PM on the first day of the study menstrual cycle, each
subject received an i.m. injection of E_2B in sesame oil at a concentration equal to one 24 hr dose (0.6, 1.20, 2.5, 5.0, 7.5, or 10
µg/kg). At 8 AM on the second day of the menstrual cycle, and
every 12 hr thereafter, additional injections of E_2B at the appropriate concentrations were administered every 12 hr for a total of
10 additional injections. GnRH, 100 µg iv at t = 0, was administered 12 hr following the last injection of E_2B. Blood samples
were drawn just prior to each E_2B injection, and at t - 14, -12,
-10, -8, -6, -4, -2 hr and t - 30, -15, 0, +5, +10, +15, +20, +25,
+30, +45, +60, +90, +120, +180 and +240 min. Each subject's gonadotropin response to GnRH after estradiol pretreatment was compared
with her own response during the control group.

Mean LH and FSH responses during the study (estradiol pretreatment) cycles and control (no estradiol pretreatment) cycles for
each group of subjects are shown in Figs. 11 and 12. Individual
and mean FSH and LH responses are presented in Table 7.

Serum estradiol values are presented in Table 8. Baseline
values at the time of GnRH administration in the control month and
individual and group mean serum estradiol levels during E_2B

Table 7.   Effects in women of varying concentrations of estradiol
pretreatment upon LH & FSH response to GnRH

Group/Subject	Maximal increase from Baseline (Δ max) (mIU/ml)				Integrated response (mIU/4hr)			
	LH		FSH		LH		FSH	
0.3µg/kg/12 hr	Control	Treat-ment	Control	Treat-ment	Control	Treat-ment	Control	Treat-ment
1	29	32	13	15	2662	3868	1865	2364
2	21	28	5	10	241	3380	779	1133
3	44	58	6	7	5680	8143	776	937
Mean	31(±7)*	39(±9)	8 (±2)	11 (±2)	2861	5130	1140	1478
					(±1573)	(±1513)	(±362)	(±447)
0.6µg/kg/12 hr								
4	17	20	4	9	1058	3458	353	669
5	16	56	6	16	1402	7058	1119	2319
6	61	50	10	15	12274	10205	702	3012
Mean	31(±15)	42(±11)	7(±2)	13(±2)	4911	6907	1076	2000
					(±3683)	(±1949)	(±203)	(±695)
1.25µg/kg/12hr								
7	54	38	9	12	7110	5873	984	1731
8	25	12	7	5	2174	1369	653	980
9	34	52	6	10	2961	9859	391	1452
10	74	184	8	36	7020	21967	1413	5892
Mean	47(±11)	72(±39)	8(±0.5)	16(±7)	3216	9767	860	2514
					(±1350)	(±4421)	(±221)	(±113)
2.5µg/kg/12hr								
5	16	151	6	34	1418	23884	1124	5173
9	34	89	6	14	2961	15122	391	1851
11	20	147	4	32	2050	22062	637	5562
Mean	23(±5)	129(±20)	5(±0.6)	27(±6)	2143	20356	717	4195
					(±448)	(±2669)	(±215)	(±1117)
3.75µg/kg/12hr								
12	27	138	3	18	1692	20907	157	8307
13	28	231	5	26	2045	31780	182	4610
14	35	374	5	40	3098	61012	575	7324
Mean	30(±2)	278(±16)	4(±0.6)	28(±6)	2278	37900	305	6747
					(±422)	(±20741)	(±135)	(±1106)
5.0µg/kg/12hr								
15	32	103	5	19	2973	17709	764	3310
14	35	331	7	30	3115	56979	484	5250
16	25	183	5	30	2174	34031	593	4916
Mean	30(±3)	206(±67)	5(±0.6)	26(±3)	2754	36240	614	4492
					(±293)	(±11390)	(±81)	(±598)

*(s.e.)

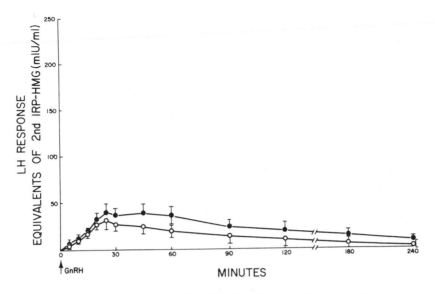

Fig. 11a.   0.3µg/kg/12 hr E$_2$B pretreatment.

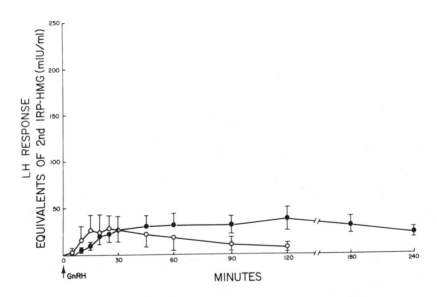

Fig. 11b.   0.6µg/kg/12 hr E$_2$B pretreatment.

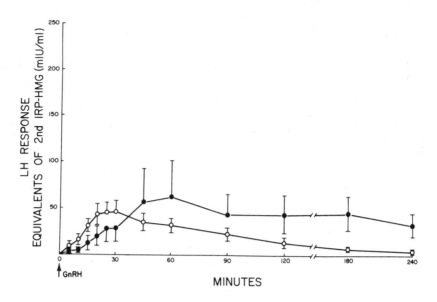

Fig. 11c.   1.25μg/kg/12 hr E$_2$B pretreatment.

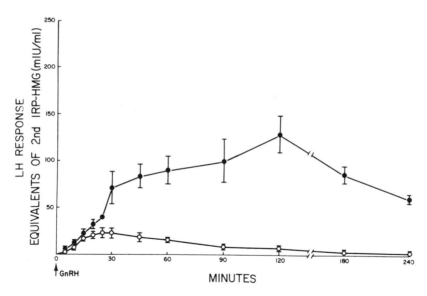

Fig. 11d.   2.5μg/kg/12 hr E$_2$B pretreatment.

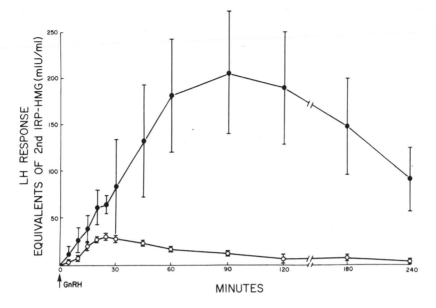

Fig. 11e. 3.75µg/kg/12 hr E$_2$B pretreatment.

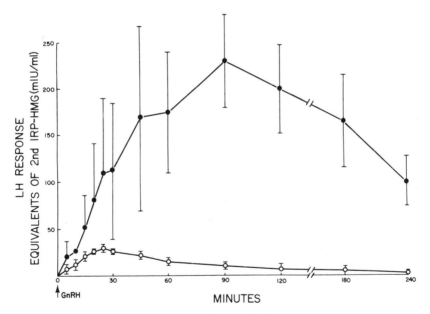

Fig. 11f. 5.0µg/kg/12 hr E$_2$B pretreatment.

Fig. 11.   Mean LH responses to Gonadotropin Releasing Hormone (GnRH) during control (no estradiol pretreatment) menstrual cycles (-o-) and during menstrual cycles in which pretreatment with varying doses of estradiol benzoate (E_2B) had been administered on menstrual cycle days 1-6 (-·-). Vertical bars represent SEM.   From: Young, J.R. and Jaffe, R.B.   J. Clin. Endocrinol. Metab.   Submitted for publication.

Table 8.   Serum estradiol concentrations in control and estradiol benzoate-treated cycles in normal women (pg/ml)

Group/Subject	t = 0 Control Cycle	t-132 to t-14* E_2B Treatment Cycle	t-12 to t-0**
0.3 µg/kg/12 hr			
1	37	50 (±4)	57 (±2)
2	40	45 (±1)	92 (±8)
3	17	34 (±4)	77 (±22)
Mean	31 (±7)***	43 (±5)	75 (±10)
0.6 µg/kg/12 hr			
4	26	55 (±4)	50 (±3)
5	25	64 (±6)	56 (±6)
6	22	40 (±2)	42 (±4)
Mean	24 (±1)	53 (±7)	50 (±4)
1.25 µg/kg/12 hr			
7	101	111 (±7)	85 (±7)
8	70	87 (±5)	108 (±9)
9	40	76 (±3)	77 (±4)
10	33	90 (±4)	85 (±3)
Mean	61 (±16)	91 (±8)	89 (±7)
2.5 µg/kg/12hr			
5	25	106 (±7)	100 (±3)
9	40	212 (±9)	188 (±12)
11	41	117 (±18)	137 (±15)
Mean	35 (±5)	145 (±33)	141 (±25)
3.75 µg/kg/12 hr			
12	28	174 (±21)	172 (±10)
13	35	235 (±20)	264 (±22)
14	56	176 (±15)	207 (±20)
Mean	40 (±8)	195 (±20)	214 (±27)
5.0 µg/kg/12 hr			
14	56	284 (±42)	306 (±27)
15	129	323 (±15)	216 (±15)
16	60	308 (±28)	449 (±26)
Mean	82 (±24)	305 (±12)	351 (±70)

*Samples drawn every 12 hr (n=12); **Samples drawn every 2 hr (n=6); ***(S.E.)   See text for details.

administration in the treatment month are given. The values are separated into mean serum estradiol during estradiol pretreatment as reflected in the samples obtained every 12 hr (120 to 14 hr prior to GnRH), and mean serum estradiol concentrations as reflected in the samples collected every 2 hr overnight prior to GnRH administration (12 to 0 hr prior to GnRH). Serum estradiol concentrations in the control month were similar to those previously reported for the early follicular phase, except for subjects 7 and 8, who had mean serum estradiol levels of 101 and 70 pg/ml respectively. However, repeat early follicular phase serum estradiol levels in other months in these two subjects demonstrated that this was a consistent phenomenon, and therefore normal for them. Control LH and FSH responses to GnRH demonstrated the marked individual variation seen in all of our previous studies.

Pretreatment of subjects with E$_2$B, 0.3 μg/kg/12 hr, resulted in a slightly augmented LH and FSH response over the control month in all three subjects, as reflected in Δmax and integrated responses (Table 7). However, the pattern of response, as seen in Figs. 11 and 12, and statistical evaluation revealed no significant changes. The apparent slightly augmented response in the group probably reflects the slightly increased serum estradiol level prior to GnRH administration in the treatment month compared to the control month (43 vs. 31 pg/ml).

At a concentration of 0.6 μg/kg/12 hr, mean Δmax FSH and integrated LH and FSH responses were slightly, but insignificantly, increased in two subjects. One subject had a slightly blunted response in all parameters except integrated FSH response. Serum estradiol concentration during E$_2$B administration (53 pg/ml) was slightly higher than that seen in the 0.3 μg/kg/12 hr group (43 pg/ml) and considerably higher than the control cycle mean value of 23 pg/ml. As seen in Figs. 11 and 12, there was a slight delay in achievement of peak FSH and LH responses and a tendency to maintain higher FSH and LH levels at 3 and 4 hr after GnRH. The latter phenomenon was presumably responsible for the increased integrated responses seen in two subjects.

Definite augmentation (increased mean Δmax LH and Δmax FSH, increased integrated response) was seen upon administration of E$_2$B 1.25 μg/kg/12 hr (Fig. 11, Table 7). However, individual responses to this dose showed marked variation. Subjects 7 and 8 had slightly diminished release of LH compared with control cycles and only a minimal increase in integrated FSH response. In contrast, subjects 8 and 10 demonstrated marked augmentation of both LH and FSH release Table 7) reflected in the group mean pattern of release seen in Fig. 11. The discrepancy in responses seen in the E$_2$B pretreatment month may be explained by the serum estradiol concentrations achieved during that month compared with the control month (Table 8). As

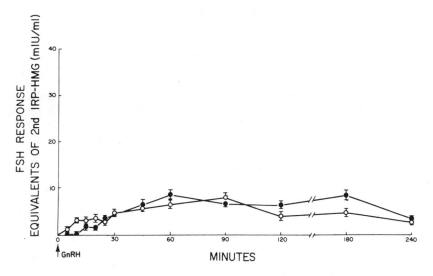

Fig. 12a.   Pretreatment with 0.3 μg/kg/12 hr E₂B.
(See p.245 for explanation of Fig. 12.)

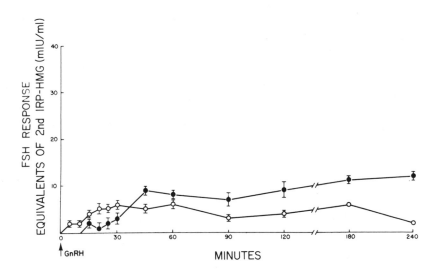

Fig. 12b.   Pretreatment with 0.6 μg/kg/12hr E₂B.

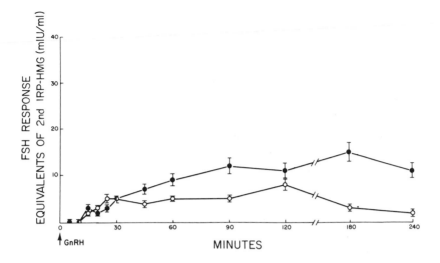

Fig. 12c.   Pretreatment with 1.25 μg/kg/12 hr E$_2$B.

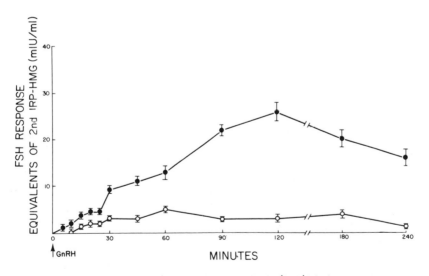

Fig. 12d.   Pretreatment 2.5 μg/kg/12 hr E$_2$B.

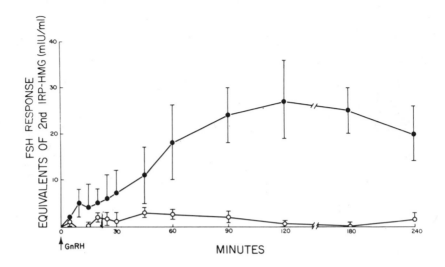

Fig. 12e.   Pretreatment with 3.75 µg/kg/12 hr E₂B.

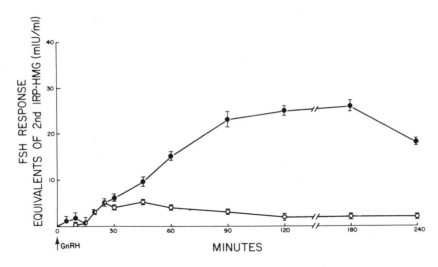

Fig. 12f.   Pretreatment with 5.0 µg/kg/12 hr E₂B.

Fig. 12. Mean FSH responses to Gonadotropin Releasing Hormone (GnRH) during control (no estradiol pretreatment) menstrual cycles (−o−) and during menstrual cycles in which pretreatment with varying doses of estradiol benzoate (E$_2$B) had been administered on menstrual cycle days 1-6 (−•−). Vertical bars represent SEM. From: Young, J.R. and Jaffe, R.B. J. Clin. Endocrinol. Metab. Submitted for publication.

previously noted, subjects 7 and 8 normally had high follicular phase estradiol concentrations (101 and 70 pg/ml), and administration of 1.25 µg/kg/12 hr E$_2$B failed to elevate serum estradiol concentrations significantly (87 and 111 pg/ml). On the other hand, subjects 9 and 10 had significant increments in serum estradiol concentrations in the treatment month compared to their control cycles.

Administration of 2.5 µg/kg/12hr E$_2$B resulted in marked augmentation in LH and FSH response to GnRH as reflected in all parameters. Augmentation was seen in all three subjects, and absolute values and pattern of release were remarkably similar to those seen in our previous studies, in which a total of 9 subjects received identical E$_2$B pretreatment (2.5 µg/kg/12 hr for 6 days).

As seen in Figs. 11 and 12 and Table 7, LH responses to GnRH after E$_2$B, 3.75 µg/kg/12 hr and 5.0 µg/kg/12 hr were further augmented over those seen with 2.5 µg/kg/12 hr, but the two groups, allowing for individual variation, were very similar in their control and treatment cycle response.

In the groups receiving 3.75 and 5.0 µg/kg/12 hr, FSH responses, in contrast to LH responses, were not appreciably augmented over those seen in subjects receiving 2.5 µg/kg/12 hr.

As was demonstrated in our previous studies, in those groups in which augmentation of LH and FSH response to GnRH was seen after E$_2$B pretreatment, there was a delay in achieving peak LH and FSH levels when compared to control cycles. In control cycles, the peak LH rise occurred 20-30 min after GnRH, whereas augmented LH peaks during the study cycles occurred at 60-90 min. The peak FSH rise in control cycles was reached at 15-60 min, and in treatment cycles was not reached until 120-180 min.

Serum LH levels during E$_2$B administration in the groups receiving 0.3 and 0.6 µg/kg/12 hr remained essentially unchanged except for normal periodicity evident in the samples obtained every 2 hr prior to GnRH administration. At other concentrations of E$_2$B, a variable LH response was seen. Within the group receiving 1.25µg/kg/12 hr, subjects 7 and 8, both of whom showed no augmentation of gonadotropin response to GnRH, had LH concentrations which remained

at pretreatment values. However, serum LH concentrations in subjects 8 and 10 were depressed to an average of 43% and 26% of pretreatment concentrations respectively. At 2.5 µg/kg/12 hr E_2B,
only in one subject, subject 9, was the LH depressed. Her mean
concentration fell to 51% of the pretreatment value. In the 3.75
µg/kg/12hr group, subject 12 maintained her LH level at a mean of
37% of pretreatment concentration and subject 13 at a mean of 85%
of pretreatment concentration. On the other hand, subject 14, after 84 hr of E_2B at 3.75 µg/kg/12 hr, manifested several LH surges
as high as 33 mIU/ml (Fig. 13). Although for the last 6 hr prior
to GnRH the serum LH concentration was 14 mIU/ml, at the time of
GnRH administration (t = 0) LH had once again risen to 52 mIU/ml
(not shown).

Fig. 13 also illustrates LH concentrations in the three subjects who received 5 µg/kg/12 hr E_2B and who subsequently received
infusions of GnRH (subjects 14, 15 and 16). All three subjects
demonstrated E_2B-induced LH surges. Subject 14 had a biphasic LH
surge, starting after 50 hr E_2B administration and lasting 66 hr,
with return to normal LH concentration prior to GnRH. Subject 15
also showed a biphasic LH peak starting after 50 hr E_2B administration and lasting approximately 60 hr. A smaller LH peak was seen
at t-12 hr. Subject 16 developed a single peak of LH after 96 hr
of E_2B. This peak only lasted 24 hr, and her circulating LH concentration returned to baseline by t = 0. Peak levels of LH (subject 14 = 45 mIU/ml, 15 = 38 mIU/ml, 16 = 34 mIU/ml) were slightly
lower than normal pre-ovulatory LH levels. The duration of LH elevations, however, was similar to the duration of the normal pre-
ovulatory LH peak.

To test the reproducibility of estrogen-induced LH discharge
during estradiol administration, three additional subjects were
given 5.0 µg/kg/12 hr E_2B according to the same protocol. No GnRH
was administered. Only one of the three developed an estrogen-induced LH discharge. Her response is also shown in Fig. 13 (subject
17). After 60 hr of E_2B at a concentration of 5.0 µg/kg/12 hr,
this subject had a large biphasic LH surge up to 82 mIU/ml from a
baseline of 6 mIU/ml. Because of the presence of three LH elevations of lesser magnitude, the duration of the peak is difficult
to judge, but appears to be approximately 36 hr. The large LH
surge is particularly reminiscent of a normal pre-ovulatory LH
discharge.

Mean serum FSH concentrations during administration of 0.3,
0.6 and 1.25 µg/kg/12 hr E_2B remained essentially unchanged. The
three subjects who received 2.5 µg/kg/12 hr E_2B showed FSH suppression to 74%, 58% and 71% of pretreatment values. Similarly, FSH
suppression to 50%, 64% and 75% of pretreatment values was seen in
the three subjects who received E_2B, 3.75 µg/kg/12 hr. In the

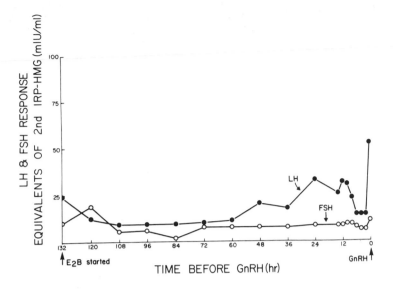

Fig. 13a.   Administration of 3.75 µg/kg/12 hr E$_2$B
(See p.249 for explanation of Fig. 13.)

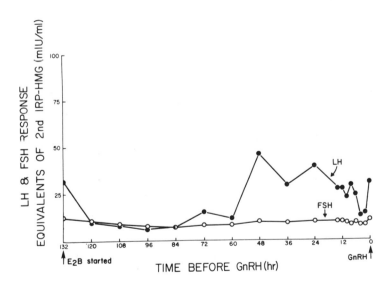

Fig. 13b.   Administration of 5.0 µg/kg/12 hr E$_2$B.

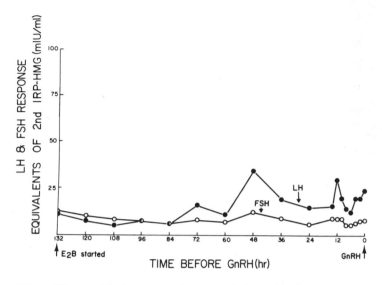

Fig. 13c.   Administration of 5.0 µg/kg/12 hr E₂B

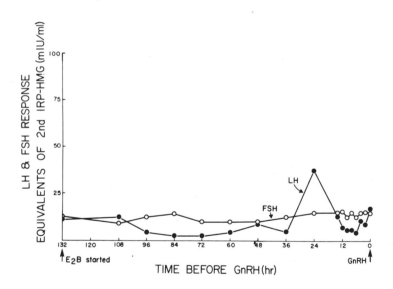

Fig. 13d.   Administration of 5.0 µg/kg/12 hr E₂B

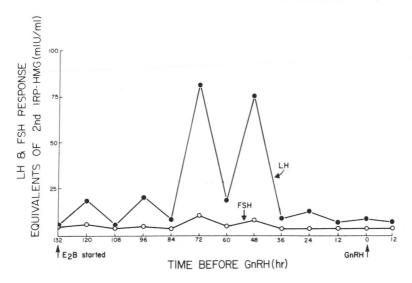

Fig. 13e.   Administration of 5.0 µg/kg/12 hr E₂B.

Fig. 13.   Circulating LH (-•-) and FSH (-o-) concentrations in
women to whom estradiol benzoate (E₂B) had been administered on
days 1-6 of the menstrual cycle prior to the administration of an
intravenous bolus of gonadotropin releasing hormone (GnRH).   Note
occurence of LH surges during E₂B administration.   From: Young,
J.R. and Jaffe, R.B.   J. Clin. Endocrinol. Metab.   Submitted for
publication.

5.0 µg/kg/12 hr E₂B group, FSH levels during E₂B were suppressed
68%, 66% and 100% of pretreatment values.

     The temporal relationships between circulating serum estradiol
and gonadotropin concentrations in the pre-ovulatory phase of the
menstrual cycle in women with normal menstrual cycles suggest that
four to six days of exposure of the hypothalamic-pituitary axis to
increasing concentrations of estradiol is necessary for initiation
of the midcycle gonadotropin surge.   These studies also demonstrate
that, in the majority of women studied, the surge of gonadotropins
begins prior to any significant decline in serum estradiol.

     In the previous studies, we demonstrated that, in normal
women in the early follicular phase, less than 60 hr exposure to
late follicular phase levels of estradiol depressed pituitary
gonadotropin responsiveness to GnRH.   In contrast, gonadotropin
responses were markedly augmented when the duration of E₂B

administration exceeded 60 hr.

The present study demonstrates that not only is pituitary responsiveness to GnRH dependent upon duration of estradiol exposure, but is also proportional to the circulating concentration of estradiol. Maintenance of circulating estradiol levels of 40-60 pg/ml for 132 hr, as achieved in the groups receiving 0.3 and 0.6 µg/kg/12 hr E_2B, did not result in any significant augmentation of gonadotropin responses to GnRH. However, when serum estradiol was maintained above 90 pg/ml for the same period, as in the group receiving 1.25 µg/kg/12 hr, significantly increased gonadotropin responses to GnRH were seen in those subjects in whom the serum estradiol level represented a major elevation over that seen in their respective control cycles. As serum estradiol levels were further elevated by progressively increasing the concentration of estradiol administered, further augmentation of LH and FSH responses were seen. A leveling trend was noted after serum estradiol concentrations of over 200 pg/ml were achieved, as seen in the groups receiving 3.75 and 5.0 µg/kg/12 hr.

Estradiol-induced LH surges seen in five instances during administration of 3.75 and 5.0 µg/kg/12 hr E_2B furnished an opportunity to study further the positive feedback effect of estradiol on the hypothalamic-pituitary system. The serum estradiol concentrations necessary to achieve this positive feedback, in general over 200 pg/ml for at least 50 hr, were similar to those described by Reiter et al (25). The strength and duration of these surges was not dissimilar to normal pre-ovulatory LH surges. These observations do not define whether positive feedback occurs primarily at the hypothalamus, pituitary or both. However, if endogenous GnRH levels were increased by estradiol administration, a rise in serum FSH and LH levels might have been expected at lower serum estradiol concentrations, even if obvious surges were not apparent. On the contrary, when serum gonadotropin levels did change during E_2B pretreatment, in the absence of discrete surges, they were always depressed.

The work of Karsch and associates in rhesus monkeys has elegantly demonstrated the strength-duration characteristics of estradiol initiation of gonadotropin surges in that animal (16). Serum estradiol concentrations below 100 pg/ml were ineffective in eliciting LH surges, even when present for 120 hr. Serum estradiol levels of 200 pg/ml elicited LH surges after approximately 42 hr and estradiol levels of 200-400 pg/ml, after only 36 hr. Supraphysiologic levels of 1200-2000 pg/ml were effective after only 24 hr. No LH surges were seen after removal of the silastic estradiol implants used to administer the estradiol.

Legan and coworkers (26,27) in studies utilizing silastic implants of estradiol 17-β in rats, have demonstrated a 5 PM daily LH surge than can be induced for up to 10 consecutive days.

The characteristics of positive estradiol feedback in our studies warrant comparison with the characteristics of hypothalamic-pituitary-ovarian relationships reported in normal women by Korenman and Sherman (18). These investigators noted that serum estradiol levels generally were increasing for 72 hr prior to any LH rise. The LH peak usually occurred after 120 hr of increasing serum estradiol concentrations. The spontaneous estradiol-induced LH surges that we observed in our subjects follow this pattern quite closely. Korenman and Sherman calculated that the endogenous estradiol secretion rate averaged 154 μg/day in women with normal cycles prior to any noticeable LH rise. The concentration of E_2B at which we achieved consistent augmentation of gonadotropin response was 2.5 μg/kg/ 12 hr, or 137.5 μg/day in a 55 kg woman. Furthermore, their studies revealed a calculated mean daily estradiol secretion of 450 μg on the day of the LH peak. In our present study, maximal augmentation of gonadotropin response to GnRH was seen at E_2B concentrations of 3.75 - 5.0 μg/kg/12 hr, or 412.5-500 μg/day in a 55 kg woman. Whereas a stepwise increment of E_2B administration in our subjects would have more closely approximated the normal estrogen milieu during the last follicular phase, we feel that the changes in pituitary sensitivity to GnRH within the physiologic range of serum estradiol concentrations have been demonstrated adequately. Stepwise increments of E_2B administration may also have eliminated some of the individual variation observed. In addition, E_2B induced FSH surges might have occurred if a stepwise dosage regime such as that employed by Reiter et al had been employed (25).

In the present study, we have demonstrated that if serum estradiol levels are maintained for 132 hr at various concentrations normally found at different stages of the last follicular phase, a dose-dependent, incremental augmentation of gonadotropin release in response to GnRH is observed.

Furthermore, estradiol-induced LH surges were seen during E_2B administration at a time when serum estradiol concentrations approached normal pre-ovulatory levels. Since gonadotropin concentrations did not rise prior to these LH surges, it is likely that no major increase in endogenous GnRH was occurring, and suggests a direct effect of estradiol upon the pituitary gland.

The magnitude of gonadotropin response to GnRH after E_2B priming, accompanied in many cases by suppression of FSH and LH levels during E_2B administration, suggests marked increase in pituitary stores and/or synthesis combined with decreased release of gonadotropins. The agumentation of gonadotropin release in response to

GhRH after E_2B pretreatment was chiefly in the form of delayed and greatly exaggerated responses when compared with control responses. This suggests that newly synthesized, as well as stored, gonadotropin is utilized in the estrogen-augmented response. In addition, estrogen may induce an increase in the GnRH receptor population in the pituitary, or bring about a change in those receptors already in existence. It is possible that membrane permeability may be altered so that the gonadotrophs are capable of releasing more gonadotropin in response to the samemagnitude GnRH stimulus. However, ginal resolution of the question of whether positive estradiol feedback occurs at the hypothalamic as well as pituitary level still awaits advances in GnRH assay techniques and further animal and human studies.

ACKNOWLEDGMENTS

    Supported, in part, by NIH Grant 08035 and a grant from the Rockefeller Foundation. Some studies were performed in the Clinical Research Unit supported by a grant from the General Clinical Research Centers Program of the Division of Research Ressources, NIH (RR-79).

    Gonadotropin determinations were performed utilizing radio-immunoassay materials furnished by the National Pituitary Agency, National Institute of Arthritis, Metabolism and Digestive Diseases.

REFERENCES

1.   Abraham, G.E., W.D. Odell, R.S. Swerdloff and K. Hopper (1972) J. Clin. Endocrinol. Metab. 34, 312.

2.   Tsai, C.C. and S.S.C. Yen (1971) J. Clin. Endocrinol. Metab. 32, 766.

3.   Yen, S.S.C. and C.C. Tsai (1972) J. Clin. Endocrinol. Metab. 34, 298.

4.   Monroe, S.E., R.B. Jaffe and A.R. Midgley, Jr. (1972) J. Clin. Endocrinol. Metab. 34, 342.

5.   Karsch, F.J., D.J. Dierschke, R.F. Weick, T. Yamaji, J. Hotchkiss and E. Knobil (1973) Endocrinology 92, 799.

6.   Yen, S.S.C., G. VanderBerg, R. Rebar and Y. Ehara (1972) J. Clin. Endocrinol. Metab. 35, 931.

7. Keye, W.R., Jr. and Jaffe, R.B. (1974) J. Clin. Endocrinol.
    Metab. 38, 805.

8. Keye, W.R., Jr., R.P. Kelch, G.D. Niswender and R.B. Jaffe
    (1973) J. Clin. Endocrinol. Metab. 36, 1263.

9. Hollander, M. and D.A. Wolfe (1973) Non-Parametric Statistical
    Methods, John Wiley and Sons, New York, p. 115.

10. Midgley, A.R., Jr. and R.B. Jaffe (1968) J. Clin. Endocrinol.
    Metab. 28, 1699.

11. Thomas, K., J. Donnez and J. Ferin (1972) Contraception 6, 55.

12. Johansson, K.N.G., B.L. Currie, K. Folkers and C.Y. Bowers
    (1973) Biochem. Biophys. Res. Commun. 50, 8.

13. Currie, B.L., K.N.G. Johansson, K. Folkers and C.Y. Bowers
    (1973) Biochem. Biophys. Res. Commun. 50, 14.

14. Bowers, C.Y., B.L. Currie, K.N.G. Johansson and K. Folkers
    (1973) Biochem. Biophys. Res. Commun. 50, 20.

15. Weick, R.F., F.J. Karsch, W.R. Butler, D.J. Dierschke, L.C.
    Krey, G. Weiss, J. Hotchkiss and E. Knobil (1972) Physiolo-
    gist 15, 300.

16. Karsch, F.J., R.F. Weick, W.R. Butler, D.J. Dierschke, L.C.
    Krey, G. Weiss, J. Hotchkiss, T. Yamaji and E. Knobil (1973)
    Endocrinology 92, 1740.

17. Keye, W.R., Jr. and R.B. Jaffe (1974) J. Clin. Endocrinol. Me-
    tab. 38, 805.

18. Korenman, S.G. and B.M. Sherman (1973) J. Clin. Endocrinol.
    Metab. 36, 1205.

19. Kohler, P.O., G.T. Ross and W.D. Odell (1968) J. Clin. Invest.
    47, 38.

20. Siler, T.M. and S.S.C. Yen (1973) J. Clin. Endocrinol. Metab.
    37, 491.

21. Monroe, S.E., R.B. Jaffe and A.R. Midgley, Jr. (1972) J. Clin.
    Endocrinol. Metab. 34, 342.

22. Libertun, C., K.J. Cooper, C.P. Fawcett and S.M. McCann (1974)
    Endocrinology 94, 518.

23.   Yen, S.S.C., G. Vandenberg and T.M. Siler (1974) J. Clin. En-
      docrinol. Metab. $\underline{39}$, 170.

24.   Taymor, M.L. (1974) Fertil. Steril. $\underline{25}$, 992.

25.   Reiter, E.O., H.E. Kulin and S.M. Hamwood (1974) Pediat. Res.
      $\underline{8}$, 740.

26.   Legan, S.J., G.A. Coon and F.J. Karsch (1975) Endocrinology
      $\underline{96}$, 57.

27.   Legan, S.J. and F.J. Karsch (1975) Endocrinology $\underline{96}$, 57.

Control of PRL and GH Secretion and Action

CONTROL OF PROLACTIN SECRETION IN MAN

H.G. Bohnet and H.G. Friesen

University of Manitoba

Winnipeg, Manitoba, R3E 0W3

METHODS OF MEASUREMENT OF hPRL

Several techniques for the detection and measurement of lactogenic activity are currently available. The specificity and the sensitivity of these assays, however, varies widely and therefore the choice of assay to be utilized--bioassay, radioimmunoassay and radioreceptor assay--is determined by the primary purpose.

The pigeon crop sac assay first was described by Riddle et al. (1933) and it became the classical assay for prolactin (PRL). Although its sensitivity was improved by several modifications this assay was not useful for estimating normal serum values since its working range is from 200 ng to 10,000 ng PRL. This bioassay, however, may still have a role in determining the potency of prolactin in pituitary extracts and standard preparations of hPRL. Two other human hormones, growth hormone (hGH) and human placental lactogen (hPL) exhibit lactogenic activity as well. They have approximately 10% the activity of prolactin standards (Forsyth and Edwards 1972, Forsyth and Parke 1973).

The in vitro bioassays using mammary tissue explants from either midpregnant mice or pseudopregnant rabbits are able to estimate lactogenic activity from 2 - 100 ng/ml plasma. These in vitro assays represented an improvement in sensitivity over the previous available pigeon crop sac assay, but hGH and hPL also exhibit some lactogenic effects, hence specificity remains a problem. Moreover, the work and expense involved is much greater than with radioimmunoassays (Forsyth and Edwards 1972, Forsyth and Parke 1973, L'Hermite 1973).

With the development of radioimmunoassays for hPRL there was an explosion of knowledge of the physiology and pathology of hPRL secretion. The first assay systems were heterologous ones utilising the cross-reaction of PRL derived from several species, in particular, primate PRLs with antiserum to ovine PRL (Guyda et al. 1971, Midgley and Jaffe 1972). Soon homologous systems were developed using primate prolactin. The development of homologous radioimmunoassays for hPRL, a highly sensitive and specific tool to measure immunoreactive hPRL in serum, greatly facilitated clinical studies (Hwang et al. 1971b, Sinha et al. 1973). Although all radioimmunoassays, heterologous as well as homologous ones, give comparable results in terms of pathophysiological findings, the absolute values and relative variations differ, suggesting that these assays do not detect the same immunoreactive component of the PRL molecule (L'Hermite 1973). Therefore, to compare results obtained by different methods and investigators, the standardized homologous systems are preferred. (Table I)

A further useful advance in studies of lactogenic hormones was the development of the radioreceptor assay (Shiu et al. 1973). It is able to detect biologically active fragments of lactogenic hormones and is nearly as sensitive as the radioimmunoassay, especially when solubilized and purified receptor from rabbit mammary gland membranes are employed. This assay is not species specific and therefore is able to detect lactogenic hormones, not only PRL, from various species. By taking advantage of this tool we were able to identify and measure various placental lactogens, i.e. mouse, rat, guinea pig, and sheep, and were also able to isolate and identify ovine placental lactogen (Chan et al. 1975) and caprine placental lactogen (Currie, to be published; personal communication, 1975). In addition, the concentrations of PRL in this system can be determined within 6 hours and they are in good agreement with those obtained by RIA and mouse mammary gland assay (Friesen et al. 1973).

HETEROGENEITY OF hPRL

Native hPRL from the pituitary gland (Hwang et al. 1973, Lewis et al. 1973) and from amniotic fluid (Ben-David and Chrambach 1974, Rogol and Chrambach 1975) is like other polypeptide hormones such as insulin (Roth et al. 1968), parathyroid hormone (Berson and Yalow 1968), gastrin (Yalow and Berson 1970), ACTH (Yalow and Berson 1971) and growth hormone (Bala et al. 1970), heterogeneous. Rogol and Rosen (1974), as well as Suh and Frantz (1974), described two components of circulating hPRL separated by gel filtration on Sephadex G 100: "little" 80-90% and "big" less than 20% in normal subjects. An additional polymer "big-big" was described by Aubert et al. (1975a) which constituted from 0.8 to 7.9% of the

TABLE I

NORMAL SERUM CONCENTRATIONS OF hPRL MEASURED BY VARIOUS RADIOIMMUNOASSAYS

Authors	System	Mean		Range	
		Male	Female	Male	Female
Friesen et al. 72	Homologous (H-H-H)	7	11	3-25	3-25
McNeilly et al. 73, 74	Homologous (H-H-H)	11	15	8-30	8-30
Sinha et al. 73	Homologous (H-H-H)	13	14	6-24	7-18
Ehara et al. 73	Homologous (H-H-H)	13	18		
Jacobs et al. 72	Heterologous (O-O-H)	6	9		
Aubert et al. 74	Heterologous (O-H-H)	5	9	1-12	4-21

total hPRL. During pregnancy, highest amounts of "big" hPRL
(16-31%) were found (Suh and Frantz 1974). Neither TRH or breast
stimulation, nor L-dopa suppression affect the distribution pattern
of the polymers of hPRL (Suh and Frantz 1974). In one study under
basal conditions the predominant form of serum hPRL was "big",
whereas after TRH the principal form was "little" hPRL, suggesting
that the nature of the secreted form varied under different
physiological circumstances (Kataoka et al. 1975).

    Freezing and thawing or urea treatment are able to convert
some but not all "big" hPRL to "little" hPRL. On the other hand,
in a comparable situation, treatment of "big" hGH with mercapto-
ethanol, an agent which dissociates noncovalent and disulfide
bonds, resulted in a 60% conversion of "big" to little hGH
(Benveniste et al. 1975). Sera from some patients with a
pituitary adenoma also display a shift to "big" and "big-big"
prolactin (Rogol and Rosen 1974, Suh and Frantz 1974, Aubert
et al. 1975a). Immediate rechromatography does not change the
previously maintained elution pattern. A comparison of RIA values
with RRA estimates, revealed that "big-big" hPRL has no activity
in the RRA (Aubert et al. 1975a)and big hPRL has about 25% less
activity in the RRA. Other investigators have not confirmed this
observation (Guyda and Whyte 1974).

    These findings suggest that the polymeric molecules of hPRL
seem to be precursor or storage forms in the pituitary and are
secreted only in low amounts in normal subjects. In states with
a high secretion rate of hPRL (pregnancy, tumours), however, a
large proportion of "big" forms are found in the circulation.
Furthermore, the lowered biological activity as judged by RRA
activity, could explain the occurrence of hyperprolactinemia
without or with little galactorrhea (vide infra) in those patients
that have a large proportion of "big-big" serum hPRL."

PHYSIOLOGICAL hPRL SECRETION

    Basal hPRL levels show random fluctuations which are referred
to as "oscillations" episodic or pulsatile secretion and therefore normal values range widely. These "bursts" are variable in
height and shape in each individual and the definition of what
constitutes an "episodic" secretion is defined somewhat arbitrarily.
It was suggested that an increase is one with an increment of
$\geq$ 4 ng/ml and either a peak of $\geq$ 14 ng/ml or as a $\geq$ 50% increase
above the value of the preceding nadir (Parker et al. 1973).

    Within 90 min. after the onset of sleep plasma hPRL concen-
trations increase episodically (Sassin et al. 1973) and sleep
peaks exceed wake peaks (Parker et al 1973) by approximately

50% (5-10 ng/ml vs 35 ng/ml deviation of the mean values) (Osterman and Wide 1975) and occur about four times more often during
sleep than during daytime (Parker et al. 1973). Such night time
elevations have been noted by Nokin et al. (1972), and are dependent on the occurrence of sleep and are not based on an inherent
rhythm (Sassin et al. 1973). Early awakening can foreshorten
this nocturnal hPRL increase (Parker et al. 1973), whereas with
extended darkness such as occurs with seasonal variation in
northern latitudes there is no apparent alteration in the waking
related decrease of hPRL levels (Osterman and Wide 1975).

Daytime naps result in clear peaks exceeding significantly
equivalent clocktime wake values and are comparable to nocturnal
ones in height (Parker et al.1973, Sassin et al. 1973). Thus,
in the human there is no nyctohemeral rhythm of PRL as in animals
(Dunn et al. 1972, Kizer et al. 1975).

A consistent hPRL release at about 1 p.m. and 6 p.m. was
observed by Sassin et al.(1973) who speculate that a possible
relationship to meals may exist. This hypothesis has not been
proven in man but apparently in rats feeding stimulates PRL secretion (Bellinger et al. 1975). However, fasting for 36 hours
accompanied by alteration of several metabolic fuels, e.g. decrease
of mean glucose and serum insulin concentrations, lowered basal
hPRL levels from about 10 ng/ml to 5 ng/ml and also significantly
decreased maximal hPRL concentrations after 100 ug TRH intravenously
(86 vs 32 ng/ml; net increase 77 vs 28 ng/ml) (Vinik et al. 1975).
Moreover, following 100 g glucose orally, patients with hPRL secreting tumors showed an increased insulin response (sum insulin
release 465 uU/ml vs 227 uU/ml) and higher serum blood glucose
concentrations (sum blood glucose 544 mg% vs 450 mg%). These
abnormalities were improved by suppression of hPRL with CB-154
(Landgraf et al. 1975).

Osmoregulatory function of PRL was first established in
amphibians. Later Horrobin et al.(1971) showed that ovine PRL
at a dose of 8 mg i.m. reduces water and sodium excretion, and
increases plasma osmolality. Water loading and infusions of
hypo- and hyperosmolar saline solutions revealed changes in hPRL
concentrations; the increases and decreases of hPRL, however,
were 5-10 ng/ml different from the starting levels (Buckman and
Peake 1973). Other carefully controlled studies using acute
water loading did not result in a consistent suppression of hPRL
and no correlation between serum hPRL and osmolality was obtained
(Archer and Josimovich 1975, Adler et al. 1975).

Psychic as well as physical stress leads to an increase in
serum hPRL concentrations; the magnitude of the increase being
considerably higher in females than in males (Hwang et al. 1971a,

Noel et al. 1972, Noel et al. 1974). The role of stress in the
genesis of menstrual disturbances and galactorrhea has been described (Foss and Short 1951, Fries and Nillius 1973). Recently
chronic psychologic disturbance (anxiety) has been suggested to
be an important factor in patients with post pill amenorrhea
galactorrhea, but more adequate controls of depression by psychological testing are required (Tyson et al. 1975). Emaciated
patients, however, suffering from anorexia nervosa were shown to
have normal hPRL levels (Beumont et al. 1974c).

Sexual intercourse even without orgasm is followed by a
marked rise in serum hPRL concentrations in only a minority of
women (Noel et al. 1972, Stearns et al. 1973). Some of these
women failed to respond to breast stimulation alone. Thus, these
two stimuli are not necessarily related (Noel et al. 1974). In
males serum hPRL levels remained unchanged during coitus and
ejaculation (Noel et al. 1974, Stearns et al. 1973). Nipple
stimulation in non-lactating females induces a rise in hPRL plasma
concentrations (Kolodny et al. 1972). On the other hand, there
are reports where serum hPRL failed to increase after mammary
stimulation in normal women as well as in men (Archer and
Josimovich 1975, Noel et al. 1974). More often, however, a
response to automanipulation was observed in women with hyper-
trophy of the breast with galactorrhea (Archer and Josimovich
1975). Whether such a response in those patients represents
a hyperresponsiveness remains unclear.

Basal hPRL levels are slightly higher in females than in
males. The irregular bursts of hPRL secretion are also somewhat greater in height in women compared to those in men. During
puberty hPRL concentrations show a wide degree of variability
which is more apparent in girls than in boys. In the latter
there is no significant change with advancing age and hPRL levels
are comparable to adult men. In girls until the age of 13 serum
hPRL concentrations are comparable to those found in boys (Daughaday et al. 1971), but rise between 14 and 15 years to reach normal
adult female levels (from 13 ng/ml to 18 ng/ml). This rise in
hPRL is paralleled by an increase in pubertal estrogens (Ehara
et al. 1975). Whether hPRL plays a role in the onset of puberty
in the human needs further investigation. Recently, however, a
model for the occurrence of puberty in the rats was offered in
which a role for PRL was postulated (Wuttke et al. 1975). At
40 days of age rats exhibited an abrupt decrease of PRL and
puberty followed. These results were obtained in experiments in
prepubertal rats. When oPRL was injected for about one week
beginning at 30 days of age, precocious puberty occurred when
PRL injections stopped.

During the reproductive lifespan in females basal hPRL
concentrations seem to be higher than after the menopause. Indeed,

Robyn and Vekemans (1975) found a progressive decline in serum
hPRL levels in females with age (from 0.234 mU/ml to 0.114 mU/ml
MRC-standard 71/222), when samples were obtained from women
between 15 and 65 years (n=86), whereas a slight increase was
found in males (n=241) (from 0.114 mU/ml to 0.169 mU/ml). These
findings, however, have not been confirmed by others (Fournier
et al. 1974). The maximal hPRL response to TRH is lower in males
than females (28 ng/ml vs 57 ng/ml). In women aged 60-79, the
peak response is lower than in those aged 40-59. In prepubertal
children, however, no sex difference is seen, suggesting that
increasing estrogens cause a greater pituitary hPRL reserve
(Jacobs et al. 1973). In psychiatric patients neuroleptic drugs
in women aged 17-45 resulted in higher serum hPRL concentrations
than in those aged 48-85 (89 ng/ml vs 46 ng/ml). On the other
hand, in male patients serum PRL levels were lower as compared
to those found in the females (aged 17-65: 35 ng/ml; aged 48-85:
10 ng/ml) (de Rivera et al. 1975).

There is still controversial evidence concerning the
existence (Robyn et al. 1973, Ehara et al. 1973) or not (Hwang
et al.1971b,Tyson and Friesen 1973, Jaffe et al. 1973, McNeilly
et al. 1973) of a midcycle elevation of hPRL. Ehara et al.(1973)
found the highest values of hPRL concentration (28 ng/ml) on the
day of the hLH surge but the values were not significantly
higher than those obtained during the follicular or luteal phase.
Furthermore, Robyn et al. (1973) found a difference in hPRL
levels between follicular and luteal phase with either higher
values or greater variation occurring in the latter phase.

Since hPRL has been shown to be present in human ovarian
follicular fluid and to influence progesterone output (McNatty et
al.1974,1975 , the problem of a luteolytic and/or luteotropic
effect of hPRL has been raised again. Neutralisation of hPRL
by an anti-hPRL antiserum in a culture of luteinized granulosa
cells decreased progesterone production significantly. Addition
of hPRL, however, to the culture medium had no effect on steroid
metabolism, if the final hPRL concentration was less than 20 ng/ml.
Increasing hPRL concentrations from 25 ng to 100 ng/ml led to a
progressive decrease in the daily progesterone production. This
inhibitory effect persisted even when hLH and/or hFSH concentrations were increased 50 fold. These experiments suggest that
high concentrations of hPRL may depress progesterone secretion
by granulosa cells, but "appropriate" normal levels are necessary
for normal progesterone secretion. In addition, it is striking
that during the late follicular phase of the cycle, hPRL concentrations were lower than at any other time of the cycle and
increased during the luteal phase (McNatty et al. 1974, 1975).

In baboons treated with TRH during the luteal phase of the cycle, serum progesterone levels were reduced. TRH administered daily during the entire cycle abolished the midcycle LH peak and thus ovulation and the luteal phase elevation of progesterone (Stevens et al. 1973). Patterns of estrone and estradiol, however, were not affected by TRH treatment in any of the baboons. Also in two women with normal menstrual cycles the administration of TRH caused increases in serum hPRL and this was accompanied by a decrease of serum progesterone compared to control cycles (Jewelewicz et al. 1974). In addition, in two of 6 normal cycling women receiving sulpiride (50 mg t.i.d.) the ovulatory LH peak was abolished and no elevation of progesterone was observed. In the remaining 4, serum hLH as well as hFSH and progesterone were significantly decreased during treatment and the luteal phase was shortened by 1 to 4 days (Delvoye et al. 1974). In another study, following discontinuation of tranquillizers, some psychiatric patients started to ovulate again (Beumont et al. 1974a,Beumont et al. 1974b).On the other hand, in Rhesus monkeys blockade of PRL by Bromocriptin severely blunted the evolution of the luteal phase serum progesterone pattern and the luteal phase increase of serum estrogen concentrations was abolished. Furthermore, treatment of lactating Rhesus monkeys with Bromocriptin caused a prompt decline in progesterone secretion as well as inducing luteal regression and abolishing lactation (Espinosa-Campos et al. 1975). However, repeated TRH injections abolished the pulsatile pattern of tonic hLH release as defined by Yen et al. (1972) in normoprolactinemic amenorrheic women (Bohnet et al. 1975a). In patients with hyperprolactinemia due to pituitary tumors a loss of episodic LH fluctuations was reported as well (Boyar et al. 1974). In conclusion, PRL seems to exert a peripheral (gonadal) effect and appears to be involved in steroid metabolism in primates as well as having a central (hypothalamic) effect.

Serum hPRL levels rise from about 8 weeks of gestation and increase continuously until term reaching mean levels of 200 ng/ml with a range from 50 to 600 ng/ml (Hwang et al. 1971b,Jacobs et al. 1971, Tyson et al. 1972, L'Hermite and Robyn 1972). This elevation of serum hPRL during pregnancy may be due to the increase in serum estrogens (Barberia et al. 1975). In rhesus monkeys, for example, serum PRL as well as estrogen concentrations remain low until the last 10 days of gestation (Josimovich et al. 1974). In addition, exogenously administered estrogens do not increase serum PRL concentrations (Butler et al. 1975).

In amniotic fluid hPRL concentrations increase until the 10th – 14th week of gestation (earliest sample studied 7th week, 8 ng/ml) (McNeilly et al., to be published; personal communication, 1975) reaching levels from 1 to 15 ug/ml and

decrease afterwards until term (Barberia et al. 1975, McNeilly
et al., to be published; personal communication, 1975). The total
amount of hPRL, however, does not decrease but remains unaltered
during gestation and the concentration falls due to the rapid
increase of amniotic fluid volume from about week 12 of pregnancy
on wards (McNeilly et al., to be published; personal communication,
1975).

   The source of amniotic fluid hPRL is still unknown. Fang
and Kim (1975) favoured a fetal origin as they found a bigger
proportion of "big" than "little" hPRL in amniotic fluid, the
first of which was shown to be stored in the pituitary and released
in smaller quantities than "little" hPRL (Rogol and Rosen 1974,
Suh and Frantz 1974). In contrast, in the Rhesus monkey PRL was
suggested to be of maternal origin. This conclusion was derived
from studies in which labelled PRL was injected into maternal
blood (Josimovich et al. 1974).

   The increase in fetal serum hPRL during gestation shows a
similar pattern as the maternal; however, the fetal increase
appears to occur later (24th week) and to reach levels as high
as 500 ng/ml. The concentration of hPRL in the umbilical vein
of babies at term ranges widely from 50 to 500 ng/ml with mean
levels about 200 ng/ml (Tyson et al. 1972b, Aubert et al. 1975b).
The hPRL concentrations obtained by Aubert et al. (1975b) of
matched samples of maternal and fetal plasma exhibited only a poor
correlation, whereas other investigators did not find any correla-
tions between fetal serum hPRL and maternal or amniotic fluid
levels, or content of fetal pituitaries or maternal serum or
amniotic fluid osmolality (McNeilly et al., to be published;
personal communication, 1975).

   During the postpartum period several hormonal as well as
psychological and physical adjustments take place. The endocrine
changes which occur in women who are breast feeding are different
from those who are not. Tyson et al. (1972a) described three types
of serum hPRL response to suckling. During the first week basal
levels were still elevated and suckling caused only a modest increase. In the following period until about 2 months postpartum,
basal hPRL levels were twice those of non pregnant women. Breast
feeding, however, caused a ten to twenty fold increase. In the
third stage basal hPRL levels were similar to those found in
non pregnant women and suckling produced a minimal increase or
none at all. Furthermore, the increase in serum hPRL after TRH
varied inversely with the basal level of serum hPRL postpartum,
suggesting that high basal levels during the first 2 weeks postpartum are associated with a smaller pituitary hPRL reserve
(Bohnet et al. 1976a). In contrast to the above findings, careful
studies of maternal plasma hPRL concentrations throughout a 24 hour

(Bunner and Vanderlaan 1975) or for a 6 hour period (Bohnet et al.
1976b) revealed that many fluctuations of serum hPRL frequently
were completely unrelated temporally to suckling.

It is well documented that ovulation is significantly delayed
in nursing mothers as compared to non lactating ones (Keettel et
al. 1961, Perez et al. 1972) and attempts have been made to
correlate changes in gonadotropin and hPRL levels. Both, during
pregnancy and in the postpartum period, high hPRL levels are
associated with decreased hLH and hFSH levels (Jaffe et al.
1973, Reyes et al. 1972, Rolland et al. 1975a, Rolland et al.
1975b). Furthermore, the baseline serum hLH concentrations do not
show characteristic episodic fluctuations during the puerperium
(Bohnet et al. 1976b), which seems to be identical with a loss of
tonic hLH release by the hypothalamus. In addition, the response
to intravenous LRH administration is impaired to a greater degree
in lactating women as compared to women who are bottle feeding
(Le Maire et al. 1974, Canales et al. 1974, Jeppsson et al. 1974,
Nakano et al. 1974).

It appears as though hPRL also exerts an inhibitory effect
on the ovaries. Within seven to eighteen days postpartum hFSH
concentrations increase to levels seen in the follicular phase
in women, but estradiol levels still remain low at that time.
These data suggest that the ovaries are refractory to endogenous
hFSH in this period (Rolland et al. 1975b). Exogenous administration
of HMG and hCG also failed to stimulate the ovaries of puerperal
women, but only in some of the cases reported by Nakano et al.
(1975). In addition, the suppression of serum hPRL post partum
was followed by an earlier rise of hFSH (Seki et al. 1974) and
of estradiol as compared to untreated women (Rolland et al. 1975b).
In conclusion, these data underline that during the postpartum
period hPRL exerts an inhibitory effect on the hypothalamo-
pituitary-gonadal axis.

Less is known about the role of hPRL in male reproductive
physiology. As mentioned above, basal serum levels of hPRL are
slightly lower and the response to TRH and other stimuli causing
hPRL elevation are less effective than in the female. During
chronic neuroleptic treatment schizophrenic patients exhibit
lower testosterone plasma concentrations than controls. Following
withdrawal of such drugs testosterone levels will increase.
Serum hPRL plasma concentrations were within the normal range for
men, but decreased after withdrawal of the tranquillizers.
Circulating levels of hLH were not affected (Beumont et al. 1974a,
Beaumont et al. 1974b). From these data it remains unclear,
however, whether lowered testosterone levels are due to a direct

effect of these drugs on the Leydig cells or due to a chronic
borderline elevation of serum hPRL concentrations.

In a short communication it was suggested that hPRL influences
the conversion of testosterone to dihydrotestosterone (Oseko et al.
1973). This inference was made from studies of the metabolic
clearance rate of testosterone and the transfer constant of
testosterone to dihydrotestosterone in patients with prostatic
cancer in whom serum hPRL was increased by treatment with chlorpromazine. Statistical analysis of data obtained by Rubin et al.
(1975) indicates that an increase in both serum hPRL and hLH
precede the nocturnal increase of plasma testosterone in male
volunteers. At present, we think that no definitive conclusion
can be stated as to the role of hPRL in testosterone metabolism
in men. However, it is well documented that male impotence
associated with hyperprolactinemia and galactorrhea can be cured
by suppressing elevated hPRL plasma concentration (Besser et al.
1972).

PHARMACOLOGICAL ASPECTS

Several drugs have been shown to either increase or decrease
serum hPRL concentration and standardized tests utilising these
responses have been developed to try to localize lesions affecting
the hypothalamic pituitary prolactin axis (Tolis et al. 1973).
The agents which have been used include TRH and CB-154 which act
directly on the pituitary to stimulate or inhibit hPRL secretion
respectively. Chlorpromazine and L-Dopa which have similar effects
appear to act via a hypothalamic mechanism, although this view is
currently under review. It is not always possible to localize
hypothalamic pituitary lesions, however, using these dynamic tests
(Archer et al. 1974, Zarate et al. 1974, Zarate et al. 1975,
Gates et al. 1973).

Clear evidence for the ability of estrogens to induce hPRL
secretion was first presented by Frantz et al. (1972) who reported
that serum hPRL levels were twice as high as normal values in
patients with prostatic carcinoma who were receiving large doses
of estrogens. In three of five male volunteers diethylstilboestrol
(15-50 mg/day) induced an increase in hPRL within one week (Frantz
et al. 1972).

In postmenopausal as well as in oophorectomized women
ethinylestradiol (1 ug/kg per day) is effective in stimulating
hPRL secretion. Within two weeks, mean concentrations of plasma
hPRL rose from 11.5 to 42.6 ng/ml (Yen et al. 1974). At the same
time plasma concentrations of gonadotropins declined from postmenopausal levels to a range found in cycling women. In another

study a lower dose of ethinylestradiol (EE) (25 ug) was given to
postmenopausal women (Robyn and Vekemans 1975) with similar
results. When estrogens were discontinued serum hPRL levels
decreased within two weeks to control levels. In volunteers with
normal menses, however, a dosage of 50 ug EE caused no consistent
changes in the basal levels of gonadotropins, whereas serum hPRL
levels were as much as two times greater during treatment than
during the control cycles. A dose of 400 ug EE was able to
abolish the midcycle surge of hLH and hFSH and to increase hPRL
4 fold (Delvoye et al.1973). Estrogen conjugates seem to be less
effective in hPRL release as shown by Robyn et al. (1973).

A number of drugs affecting the concentration or metabolism
of cerebral neurotransmitters such as catecholamines, dopamine
and several other amines, cause a marked change of hPRL secretion,
presumably by a hypothalamic mechanism.

Several authors described elevated hPRL levels in patients
receiving psychoactive agents including, e.g. fluphenazine,
perphenazine chlorpromazine, imipramine, haloperidol, sulpiride,
meprobamate (Kleinberg et al. 1971b,Friesen et al. 1972,
Apostalakis et al. 1972, Frantz et al. 1973). Such a rise of
circulating hPRL can be accompanied by hypogonadism with or without
galactorrhea. Treatment with such drugs, however, does not
consistently increase serum hPRL (Beumont et al. 1974a,Beumont et
al. 1974b). The response to phenothiazine and its derivatives
depends on the duration of the treatment and on the age of the
subjects (de Rivera et al. 1975). Similar age dependent changes
were observed in rats aged 25-60 days who exhibited a maximal
PRL response to chlorpromazine (25 mg/kg), but the elevation in
young rats lasted about 2 hr. whereas in the old ones, PRL remained
elevated for as long as 4 hr. (Bohnet et al. 1975).

L-tryptophan, methyltyrosine and monoiodotyrosine stimulate
PRL secretion, without affecting the thyroid axis. The mechanism
involved is unclear, but is thought to involve the hypophysis as
well as the hypothalamus (Smythe et al. 1975). In a recent report,
however, 5 OH-tryptophan failed to increase serum hPRL (Handwerger
et al. 1975).

Recent studies in rodents showed PRL release after prostaglandin E_1 was administered into the third ventricle (Harms et al.
1973), but PGE_2, PGF_1, and PGF_2 were ineffective (Ojeda et al.
1974). By contrast intravenous injections of PGE_1, PGE_2 and
PGF_2 increased PRL levels in all cases (Sato et al. 1975). In
humans, administration of PGF_2 α for the induction of therapeu-

tic abortion was associated with a significant increase in serum
hPRL (Yue et al. 1974). In our opinion, more work is needed to
elucidate further the interaction of hPRL and the prostaglandins
as this topic seems to be important for human reproduction.

In contrast to the great number of stimulatory compounds,
relatively few agents inhibit the secretion of hPRL. Among these
L-Dopa was first applied in the treatment of hyperprolactinemia
(Kleinberg et al. 1971a, Malarkey et al. 1971, Turkington 1972).
This drug is also able to decrease hPRL secretion in normal
subjects (Friesen et al. 1972) and it was suggested that it might
be useful in differentiating hypothalamic from pituitary disorders (vide supra).

The ergot alkaloids have become most important for their
PRL-suppressive action. The efficacy of the various derivatives
varies widely but all appear to act by the same basic mechanism,
namely by inhibiting PRL secretion by a direct action on the
pituitary lactotrophs and in addition, it is possible that some
of their actions may be attributed to an increased dopamine turnover in the tubero-infundibular dopaminergic neurons (Hökfelt
and Fuxe 1972, Flückiger 1975). Furthermore, treatment with
Bromocriptin caused a decline of dopamine $-\beta-$ hydroxylase activity
in sera of patients with post pill galactorrhea-amenorrhea syndrome.

Although the naturally occurring ergots are potent inhibitors
of PRL secretion as numerous studies have demonstrated, they are
toxic substances. Of the alkaloids 2-bromo-α-ergocryptine
(Bromocriptin R, CB-154), a synthetic derivative, has proved to
be most useful in treatment of human hyperprolactinemia. More
recently, it was shown that dihydrogenated ergots (i.e. dihydro-
ergocornine, dihydroergocristine, dihydroergocryptin) without the
toxic vasoconstrictive properties suppress PRL effectively
(Clemens et al. 1974). Hydergin containing three hydrogenated
alkaloids has been used in the treatment of vascular diseases
some years ago. Ergolines which lack the peptide chain of the
ergot alkaloids have also been shown to suppress PRL and current
clinical trials are underway to assess their usefulness (Clemens
et al. 1975).

hPRL SECRETION UNDER PATHOLOGICAL CONDITIONS

Although there is a wide range of plasma concentrations of
hPRL, levels over 200 ng/ml are suspicious of a PRL secreting
tumor. However, a high degree of variation of hPRL plasma
concentrations are observed in patients with pituitary tumors

(Tolis et al. 1975, Daughaday et al. 1973, Beauregard et al.
1974). Whether such tumors result from hypothalamic dysfunction,
i.e., hyperstimulation of PRF, or hypostimulation of PIF, or if
they are autonomous is still unclear. Other tumors associated
with hyperprolactinemia include craniopharyngiomas, metastases
or pituitary stalk compression. The elevated prolactin levels
presumably result from pressure on hypothalamic centres which
regulate PRL secretion.

Other disorders leading to increased PRL secretion include
thyroid dysfunction either hypo- or hyperthyroidism, chronic
renal failure, Nelson's syndrome and ectopic PRL production by
malignant tumors. Nevertheless, some cases remain in the
"idiopathic" category.

The traditional classification of galactorrhea based on
eponyms is unsatisfactory (Zarate et al. 1974, Zarate et al.
1975, Rolland et al. 1975, Bohnet et al. 1976). We prefer to
designate disturbances accompanied by hyperprolactinemia as
"Hyperprolactinemic Anovulatory Syndromes". Female hyperprolactinemic hypogonadism is reported to occur in about 15% of patients
with secondary amenorrhea (Fries and Nillius 1975, Bohnet et al.
1976). Baseline gonadotropin levels are normal or decreased,
but in longstanding hyperprolactinemia a decrease in serum hLH
precedes the decrease in serum hFSH. Furthermore LRH stimulation
tests more frequently reveal an impaired or absent hLH response
rather than a normal one (Tyson et al. 1975, Zarate et al. 1975,
Bohnet et al. 1976c)and hLH secretion seems to be a more reliable
index of the gonadotropic reserve than FSH (Zarate et al. 1975,
Bohnet et al. 1976d). In addition, tonic hLH release, as judged
by pulsatile baseline fluctuation, is impaired (Boyar et al. 1974,
Bohnet et al.1976b,c) and during sleep a further rise of hPRL was
observed with an accompanying fall of serum gonadotropins
(Kapen et al. 1975). Endogenous estradiol concentrations are
lowered, but in most cases reach early follicular phase levels
(Tyson et al. 1975), so that patients do respond to exogenous
gestagens with withdrawal bleeding (Bohnet et al.1976c). In
contrast, most of the patients do not ovulate following clomiphene
treatment (Forsyth and Edwards 1972, Bohnet et al.1976c), although
a rise in gonadotropins can be observed (Kapen et al. 1975).
Furthermore, LRH treatment is not able to convert the clomiphene
unresponsiveness into a positive response as one can in patients
with functional amenorrhea without hyperprolactinemia (Bohnet et
al.1976d) . In short-lived hyperprolactinemia, however, ovulation
can be induced by clomiphene, but it is followed by corpus
luteum insufficiency (Bohnet et al. 1976c).

In the last few years a large number of publications on the
association of hyperprolactinemia and amenorrhea have appeared.

One of the most consistent findings in this group of patients is
that with appropriate suppression of serum hPRL, all impaired
endocrine parameters can be restored and hypogonadism is terminated.

ROLE OF PROLACTIN IN GALACTORRHEA

Despite the fact that hPRL is a necessary factor in lactation,
it is well established that many patients with elevated hPRL
levels do not have galactorrhea, in particular, those bearing a
pituitary adenoma (Fournier et al. 1974, Zarate et al. 1975).
Paradoxically, a large number of patients with galactorrhea have
serum hPRL concentrations in the normal range. This finding
emphasizes the fact that lactation is a complex process.

A number of hypotheses may be advanced to explain the above
paradox. With the demonstration of the heterogeneity of hPRL
in serum (Vide Supra) it was shown that "big-big" hPRL has little
or no biological activity in radioreceptor assays and "big" hPRL
may have a decreased one. Therefore, one could explain the
absence of galactorrhea in some patients with hyperprolactinemia
if one postulated that some tumors secrete predominantly "big-
big" or "big" rather than "small" hPRL. Indeed, several tumors
of this kind have been reported (Rogol and Rosen 1974, Suh and
Frantz 1974, Aubert et al. 1975a).

In addition, studies in our lab (Kelly et al. 1974) have
indicated that the number of PRL receptors in tissues varies
greatly under different physiological conditions. It is conceivable that in some subjects there may be an absence or deficiency
of PRL receptors. Hence despite the high serum PRL levels, no
biological effects would be initiated. The fact that PRL receptors
are critically involved in mediating the action of PRL was
demonstrated by experiments in which antibodies to the PRL receptor
were incubated with mammary gland explants. In the presence of
antiserum to the PRL receptor but not in the presence of control
serum, PRL stimulated casein synthesis, glucose oxidation and
aminoisobutyric acid transport was completely blocked. The latter
two functions are also stimulated by insulin but in this case
antiserum to the PRL receptor had no effect.

HUMAN BREAST CANCER AND PROLACTIN

In experimental mammary tumors in animals an important role
of PRL is well established (Hobbs et al. 1973). The first indirect evidence that hPRL might play a role in human breast cancer
was gained from clinical experience. Following hypophysectomy
human breast cancer may remit although previous oophorectomy as

well as adrenalectomy failed to effect any improvement in the
disease. Attempts have been made to treat human breast cancer
by decreasing serum hPRL. In a few cases an improvement followed
treatment with L-Dopa (Frantz et al. 1972) and with bromocriptin
with only limited success (Schulz et al. 1973). Only exceptionally
are hPRL levels increased in patients bearing a mammary cancer
(Berle and Voigt 1972, Franks et al. 1974) and the role of
reserpine (Boston Collaborative Study 1974, Armstrong et al.
1974, Heinaren et al. 1974) and other agents which stimulate
hPRL secretion (Wilson et al. 1973) in human mammary tumorigenesis
needs further elucidation.

A provocative study by Kwa et al. (1974) should be mentioned.
These investigators also found no mean elevation of serum prolactin
levels in patients with breast cancer, but in a population of
patients with a high risk of developing breast cancer there was
a much greater frequency of elevated serum prolactin levels than
in the control population. Using our radioreceptor assay, serum
hPRL concentrations correlated well with values determined by
radioimmunoassay suggesting that no other lactogenic substances
are present in (Friesen et al. 1973) patients with breast cancer.

Direct studies to demonstrate an effect of prolactin on the
human mammary gland derive from 2 approaches. The first depends
on cytochemical changes in mammary tissue after short-term
incubations in the presence of prolactin or other hormones. With
this technique, Hobbs et al. (1973) have found that approximately
32% of tumors respond to the addition of prolactin.

In studies on PRL receptors in our laboratory Holdaway and
Friesen (1975) found that 20% of mammary tumors exhibit specific
binding sites for PRL. In all cases, however, the binding of
PRL is very low compared with that found in rabbit mammary tissue
or experimental mammary tumors.

In summary, there is convincing evidence for an important
role of PRL in mammary tumors in mice and rats but in humans the
data supporting such an association is still very limited.

REFERENCES

Adler, R.A., Noel, G.L., Wartofsky, L., and Frantz, A.G. (1975)
J. Clin. Endocrinol. Metab. 41, 383-389.

Apostalakis, M., Kapesanakis, S., Lazos, G., and Pyngaki, A. M.
(1972) In: Lactogenic Hormones (G.E.W. Worstenholme and J. Knight,
eds.) Churchill Livingstone, Edinburgh and London, pp. 349-356.

Archer, D.F., Nankin, H.R., Gabos, P.F., Maroon, J.,Nosetz, S.,
Wadhwa, S.R., and Josimovich, J.B. (1974) Am. J. Obstet. Gynecol.
119, 465-472.

Archer, D.F. and Josimovich, J.B. (1975) Fert. Steril. 26, 627-633.

Armstrong, B., Stevens, N., and Doll, R. (1974) Lancet II, 672-674.

Aubert, M.L., Grumbach, M.M., and Kaplan, S.L. (1974) Acta Endocr.
77, 460-476.

Aubert, M.L., Garnier, P.E., Kaplan, S.L., and Grumbach, M.M.
(1975a) Fifty-seventh annual meeting of the Endocr. Soc. A-59.
(Abstract).

Aubert, M.L., Grumbach, M.M., and Kaplan, S.L. (1975b) J. Clin.
Invest. 56, 155-164.

Bala, R.M., Ferguson, K.A., and Beck, J.C. (1970) Endocrinology
87, 506-516.

Barberia, J.M., Abu-Fadil, S., Kletsky, O.A., Nakamina, R.M.,
and Mishell, D.R. (1975) Am. J. Obstet. Gynecol. 121, 1107-1110.

Beauregard, H., Hardy, J., and Lanthier, A. (1974) Clin. Res.
22, 729A.

Bellinger, L.L., Moberg, G.P., and Mendel, V.E. (1975) Horm.
Metab. Res. 7, 43-45.

Ben-David, M. and Chrambach, A. (1974) Endocr. Res. Comm. 1,
193-210.

Benveniste, R., Stachura, M.E., Szabo, M., and Frohmann, L.A.
(1975) J. Clin. Endocrinol. Metab. 41, 422-425.

Berle, P. and Voigt, K.D. (1972) Am. J. Obstet. Gynec. 114,
1101 - 1102.

Berson, S.A. and Yalow, R.S. (1968) J. Clin. Endocrinol. Metab. 28, 1037-1047.

Besser, J.M., Parke, L., Edwards, C.R.W., Forsyth, I.A. and McNeilly, A.S. (1972) Brit. Med. J. 3, 669-672.

Beumont, P.J.V., Corker, C.S., Friesen, H.G., Gelder, M.G., Harris, G.W., Kolakowska, T., MacKinnon, P.C.B., Mandelbrote, B.M., Marshall, J., Murray, M.A.F., and Wiles, D.H. (1974a) Brit. J. Psychiat. 124, 413-419.

Beumont, P.J.V., Corker, C.S., Friesen, H.G., and Kolakowska, T. (1974b) Brit. J. Psychiat. 124, 420-430.

Beumont, P.J.V., Friesen, H.G., Gelder, M.G., and Kolakowska, T. (1974c) Psychol. Med. 4, 219-221.

Bohnet, H.G., Aragona, C., and Friesen, H.G. (1975) Endocrinology, Submitted for publication.

Bohnet, H.G., Dahlen, H.G., Keller, E., Friedrich, E., Schindler, A.E., Wyss, H.I., and Schneider, H.P.G. (1975d) J. Clin. Endocrinol. In press.

Bohnet, H.G., Heuberger, L.W.L., Dahlen, H.G., and Schneider, H.P.G. (1976a) Endokrinologie, In press.

Bohnet, H.G., Wiest, H.J., Dahlen, H.G., and Schneider, H.P.G. (1976c) Endokrinologie, In press.

Bohnet, H.G., Dahlen, H.G. Wuttke, W., and Schneider, H.P.G. (1976   J. Clin. Endocrinol. Metab., In press.

Boston Collaborative Drug Surveillance Program (1974) II, 669-71.

Boyar, R.M., Kapen, S., Finkelstein, J.W., Perlow, M., Sassin, J. F., Fukushima, D.K., Weitzman, E.D., and Hellman, L. (1974) J. Clinical Invest. 53, 1588-1598.

Buckman, M.T. and Peake, G.T. (1973) Science 181, 755-757.

Bunner, D.L. and Vanderlann, W.P. (1975) Clin. Res. 23, A387.

Butler, W.R., Krey, L.C., Lu, K.H., Peckham, W.D., and Knobil, E. (1975), Endocrinology, 96, 1099-1105.

Canales, E.S., Zarate, A., Garoido, J., Leon, C., Soria, J., and Schally, A.V. (1974) J. Clin. Endocrinol. Metab. 38, 1140-1142.

Chan, J.S.D., Robertson, H.A., and Friesen, H.G. (1976) Endocrinology, In press.

Clemens, J.A., Shaar, C.J., Smalstig, E.B., Bach, N.J., and Kornfeld, E.C. (1974) Endocrinology 94, 1171-1176.

Clemens, J.A., Smalstig, E.G., and Shaar, C.J. (1975) Acta Endocr. 79, 230-237.

Daughaday, W.H., Loewenstein, J.E., Jacobs, L.S., Malarkey, W.B., and Mariz, I.K. (1971) In: Gonadotropins (Saxena et al., eds.) John Wiley and Sons, Inc., New York, pp.460-501.

Daughaday, W.H., Cryer, P.C., and Jacobs, L.S. (1973) In: Excerpta Medica (P.O. Kohler and G.T. Ross, eds.) Amsterdam, pp. 26-34.

Delvoye, P., Hasau, S.H., L'Hermite, M., Neumann, F., and Robyn, C. (1973) Acta endocr. Suppl. 177, Abstract No. 132.

Delvoye, P., Taubert, H.D., Jurgensen, O., L'Hermite, M., Delogne, J., and Robyn, C. (1974) C.R. Acad. Sc. Paris, t. 279, Serie D., 1463-1466.

de Rivera, J.L., Ettigi, P., Honkela, S., Muller, H.F., and Friesen, H.G. (1975), submitted for publication.

Dunn, J.D., Arimura, A., and Schering, L.E. (1972) Endocrinology 90, 29-33.

Ehara, Y., Siler, T.M., Vanden Berg, G., Sinha, Y.N., and Yen, S.S.C. (1973) Am. J. Obstet. Gynecol. 117, 962-970.

Ehara, Y., Yen, S.S.C., and Siler, T.M. (1975) Am. J. Obstet. Gynecol. 121, 995-997.

Epinosa-Campos, J., Butler, W.R., and Knobil, E. (1975) Fifty-seventh Annual Meeting of the Endocr. Soc. A-63 (Abstract).

Fang, V.S. and Kim, M.H. (1975) Fifty-seventh Annual Meeting of the Endocr. Soc. A- 353 (Abstract).

Fluckiger, E. (1975) Acta Endocr. Supplement 193, 78-79.

Forsyth, I.A. and Edwards, C.R.W. (1972) Clin. Endocr. 1, 293-314.

Forsyth, I.A. and Parke, L. (1973) In: Human Prolactin (J.L. Pasteels and C. Robyn, eds.) Excerpta Medica Amsterdam, pp.71-81.

Foss, G.L. and Short, D. (1951) J. Obstet. Gynacol. Br. Emp. 58, 35 -46.

Fournier, P.J.R., Desjardins, P.D., and Friesen, H.G. (1974) Am. J. Obstet. Gynecol. 118, 337-343.

Franks, S., Ralphs, D.W.L., Seagrott, V. and Jacobs, H.S. (1974) Brit. Med. J. 4, 320-21.

Frantz, A.G., Kleinberg, D.L., and Noel, G.L. (1972) Rec. Prog. Horm. Res. 28, 527-590.

Frantz, A.G., Habif, D.V., Hyman, G.A., Suh, H.K., Sassin, J.F., Zimmermann, E.A., Noel, G.L., and Kleinberg, D.L. (1973) In: Human Prolactin (J.L. Pasteels and C. Robyn, eds) Excerpta Medica Amsterdam, p. 273-291.

Fries, H. and Nillius, S.J. (1973) Acta Psychiat. Med. 273, 897-901.

Friesen, H.G., Guyda, H., Hwang, P., and Tyson, J.E. (1972) J. Clin. Invest. 51, 706-709.

Friesen, H.G., Tolis, G., Shiu, R., and Hwang, P. (1973) In: Human Prolactin (J.L. Pasteels and C. Robyn, eds.) Excerpta Medica Amsterdam, pp.11-23.

Gates, R.B., Friesen, H.G., and Samaan, N.A. (1973) Acta Endocr. 72, 101-114.

Guyda, H., Hwang, P., and Friesen, H.G. (1971) J. Clin. Endocrinol. Metab. 32, 120-123.

Guyda, H. and Whyte, S. (1974) Clin. Res. 22, 341A (Abstract).

Handwerger, S., Plonk, J.W., Lebovitz, H.E., Bivens, C.H., and Feldmann, J.M. (1975) Horm. Metab. Res. 7, 214-216.

Harms, P.G., Ojeda, S.R., and McCann, S.M. (1973) Science 181, 760-761.

Heinanen, O.P., Shapiro, S. Tuominen, L. and Turner, M.I. (1974) Lancet II, 675-677.

Hobbs, J.R. Salih, H., Flax, H., and Brander, W. (1973) In: Human Prolactin (J.L. Pasteels and C. Robyn, eds.) Excerpta Medica Amsterdam, pp.249-258.

Hokfelt, T. and Fuxe, K. (1972) Neuroendocrinology 9, 100-122.

Holdaway, I.M. and Friesen, H.G. (1976) J. Nat. Canc. Inst., Submitted for publication.

Horrobin, D.F., Lloyd, I.J., Lipton, A., Burstyn, P.G., Durkin, N., and Muiruri, K.L. (1971) The Lancet, 352-356.

Hwang, P., Friesen, H.G., and Hardy, J. (1971a) J. Clin. Endocrinol. Metab. 33, 1-7.

Hwang, P., Guyda, H., and Friesen, H.G. (1971b) Proc. Nat. Acad. U.S.A. 68, 1902-1906.

Hwang, P., Robertson, M., Guyda, H., and Friesen, H.G. (1973) J. Clin. Endocrinol. Metab. 36, 1110-1118.

Jacobs, L.S., Mariz, I.K. and Daughaday, W.H. (1971), J. Clin. Endocrinol. Metab. 34, 484-490.

Jacobs, L.S., Snyder, P.S., Utiger, R.D., and Daughaday, W.H. (1973) J. Clin. Endocrinol. Metab. 36, 1069-1073.

Jaffe, R.B., Yuen, B.H., Keye, W.R., Midgley, A.R. (1973) Am. J. Obstet. Gynecol. 117, 757-773.

Jeppsson, S., Rannevik, G., and Kullander, S. (1974) Am. J. Obstet. Gynecol. 120, 1029-1034.

Jewelewicz, R., Dyrenfurth, I., Warren, M., Frantz, A.G., and Vande Wiele, R.L. (1974) J. Clin. Endocrinol. Metab. 39, 387-389.

Josimovich, J.B., Weiss, G., and Hutchinson, D.L. (1974) Endocrinology 94, 1364-1371.

Kapen, S., Boyar, R.M., Freeman, R., Frantz, A., Hellman, L., and Weitzman, E.D. (1975) J. Clin. Endocrinol. Metab. 90, 234-239.

Kataoka, K., Imai, Y., and Hollander, C.S. (1975) Clin. Res. 23, 238A (Abstract).

Keettel, W.C. and Bradbury, J.T. (1961) Am. J. Obstet. Gynecol. 82, 995-1002.

Kelly, P.A. Posner, B.I., Tsushima, T., and Friesen, H.G. (1974) Endocrinology 95, 532-539.

Kizer, J.S., Zivin, J.A., Jacobowitz, D.M., and Kopin, I.J. (1975) Endocrinology 96, 1230-1240.

Kleinberg, D.L., Noel, G.L., and Frantz, A.S. (1971a) J. Clin. Endocr. Metab. 33, 873–876.

Kleinberg, D.L., Wharton, R.N., and Frantz, A.G. (1971b) Fifty-third Annual Meeting of the Endocrine Soc. A-126 (Abstract).

Kolodny, R.C., Jacobs, L.S., and Daughaday, W.H. (1972) Nature 238, 284-285.

Kroa, H.G., De Jong-Bakker, M., Engelsman, E., Cleton, I.J. (1974) Lancet I, 433–434.

Landgraf, R., Weissmann, A., Landgraf-Leuvs, M., von Werder, K. (1975) Acta Endocr. Suppl. 193 65 (Abstract).

LeMaire, W.J. Shapiro, A.G., Riggall, F., and Yong, N.S.T. (1974) J. Clin. Endocrinol. Metab. 38, 916–918.

Lewis, U.J. and Singh, R.N.P. (1973) In: Human Prolactin (J.L. Pasteels and C. Robyn, eds.) Excerpta Medica Amsterdam, p. 1–10.

L'Hermite, M. and Robyn, C. (1972) Am. d'Endocr. 33, 357–360.

L'Hermite, M. (1973) Clinics in Endocrinol. Metab. 2, 423–449.

Malarkey, W.B., Jacobs, L.S., and Daughaday, W.H. (1971) New Engl. J. Med. 285, 1160-1163.

McNatty, K.P., Sawers, R.S., and McNeilly, A.S. (1974) Nature 250, 653–655.

McNatty, K.P., Hunter, W.M., McNeilly, A.S., and Saivers, R.S. (1975) J. Endocrinol. 64, 555–571.

McNeilly, A.S., Evans, G.E., Chard, T. (1973) In: Human Prolactin (J.L. Pasteels and C. Robyn, eds.) Excerpta Medica Amsterdam, pp.231–232.

McNeilly, A.S., Sturdy, J., Evans, D.G., and Chard, T. (1974) J. Endocr. 61, 301–302.

Midgley, A.R., Jr., and Jaffe, R.B. (1973) In: Proceedings of the Fourth International Congress of Endocrinology (R.O. Scow et al., eds.) Excerpta Medica Amsterdam, pp.629–634.

Nakano, R., Kayashima, F., Mori, A., Kotsuji, F., Hashiba, N., and Tojo, S. (1974) Acta Obstet. Gynecol. Scand. 53, 303–307.

Nakano, R., Mori, A., Kayashima, F., Washio, M., and Tojo, S. (1975) Am. J. Obstet. Gynecol. 121, 187-192.

Noel, G.L., Suh, H.K., Stone, J., and Frantz, A.G. (1972) J. Clin. Endocrinol. Metab. 35, 840-851.

Noel, G.L., Suh, H.K., and Frantz, A.G. (1974) J. Clin. Endocrinol. Metab. 38, 413-423.

Nokin, J., Vekemans, N., L'Hermite, M., and Robyn, C. (1972) Br. Med. J. 3, 561-562.

Ojeda, S.R., Harms, P.G., and McCann, S.M. (1974) Endocrinology 95, 613-618.

Oseko, F., Slaunwhite, W.R., Farnsworth, W.E., Gonder, M.J., and Seal, U.S. (1973) Fifty-fifth Annual Meeting of the Endocr. Soc. A-51 (Abstract).

Ostermann, P.O. and Wide, L. (1975) Acta Endocr. 78, 675-682.

Parker, D.C., Rossman, L.G., and VAnderlaan, E.F. (1973) J. Clin. Endocrinol. Metab. 36, 1119-1124.

Perez, A., Vela, R., and Masnick, G.S. (1972) Am. J. Obstet. Gynecol. 114, 1041-1047.

Reyes, F.I., Winter, J.S.D., and Faiman, C. (1972) Am. J. Obstet. Gynecol. 114, 589-594.

Riddle, O., Bates, R.W., and Dykshorn, S.W. (1933) Am. J. Physiol. 105, 191-216.

Robyn, C., Delvoye, P., Nokin, J., Vekemans, M., Badawi, M., Perez-Lopez, F.R., and L'Hermite, M. (1973) In: Human Prolactin (J.L. Pasteels and C. Robyn, eds.) Excerpta Medica Amsterdam, pp. 167-188.

Robyn, C. and Vekemans, M. (1975) In: Estrogens in the Post-menopause (P.A. van Keep and C.H. Lauritzen, eds.) Karges Verlag, Basel, In press.

Rogol, A.D. and Rosen, S.W. (1974) J. Clin. Endocrinol. Metab. 38, 714-717.

Rogol, A.D. and Chrambach, A. (1975) Endocrinology 97, 406-417.

Rolland, R., Schellekens, L.A., and Lequin, R.M. (1974) Clin. Endocr. 3, 155-165.

Rolland, R., de Jong, F.H., Schellekens, L.A., and Lequin, R.M. (1975a) Clin. Endocr. 4, 27-38.

Rolland, R., Lequin, R.M., Schellekens, L.A., and de Jong, F.H. (1975b) Clin. Endocr. 4, 15-25.

Roth, J., Gorden, P., and Pastan, I. (1968) Proc. Natl. Acad. Sci. U.S.A. 61, 138-146.

Rubin, R.T., Gouin, P.R., Lubin, A., Poland, R.E., and Pirke, K.M. (1975) J. Clin. Endocrinol. Metab. 40, 1027-1033.

Sassin, J.F., Frantz, A.G., Kapen, S., and Weitzman, E.D. (1973) J. Clin. Endocrinol. Metab. 37, 436-440.

Sato, T. Hirono, M., Jyujo, T., Lesaka, T., Taya, K. and Igarashi, M. (1975) Endocrinology 96, 45-49.

Schulz, K.D., Zygan, P.J., del Pozo, E. and Friesen, H.G. (1973) In: Human Prolactin (J.L. Pasteels and C. Robyn, eds.) Excerpta Medica Amsterdam, pp. 268-272.

Seki, K. Seki, M., and Okumura, T. (1974) J. Clin. Endocrinol. Metab. 39, 184-186.

Shiu, R.P.C., Kelly, P.A., and Friesen, H.G. (1973) Science 180, 968-971.

Sinha, Y.N., Selby, F.W., Lewis, U.J., and Vanderlaan, W.P. (1973) J. Clin. Endocrinol. Metab. 36, 509-516.

Smythe, G.A., Compton, P.J., and Lazarus, L. (1975) J. Clin. Endocrinol. Metab. 40, 714-716.

Stearns, E.L., Winter, J.S.D., and Faiman, C. (1973) J. Clin. Endocrinol. Metab. 37, 687-691.

Stevens, V.C., Powell, J.E., and Sparks, S.J. (1973) Fifty-fifth Annual Meeting of the Endocr. Soc., A-64 (Abstract).

Suh, H.K. and Frantz, A.G. (1974) J. Clin. Endocrinol. Metab. 39, 928-935.

Tolis, G. Goldstein, M., and Friesen, H.G. (1973) J. Clin. Invest. 52, 783-788.

Tolis, G., Hardy, J., Bernard, G., and McKenzie, J.M. (1975) Fifty-seventh Annual Meeting of the Endocr. Soc., A347 (Abstract).

Turkington, R.W. (1972) J. Clin. Endocrinol. Metab. 34, 306-311.

Tyson, J.E., Friesen, H.G., and Anderson, M.S. (1972a) Science 177, 897-899.

Tyson, J.E., Hwang, P., Guyda, H., and Friesen, H.G. (1972b) Am. J. Obstet. Gynecol. 113, 14-20.

Tyson, J.E. and Friesen, H.G. (1973) Am. J. Obstet. Gynecol. 116, 377-387.

Tyson, J.E., Andreasson, B., Huth, J., Smith, B., and Facur, H. (1975) Obst. Gynec. 46, 1-11.

Vinik, A.I., Kelk, W.J., McLaren, H., and Paul, M. (1976) Horm. Metab. Res. 6, 499-501.

Wilson, R.G., Forrest, A.P.M., Boyns, A.R., and Griffiths, K. (1973) In: Human Prolactin (J.L. Pasteels and C. Robyn, eds.) Excerpta Medica Amsterdam, pp. 266-268.

Wuttke, W., Dohler, K.D., and Gelato, M. (1975) J. Endocr., In press.

Yalow, R.S. and Berson, S.A. (1970) Gastroenterology 58, 609-615.

Yalow, R.S. and Berson, S.A. (1971) Biochem. Biophys. Res. Commun. 44, 439-445.

Yen, S.S.C., Tsai, C.C., Naftolin, F., Vandenberg, G., and Ajabor, L. (1972) J. Clin. Endocrinol. Metab. 34, 671-675.

Yen, S.S.C., Ehara, Y., and Siler, T.M. (1974) J. Clin. Invest. 53, 652-655.

Yue, D.K., Smith, I.D., Turtle, J.R. and Sherman, R.P. (1974) Prostaglandins 8, 387-395.

Zarate, A., Canales, E.S., Soria, J., Ruiz, F. and MacGregor, C. (1972) Am. J. Obstet. Gynecol. 112, 1130-1133.

Zarate, A., Canales, E.S., Soria, J., Garrido, J., Jacobs, L.S. and Schelly, A.V. (1974) Ann. d'Endocrinol. 35, 535-545.

Zarate, A., Canales, E.S., Villahobos, H., Soria, J., Jacobs, L.S., Kastin, A.J., and Schally, A.V. (1975) J. Clin. Endocrinol. Metab. 40, 1034-1037.

NEUROPHARMACOLOGICAL ASPECTS OF THE NEURAL CONTROL

OF PROLACTIN SECRETION

James A. Clemens

The Lilly Research Laboratories (Eli Lilly and Co.)

Indianapolis, Indiana 46206

In recent years, an increasing number of studies have appeared in which neuropharmacological agents were used in attempts to clarify which of the putative neurotransmitters are involved in the control of prolactin secretion. Some of the more recently developed drugs and pharmacological agents can be expected to demonstrate a high degree of specificity if used judiciously. The use of these agents in neuroendocrine studies has led to the identification of several neurotransmitters that are involved in the control of prolactin secretion. Few reviews have been totally devoted to the effects of pharmacological agents on prolactin secretion, therefore, a few aspects of the neuropharmacology of prolactin control are considered in some detail, and integration of data from a variety of sources is attempted.

Before embarking on a discussion of drug-related studies on prolactin control, it might be appropriate to consider a list of general guidelines which could be followed in any neuroendocrine study involving the use of neuropharmacological agents. The following list was prepared with the intention of providing the investigator with a number of important criteria that need to be taken into consideration before undertaking any neuroendocrine study with drugs and chemical agents.

1. Some measure of the desired drug effect should be available to determine if the drug is being effective. If no measure is available, a dose should be used that has been reported to be effective in the particular species concerned in the study.

2. Determine if the drug acts in the CNS as well as at the
    periphery. Many monoamines and compounds containing
    quaternary nitrogen exert mainly peripheral effects and
    do not act directly on the CNS to a significant extent.
    Most of the structure-activity profiles were obtained
    using peripheral receptor models.

3. Very few drugs are selective. However, some demonstrate
    selectivity over a limited dose range. The upper limits
    of this dose range should not be exceeded.

4. All experimental measurements should be performed before
    the pharmacological agent is inactivated. It is impor-
    tant to know the biological half-life.

5. Although all of the above criteria are satisfied, the
    same experimental result should be obtained with more
    than one pharmacological agent with a similar selecti-
    vity profile before firm conclusions can be reached.

In the ensuing discussion, drugs affecting prolactin secretion
are grouped into categories according to the putative neurotransmitter that is affected by the drug.

DOPAMINE

Neuropharmacological studies have amply demonstrated that dopamine has an inhibitory role in the control of prolactin release.
Studies with catecholamine synthesis inhibitors have unequivocally
demonstrated that a catecholamine is involved in the inhibitory
control of prolactin release. Table I summarizes these studies.
Studies with synthesis inhibitors alone can not be definitive, because the synthesis of all catecholamines is inhibited.

Somewhat more definition was added by the use of catecholamine
antagonists. The catecholamine antagonists block the action of the
catecholamine on its receptor. The antipsychotic drugs were a good
source of catecholamine receptor blockers, because among most antipsychotic drugs, a positive correlation between dopamine receptor
blocking ability and antipsychotic potency exists. Table 2 summarizes the studies performed with the receptor blocking drugs. One
can feel confident that all of the drugs listed in Table 2 are acting on CNS receptors as well as peripheral receptors, because all
of the drugs listed except cyproheptadine and promethazine are
antipsychotic agents.

TABLE I. Effect of Catecholamine Synthesis Inhibitors on Prolactin Release.

Drug	Primary Action	Effect on serum prolactin	Reference
Alpha-methyl-p-tyrosine	Inhibits tyrosine hydroxylase		
(200 mg/kg)		Increase	Lu, et al. (1970)
(320 mg/kg)		Increase	Chen and Meites (1975)
(100 mg/kg)		Increase	Donoso, et al. (1971)
Alpha-methyldopa	Inhibits DOPA decarboxylase		
(32 mg/kg)		Increase	Lu and Meites (1971)
3-Odotyrosine	Inhibits tyrosine hydroxylase		
(100 mg/kg)		Increase	Smythe, et al. (1974)

TABLE 2. Effect of Catecholamine Receptor Blocking Drugs on Prolactin Secretion.

Drug	Receptors blocked	Effect on prolactin secretion	Reference
Chlorpromazine	Dopamine Norepinephrine Histamine 1	Increase	Lu, et al.(1970) Kleinberg, et al (1971)
Perphenazine	Dopamine Norepinephrine Histamine 1	Increase	Ben-David, et al. (1971) Ben-David, et al. (1970) MacLeod, et al. (1970)
Haloperidol	Dopamine Norepinephrine	Increase	Dickerman, et al (1972)
Cyproheptadine	Dopamine Serotonin	Increase	Clemens, unpublished
Promethazine	Histamine 1 Serotonin	Decrease	Clemens, et al.(1974)
Pimozide	Dopamine	Increase	Clemens, et al. (1974)
Sulpiride	Dopamine ?	Increase	Clemens, et al. (1974)

Out of this group of drugs, only pimozide is known to be a specific blocker of dopamine receptors over a limited dose range. While all of the drugs listed appear to implicate some monoamine as being involved in the inhibitory control of prolactin secretion, only the studies with pimozide clearly focus on dopamine as a monoamine that is involved in inhibiting prolactin release.

Fortunately, specific centrally-acting dopamine agonists are available and have helped to further clarify the role of dopamine as a regulator of prolactin secretion. Apomorphine has been shown to be a selective dopamine agonist (Ferrini and Miragoli, 1972; Repper et al., 1972; Patel et al., 1973; Lal et al., 1972; Pinder et al., 1972). Recently, various ergolines have been shown to be selective dopamine agonists (Corrodi et al., 1973; Stone, 1973; Woodruff et al., 1974). Apomorphine inhibits prolactin secretion in the rat (Smalstig and Clemens, 1974; MacLeod and Lehmeyer, 1974) and in humans (Martin et al., 1974). Ergot alkaloids and various ergoline derivatives have been shown to inhibit prolactin secretion in rats (Nicoll, C.S. et al., 1970; Nagasawa and Meites, 1970; Wuttke et al., 1971; Malven and Hoge, 1971; Shaar and Clemens, 1972; Cassady et al., 1973), in the bovine (Schams et al., 1973; Smith et al., 1973), in sheep (Niswender, 1974), in dogs (Mayer and Schutze, 1973), and in humans (Besser et al., 1972; Del Pozo et al., 1972; Brun del Re et al., 1973; Del Pozo et al., 1973; Lemberger et al., 1974; Rolland et al., 1974).

We have had the opportunity to examine a variety of potent dopamine receptor agonists from different structural classes. The structures of these agonists are shown in Fig. 1. They represent dissimilar structural classes. However, they all possess a tertiary nitrogen and a phenylethylamine nucleus. The effects of these compounds on serum prolactin levels were determined in male rats. Each rat received an aqueous suspension of 2.0 mg of reserpine 24 hours before administration of the receptor agonists. Animals were killed by decapitation 1 hr after i.p. administration of the drugs. Blood was collected and the serum was assayed for prolactin by radioimmunoassay. All of the dopamine agonists significantly lowered prolactin levels (Table 3). Apomorphine was the least potent inhibitor while (-)6-prolyl-10, 11-norapomorphinediol hydrochloride (6-propyl-apomorphine) was much more potent. The potency of M-7 could not be determined because only one dose level was administered. The ergoline derivative, lergotrile mesylate, was found to be a very potent inhibitor of prolactin release.

The site of action of dopamine and its agonists has been the subject of intense study. Shaar and Clemens (1974) reported that biochemical extraction of catecholamines from hypothalamic extracts resulted in loss of prolactin inhibiting activity from the extracts. In addition, they reported that extremely small amounts of catecholamines were able to inhibit release of prolactin from pituitaries

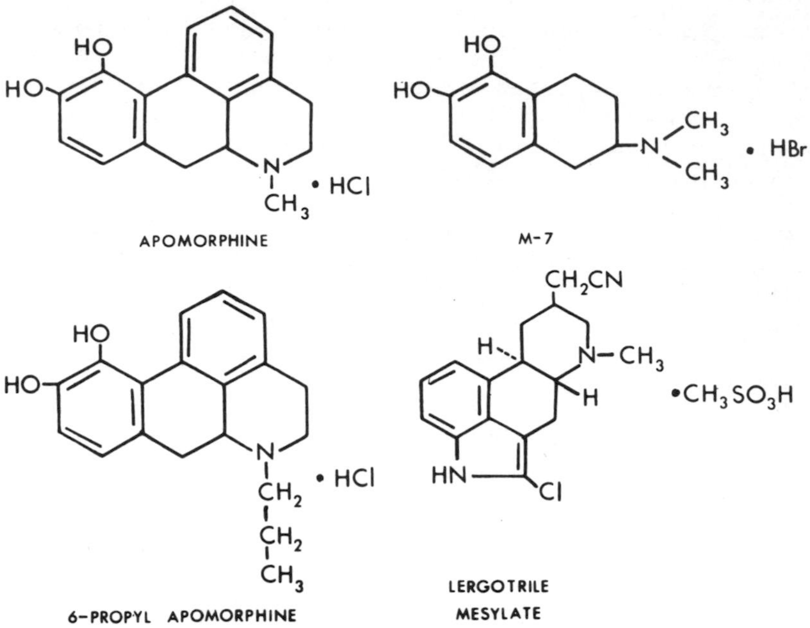

Fig. 1: Chemical structures of various dopamine agonists

incubated in vitro. Paired pituitary halves were incubated in medium 199 and various amounts of catecholamines were added to one
of the paired halves, while the other half of the pair was incubated with vehicle. After 4 hours of incubation at $37^{\circ}C$, the incubation medium was collected and assayed for prolactin by radioimmunoassay. Fig. 2 shows the mean difference in prolactin released
between treated and control pituitary halves vs log of the amount
of catecholamine added.

It appears that dopamine is a much more potent inhibitor of
prolactin release than either norepinephrine or epinephrine. This
study demonstrated that dopamine, in amounts much less than that
found in the basal hypothalamus, was able to inhibit the release
of prolactin by a direct action on the pituitary. Others have
shown that dopamine could inhibit prolactin release from the pituitary by a direct action, however, the amounts needed to demonstrate inhibition were greater than the total amount present in the
basal hypothalamus (MacLeod et al., 1970; MacLeod and Lehmeyer,
1974; Koch et al., 1970).

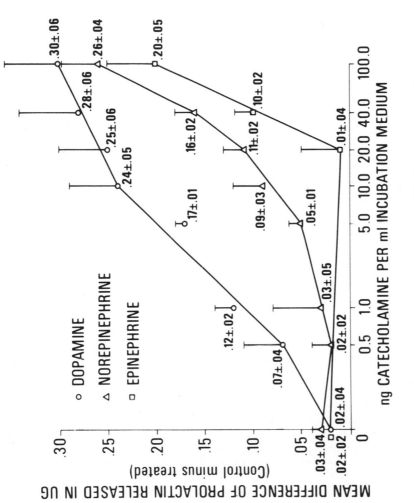

Figure 2. Log dose response curve for the inhibition of prolactin secretion by catecholamines.

TABLE 3.   Effects of Various Dopamine Agonists on Prolactin
           Secretion in male rats

Agonist	Dose/Rat	Serum Prolactin levels ng/ml
Control, saline	1.0 ml	28.7 ± 2.8[a]
Apomorphine	1.0 mg	18.3 ± 3.1[b]
6-propyl-apomorphine	100 ug	10.9 ± 1.5[c]
	10 ug	9.6 ± 0.6[c]
	1 ug	23.3 ± 2.8
M-7	1.0 mg	9.1 ± 0.3[c]
Lergotrile Mesylate	10 ug	12.7 ± 0.6[c]

a. Mean ± standard error
b. $p < 0.5$;
c. $p < 0.001$

MacLeod and Lehmeyer (1974) reported that drugs possessing
both dopaminergic and alpha-adrenergic blocking capabilities were
able to block the inhibitory action of dopaminergic agonists on
prolactin release in vitro. In their study, phentolamine (4×10^{-5} M)
was able to partially reverse the inhibitory effect of 5×10^{-7} M
dopamine. In view of the large amount of phentolamine needed to
partially inhibit the action of dopamine, alpha-adrenergic receptors on the pituitary cells do not appear to be involved in the action of dopamine agonists as they had suggested. Smalstig and Clemens (1974) had reported that the more specific dopamine receptor
blocker, pimozide, was able to antagonize the inhibitory action of
apomorphine on prolactin release. We recently undertook a study
to compare the effects of alpha and beta-adrenergic antagonists
and pimozide on the inhibitory action of apomorphine on prolactin
release in vitro. In this study, the paired pituitary incubation
system (Shaar and Clemens, 1974) was used. In order to determine
if the antagonists could reverse the effects of apomorphine, one
half of the pair was incubated with 25 ng/ml of apomorphine (2.0
ml, total volume), while the other half of the pair was incubated
with the same dose of apomorphine plus an equimolar amount of the
antagonist. The results are shown in TABLE 4.

An identical in vitro incubation was performed using the dopamine agonist, lergotrile mesylate. Once again, phentolamine, pro-

TABLE 4. Effects of Neurotransmitter Antagonists on the Ability
of Apomorphine to Inhibit Prolactin Release In Vitro.

Conditions	Prolactin Released (ng/mg AP)	
	Average	Mean Difference
Saline	381.9	
APO (25 ng/ml)[a]	133.5	284.4 ± 47.4
		(p < .01)
APO (25 ng/ml)	112.2	
		0.3 ± 18.1
APO (25 ng/ml) - Propranolol (20 ng/ml)	111.9	
APO (25 ng/ml)	153.8	
APO (25 ng/ml) - Phentolamine (30 ng/ml)	132.5	21.3 ± 20.8
APO (25 ng/ml)	128.9	
		248.2 ± 59.6
		(p < .01)
APO (25 ng/ml) - Pimozide (32 ng/ml)	377.1	

[a]APO = Apomorphine

pranolol and pimozide were used as blocking agents. Fig. 3 clearly shows that the inhibitory action of lergotrile mesylate on prolactin release was reversed only by the dopamine antagonist, pimozide. Therefore, dopamine and its agonists appear to exert their
inhibitory influence on prolactin secretion by a direct action on
dopamine receptors located on the prolactin-secreting cells in the
anterior pituitary.

The close proximity of the tuberoinfundibular dopaminergic
nerve endings to the capillary plexus of the portal vessels in the
median eminence and the lack of neuronal monoaminergic synapses in
this area (Ajika and Hokfelt, 1975) suggest that prolactin secretion might, at least in part, be regulated by dopamine released
from the nerve endings in the median eminence. This can not exclu-
de the possibility that there might be polypeptides that inhibit
prolactin secretion, or perhaps dopamine might be released complexed with a polypeptide. Dupont and Redding (1975) and Greibrokk et

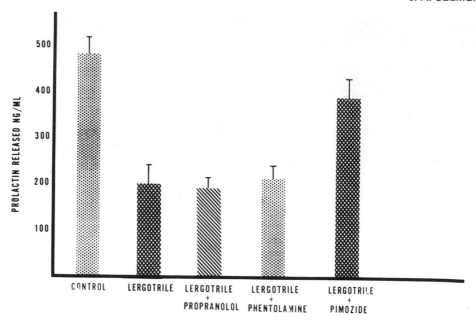

Fig. 3:   Effects of various receptor-blockers on the ability of
          lergotrile mesylate to inhibit prolactin release

al. (1974) claimed to have purified non-dopamine containing hypothalamic fractions with PIF activity.

   Neuroendocrine studies using neuropharmacological agents have
clearly demonstrated an inhibitory role for dopamine in the control
of prolactin secretion. There are several instances, however, when
surges of prolactin occur, e.g., proestrous surge, suckling-induced
surge, rise in response to stress, rise after cervical stimulation.
Little is known about the participation of dopaminergic neurons in
the initiation of these surges. We became interested in investigating the possible participation of dopamine in the surges of hormones on the afternoon of proestrus. Apomorphine appeared to be
ideal for this purpose because it is a short-acting dopamine agonist. Thus, if dopamine participated in the chain of neural events
leading up to the surge of hormones on the afternoon of proestrus,
apomorphine might be able to facilitate these events and be gone
from the system by the time of the surge. In our animal colony,
the lights are on from 4 a.m. to 6 p.m., and serum prolactin levels
are substantially elevated after 3 p.m. Normal adult female rats

with 4-day estrous cycles were chosen for experimentation on the day of proestrus. One group of rats was treated with 15.0 mg/kg of apomorphine at 12:30 p.m., another group was treated with the same dose of apomorphine at 2:30 p.m., corresponding control groups were treated with saline, and all rats were killed by decapitation at 3:30 p.m. The serum was assayed for prolactin by radioimmunoassay. The results are shown in TABLE 5.

This study provides evidence that there may be dopaminergic synapses in the CNS that facilitate or stimulate the rise of hormones on the afternoon of proestrus. In future studies, it should be possible to discover the neuronal pathways where dopamine is involved in the control of all aspects of prolactin secretion by coupling the use of proper neuropharmacological agents and neurophysiological techniques.

SEROTONIN

Not nearly as many studies implicate serotonin in the control of prolactin release as implicate dopamine. Most of the reports indicate that serotonin is stimulatory to prolactin release presumably by exerting an inhibitory influence on PIF release. Kambari et al. (1971) induced prolactin release by the injection of serotonin into the third ventricle. No effect on prolactin release was noted by Lu et al. (1970) after systemic administration of serotonin, while a significant increase in serum prolactin levels after systemic administration of serotonin was reported by Lawson and Gala (1975). It is noteworthy, however, that the difference bet-

TABLE 5. Effects of Apomorphine Administration at Different Times of Day on Serum Prolactin Levels

Treatment	Time	Serum Prolactin Levels (ng/ml) at 3:30 p.m.
Saline	12:30 p.m.	272.5 ± 15.6[a]
Apomorphine (15 mg/kg)	12:30 p.m.	443.3 ± 52.0 (p < .01)
Saline	2:30 p.m.	282.4 ± 26.7
Apomorphine (15 mg/kg)	2:30 p.m.	33.8 ± 8.8 (p < .001)

[a]Mean ± standard error

ween these two studies can be accounted for by the length of the
sampling intervals. Lawson and Gala (1975) saw the increase in
prolactin levels during the first 30 minutes, and the levels had
returned to normal at one hour which was the time the first sample
was collected by Lu et al. (1970).

Caligaris and Taleisnik (1974) reported that the serotonin
precursor, 5-hydroxytryptophan (5-HTP) as well as serotonin was
able to cause a significant rise in serum prolactin levels in estrogen-primed rats. In addition, they found that the effects of
estrogen on prolactin release could be blocked by para-chlorophe-
nylalanine. This implied that estrogen acted via serotonin neurons
to stimulate prolactin release. Interestingly, they observed that
picrotixin blocked the action of serotonin on prolactin release,
whereas strychnine was not as effective in blocking the action of
serotonin. They proposed that serotonin was acting to stimulate
an unidentified inhibitory interneuron that synapsed with the catecholamine neuron responsible for stimulating PIF release. In
view of the greater ability of picrotixin to block the increase in
serum prolactin, the identity of the inhibitory interneuron is probably a gamma-aminobutyric acid (GABA) neuron. Picrotoxin is a
more potent GABA blocking agent than strychnine. Strychnine is
mainly regarded as a glycine blocker.

More recently, Chen and Meites (1975) reported that para-chlo-
ro-amphetamine (PCA) was able to reduce serum prolactin levels in
estrogen-primed ovariectomized rats. PCA inhibits serotonin synthesis for more than a month (Fuller and Snoddy, 1974), and also
exerts a neurotoxic effect on certain serotonin neurons (Bertil-
son et al., 1975; Harvey et al., 1975). The finding that PCA was
able to inhibit prolactin secretion fits well with the concept
that serotonin neurons stimulate prolactin release, either by inhibiting PIF (dopamine?) release or by stimulating PRF release. Mac-
Indoe and Turkington (1973) reported that human prolactin secretion
was stimulated by intravenous infusions of L-tryptophan. Kato et
al. (1974) reported that 5-HTP infusion to humans results in elevated prolactin levels. Handwerger et al. (1975), however, found no
effect of 5-HTP on prolactin secretion in humans and criticized
the above human studies for being improperly controlled.

The suckling-induced rise in serum prolactin levels appears
to be dependent on serotonergic pathways. Kordon et al. (1973)
have blocked the suckling-induced rise in serum prolactin with PCPA
and Rabbi and Gallo (1975) have blocked it with methysergide.

The use of high doses of 5-HTP and PCPA may not be selective for serotonin neurons. Exogenous 5-HTP can ether catecholamine terminals, be decarboxylated to 5-HT and displace endogenous catecholamine. PCPA is a neutral amino acid and
can compete with tyrosine for uptake into catecholamine neurons

(Wurtman, 1975). One way to determine if a substance such as 5-HTP is exerting a selective effect on serotonin neurons is to adminis- ter it in animals pretreated with a compound that blocks the amine uptake pump of serotonin neurons. One such agent is Lilly 110140 (Wong et al., 1974). This compound is a more potent and specific inhibitor of serotonin uptake by serotonergic neurons in vivo in rats than is any previously known drug. Based on the assumption that reuptake is a major means by which serotonin is inactivated at the neuronal synapse, Lilly 110140 should facilitate transmis- sion via serotonergic pathways. Input through a serotonergic neu- ral system controlling prolactin release would thereby be enhanced. The serotonergic response to 5-HTP should be greatly enhanced by 110140 if the 5-HTP is exerting its effect on prolactin secretion via serotonin neurons. The following experiment was performed to determine if the elevation of serum prolactin levels observed af- ter 5-HTP was in fact due to increased serotonergic activity. A- dult female Sprague-Dawley rats were selected for experimentation on the first or second day of diestrus. The control group received saline while other groups received 5-HTP, Lilly 110140 or a combi- nation of the two compounds. In the group where the combination was used, the rats were pretreated with 10 mg/kg of Lilly 110140 (i.p.) one hour before 5-HTP treatment. In this study, a low dose of 5-HTP (30 mg/kg i.p.) was utilized. The rats were killed by decapitation one hour after 5-HTP treatment, and the serum was col- lected for radioimmunoassay of prolactin. The results of this study are shown in TABLE 6. Lilly 110140 alone was unable to change serum prolactin levels when administered to diestrous rats. The small dose of 5-HTP (30 mg/kg) was unable to elevate serum prolactin levels, but when the same dose of 5-HTP was given to rats pretreated with Lilly 110140, a dramatic rise in serum pro- lactin was observed.

These results add strong support to the hypothesis that sero- tonin neurons in the CNS are stimulatory to prolactin release. The remarkable elevation of serum prolactin seen in the rats treated with the combination of 5-HTP and Lilly 110140 could not have been due a non-specific influence of 5-HTP on non-serotonin neurons, because Lilly 110140 only inhibits uptake of amines into serotonin- ergic neurons.

Other pharmacological agents are available that one can use to study the participation of serotonin on the control of prolac- tin secretion. Two of these agents, 2-(1-piperazinyl) quinoline maleate (quipazine) and N,N-Dimethyl-5-methoxytryptamine, are ca- pable of directly stimulating serotonin receptors in the CNS. The pharmacology of quipazine was reported by Hong and Pardo (1966), and its serotonin-like action on the CNS was reported recently by Rodriguez et al. (1973). One advantage of an agent such as quipa- zine is that it can easily cross the blood-brain barrier and is not subject to metabolism by monoamine oxidase. We decided to determine the effects of quipazine on prolactin secretion in male rats. Adult male Sprague-Dawley rats were used in this study. One group of 7 rats received an i.p. injection of saline, while another group of 7 rats received an i.p. injection of 40 mg/kg of quipazine. One hour after treatment, the rats were killed by decapitation, and serum was collected and assayed for prolactin by radioimmunoassay. The results are shown in TABLE 7. Quipazine administration induced a nearly three-fold increase in serum prolactin levels one hour after treatment. This finding supplies additional evidence for the hypothesis that serotonin neurons can exert a stimulatory influence on prolactin secretion.

While investigating serotonergic influences on prolactin release, we also discovered that there can also be inhibitory influences of serotonin on prolactin release (Clemens et al., unpublished). The expression of the inhibitory influence appears to depend on the stage of the estrous cycle during which the drug is administered. Administration of Lilly 110140 to rats on the afternoon of estrous causes a dramatic reduction in serum prolactin. In conclusion, the evidence appears very convincing that serotonin neurons can exert a stimulatory influence on prolactin secretion.

TABLE 6. Effects of 5-HTP and Lilly 110140 individually or in combination on serum prolactin levels in diestrous rats

Treatment	No. of Rats	Serum Prolactin levels (ng/ml)
Saline	14	20.5 ± 1.4[a]
110140 (10 mg/kg)	9	17.5 ± 2.0
Saline	7	14.3 ± 1.8
5-HTP (30 mg/kg)	7	18.2 ± 4.8
5-HTP (30 mg/kg)	7	205.8 ± 24.1
110140 (10 mg/kg)		(p < .001)

[a]Mean   standard error

TABLE 7. Effects of quipazine on serum prolactin levels in male rats

Treatment	Number of Rats	Serum Prolactin Levels (ng/ml)
Saline	7	16.3 ± 2.5[a]
Quipazine	7	45.1 ± 8.4 ($p < .01$)

[a]Mean ± standard error

NOREPINEPHRINE AND ACETYLCHOLINE

Very little is presently known about the participation of norepinephrine in the control of prolactin secretion. Disulfiram,
a drug that inhibits norepinephrine synthesis, reduced serum prolactin levels in rats (Clemens et al., unpublished). Donoso et al.
(1971) presented evidence that norepinephrine may act to increase
prolactin release. They found that administration of L-DOPS to
rats treated with α-methyl-p-tyrosine increased serum prolactin levels to a greater extent than α-methyl-p-tyrosine increased serum
prolactin levels to a greater extent than α-methyl-p-tyrosine alone. Recently, Wuttke and Fenske (1974) reported that prolactin levels were elevated for several days after 7-hydroxydopamine administration, but were depressed 37 and 71 days after treatment. More
work needs to be done with specific alpha agonists and antagonists
before the role of norepinephrine in the control of prolactin secretion can be determined.

Grandison et al. (1974) presented convincing evidence that
acetylcholine was involved in the regulation of prolactin release.
Cholinergic agonists and cholinesterase inhibitors decreased serum
prolactin levels. They suggested that acetylcholine may act on the
dopaminergic nerve endings in the median eminence to promote dopamine release or may possibly act on the anterior pituitary. Libertun and McCann (1974) reported similar findings with cholinergic
agonists and cholinesterase inhibitors, but several hours after
the initial depression, a significant stimulation of prolactin re-

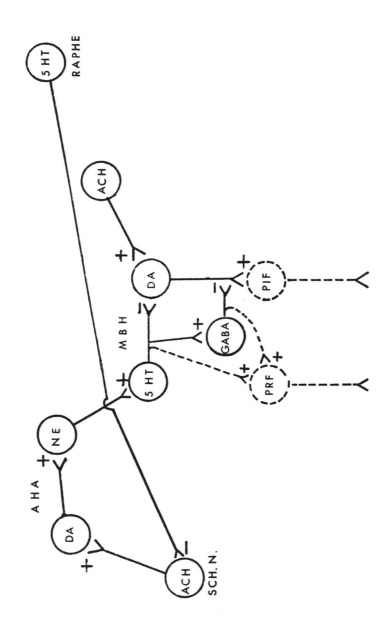

Figure 4.   Hypothetical neuronal network for the control of the tonic and cyclic components of prolactin release. Tonic components are in the medial basal hypothalamus (MBH). DA = dopamine, NE = norepinephrine, ACH = acetylcholine, 5 HT = serotonin, SCH.N. = suprachiasmatic nucleus, AHA - anterior hypothalamic area.

lease occurred. They suggested that the elevation in serum prolactin levels several hours after cholinergic agonists appeared to be
triggered by a circadian clock mechanism. They concluded that cholinergic drugs may sensitize the animals so that the firing of the
cyclic clock mechanism precipitates hormonal discharge. Much more
work needs to be done in the area of cholinergic influences on prolactin release before we can begin to understand how the cholinergic system influences or is influenced by serotonergic, adrenergic
or dopaminergic systems also involved in the regulation of prolactin secretion.

SUMMARY

The use of neuropharmacological agents in neuroendocrine studies has had a significant impact on our knowledge about the neurotransmitter systems that are involved in the control of prolactin
secretion. Selective drugs have played a key role in the identification of the dopaminergic inhibitory and serotonergic stimulatory
influences. With the development of additional specific neuropharmacological agents in the future, we can expect to gain a better
understanding of the complex neural interrelationships involved in
the control of anterior pituitary hormone secretion.

In view of what we already know about the neurotransmitters
involved in the control of prolactin release, a tentative neuronal
configuration can be proposed. The following neuronal network
most probably does not include several components that may be shown
by future studies to be involved in prolactin control, but it does
represent a possible functional network based on what knowledge is
at the present time (Fig. 4).

REFERENCES

1. Ben-David, M., Davon, A., Benveniste, R., Weller, C.P. and
    and Sulman, F.G.(1971) J. Endocrinol. 50, 599-606.

2. Bertilsson, L., Koslow, S. and Costa, E. (1975) Brain
    Research 91, 348-350.

3. Besser, G.M., Parke, L., Edwards, C.R.W., Forsyth, I.A. and
    McNeilly, A.S. (1972) Brit. Med. J. 3(5828), 669-672.

4. BrunDelRe, R., del Pozo, E., de Grandi, P., Friesen, H.,
    Hinselmann, M. and Wyss, H. (1973) Ob. Gyn. 41, 884-890.

5. Caligaris, L. and Taleisnik, S. (1974) J. Endocrinol. 62,
    25-33.

6. Cassady, J.M., Li, G., Spitzner, E., Floss, H. and Clemens,
    J.A. (1974) J. Med. Chem. 17, 300-307.

7. Chen, H. J. and Meites, J. (1975) Endocrinology 96, 10-14.

8. Clemens, J.A., Smalstig, E. B and Sawyer, B.D. (1974)
    Psychopharmacologia 40, 123-127.

9. DelPozo, E., Friesen, H. and Burmeister, P. (1973) Schweig.
    Med. Wschr. 103, 847-848.

10. DelPozo, E., Brun del Re, R., Varga,L. and Friesen, H. (1972)
    J. Clin. Endocrinol. Metab. 35, 768-771.

11. Dickerman, S.,Clark, J. Dickerman, E. and Meites, J. (1972)
    Neuroendocrinology 9, 332-340.

12. Donoso, A.O., Bishop, W., Fawcett, C.P., Krulich, L. and
    McCann, S.M. (1971) Endocrinology 89, 774-784.

13. Dupont, A. and Redding, T.W. (1975) Program of the 57th
    Meeting of the Endocrine Society, New York, Abstract No. 85.

14. Ferrini, R. and Miragoli (1972) Pharmacol. Res. Commun. 4,
    347-352.

15. Fuller, R. W., and Snoddy, H. D. (1974) Neuropharmacology 13,
    85-90.

16. Greibrokk, T., Currie, B.L. Johnansson, K.N.G., Hansen, J.J.,
    Folkers, K. and Bowers, C. Y. (1974) Biochem. Biophys. Res.
    Commun. 59, 704-709.

17. Handwerger, S., Plank, J.W., Lebowitz, H. E., Bivens, C. H. and Feldman, J. U. (1975) Horm. Metab. Res. 7, 214-216.

18. Harvey, J. A., McMaster, S.E. and Yunger, L.M. (1975) Science 187, 841-843.

19. Kambari, I. A., Mical, R.S. and Porter (1971) Endocrinology 88, 1288-1293.

20. Kato, Y., Nakai, Y., Imura, H., Chihara, K. and Ohgo, S. (1974) J. Clin. Endocrinol. Metab. 38, 695-697.

21. Kleinberg, D.L., Noel, G.L. and Frantz, A.G. (1971) J. Clin. Endocrinol. Metab. 33, 873-876.

22. Koch, Y, Lu,K.H. and Meites, J. (1970) Endocrinology 87, 673-675.

23. Kordon, E., Blake, C.A., Terkel, J. and Sawyer, C. H. (1973) Neuroendocrinology 13, 213-223.

24. Lal. S., Sourkes, T. L., Misscala, K. and Belendkink, G. (1972) Europ. J. Pharmacol. 20, 71-80.

25. Lawson, D.M. and Gala, R.R. (1975) Endocrinology 96, 313-318.

26. Lemberger, L., Crabtree, R., Clemens, J., Dyke, R. and Woodburne (1974) J. Clin. Endocrinol. Metab. 39, 579-584.

27. Lu, K. H., Amenomori, Y., Chen, C. L. and Meites, J. (1970) Endocrinology 87, 667-672.

28. Lu, K. H. and Meites, J. (1971) Proc. Soc. Exp. Biol. Med. 137, 480-483.

29. MacLeod, R. M. and Lehmeyer, J. E. (1974) Endocrinology 94, 1077-1085.

30. Malven, P. R. and Hoge, W. R. (1971) Endocrinology 88, 445-449.

31. Martin, J. B., Lal, S., Tolis, G. and Friesen, H. (1974) J. Clin. Endocrinol. Metab. 39, 180-182.

32. Mayer, P. and Schütze, E. (1973) Experentia 29, 484-485.

33. Nagasawa, H. and Meites, J.(1970) Proc. Soc. Exp. Biol. Med. 135, 469-472.

34. Nicoll, C.S., Yaron, Z., Nutt, N. and Daniels, E. (1970) Biology of Reproductive 5, 59-66.

EPISODIC GH SECRETION: EVIDENCE FOR A HYPOTHALAMIC DOPAMINERGIC

MECHANISM

John O. Willoughby and Joseph B. Martin

Division of Neurology, Department of Medicine

Montreal General Hospital, McGill University, Montreal

HUMAN ANTERIOR PITUITARY HORMONE SECRETION

With the development of specific radioimmunoassays for human anterior pituitary (AP) hormones, it became apparent that concentrations of the various hormones in random blood samples often varied widely. It was subsequently recognized by frequent sampling, that blood levels of the AP hormones fluctuated abruptly. This phenomenon, originally described for growth hormone (GH) and adrenocorticotrophic hormone (ACTH) is also demonstrated by other AP hormones, and is presumed to be due to intermittent rather than continuous hormonal secretion. Abrupt changes in hormonal clearance rate, peripheral storage, or excretion which might contribute to such a phenomenon have not been sought extensively, but would appear to be unlikely factors.

The daily pattern of human GH (h-GH) secretion was first described in 1966 (Quabbe et al., 1966). Sporadic daytime bursts with unmeasurable interval levels, and prominent secretory episodes shortly after sleep onset were described. Large h-GH secretory episodes during waking hours have also been demonstrated in fasted (Glick and Goldsmith, 1968) and adolescent (Finkelstein et al., 1972) subjects. The major h-GH secretory episodes which follow sleep onset are dependent on it (Takahashi et al., 1968; Honda et al., 1969; Parker et al., 1969) but their relationship to slow wave sleep is not completely established.

ACTH (h-ACTH) secretory profiles obtained in human subjects using a 5 minute sampling frequency dramatically demonstrate the phenomenon of pulsatile release and enable close correlation with

concurrent cortisol levels (Gallagher et al., 1973). Typically,
h-ACTH levels rise abruptly from unmeasurable values to produce
secretory episodes of varying sizes. A change in the frequency
and size of h-ACTH secretory episodes determines the diurnal pattern of episodic cortisol secretion concurrently observed (Gallagher et al., 1973). This variation in daily cortisol secretion
has been shown to persist in sleep deprived subjects but to syn-
chronise in several days with reversed sleep patterns (Hellman
et al., 1970).

Human prolactin (h-PRL) levels fluctuate continually though-
out the day and night (Sassin et al., 1972) and also exhibit
secretory bursts related to Rapid Eye Movement (REM) - NonREM sleep
cycles (Parker et al., 1973) although evidence on this point is
not completely consistent (Vanhaelst et al., 1973).

Human Follicle Stimulating Hormone (h-FSH) and luteinizing
hormone (h-LH) both fluctuate continually, apparently independently
and without a definite 24 hour variation (Krieger et al., 1972).
However, in pubertal subjects LH exhibits a definite sleep associated rise related to REM-NonREM sleep cycles (Boyar et al.,
1972a). An 18% increase in h-LH during REM sleep has been reported
in adults, but there is some conflicting evidence (Rubin et al.,
1972; Boyar et al., 1972b).

Human thyroid stimulating hormone (h-TSH) displays only small
fluctuations throughout the day, but some individuals do demonstrate prominent nocturnal secretory episodes usually between 0300
and 0700 hours. However, there is no clear 24 hour variation
(Vanhaelst et al., 1973).

Thus, while all human AP hormones exhibit physiological pulsatile release on some occasions, for h-ACTH, h-GH, possibly h-PRL,
and h-LH, hormone release occurs entirely in episodic bursts. The
more broadly based variations in AP hormone secretion (diurnal,
sleep related, and reproductive cyclic variations) probably represent superimposed neural and hormonal influences on this basic
secretory mechanism.

ANTERIOR PITUITARY HORMONE SECRETION IN EXPERIMENTAL ANIMALS

The application of frequent sequential blood sampling methods
to experimental animals followed recognition that human AP hormones exhibited pulsatile release.

Circhoral (about 1 hour) oscillations of LH levels have been
described in ovariectomised monkeys (Dierschke et al., 1970) and
ewes (Nett et al., 1974), while pulsatile secretion of LH and FSH

occurs in castrated male and female rats (Gay and Sheth, 1972).
In our laboratory, episodic release of PRL and TSH has been demonstrated in the rat (unpublished observations).

For GH, data in laboratory animals is abundant. Pulsatile
release of GH has been demonstrated in rat (Martin et al., 1974;
Tannenbaum and Martin, 1975a; Tannenbaum, 1975), rabbit (McIntyre
and Odell, 1974), rhesus monkey (Sassin et al., 1971), and baboon
(Parker et al., 1972), while strongly suggestive evidence is
available for the mouse (Schindler et al., 1972).

In addition to demonstrated pulsatile release of AP hormones
in animals, more broadly based variations are evident in the
oestrus cycle surges of PRL and LH (Neill, 1972), the diurnal
rhythm of corticosterone, and sleep related GH release in the
baboon (Parker et al., 1972), while non-episodic secretion is
likely to be an additional mechanism for some hormones.

GROWTH HORMONE SECRETION IN THE RAT

In the studies to be described, an experimental design was
used which permitted frequent removal of blood samples from un-
disturbed animals. Results indicate that physiological r-GH
secretion in this species is entirely episodic, and that the
phenomenon depends on a hypothalamic mechanism.

Male 350-450 g Sprague-Dawley rats were prepared after the
method of Brown and Hedge (1972) with right atrial cannulae
exteriorised through an acrylic headpiece. Animals were subsequently adapted to sampling cages which were contained within
isolation boxes, arranged so that tubing attached to the cannula
opening on the headpiece could be led to the outside through a
swivel-mounted flexible steel spring. Using this system, and with
reinjection of red cells resuspended in 0.9% saline replacing
plasma removed, it was possible to withdraw blood at 15 minute
intervals for up to 24 hours without stress effects, or to sample
the same animal on several occasions. Plasma samples were subsequently analysed for r-GH by radioimmunoassay using materials
supplied by NIAMDD.

Using this model, pulsatile secretion of r-GH was first described in 1974 (Martin et al., 1974), and evidence for a hypothalamic mechanism was presented (see below). Subsequent investigation has revealed that secretory episodes usually contain
2 or 3 peaks and often exceed 200 ng/ml while trough values are
unmeasurable often for longer than 1 hour. Tannenbaum and Martin
(1975b) have recently determined that the mean periodicity of

secretory episodes is 3.3 hours. A representative 24 hour r-GH
profile obtained from 1 rat is shown in Figure 1, and agrees with
the earlier observations of Tannenbaum and Martin (1975b). Secretory episodes consist of an abrupt rise of r-GH from unmeasurable
levels to over 200 ng/ml. Often 2 or 3 peaks are contained within
an episode, and r-GH levels decline at a rate consistent with the
half-life of r-GH in this species (Frohman and Bernardis, 1970).

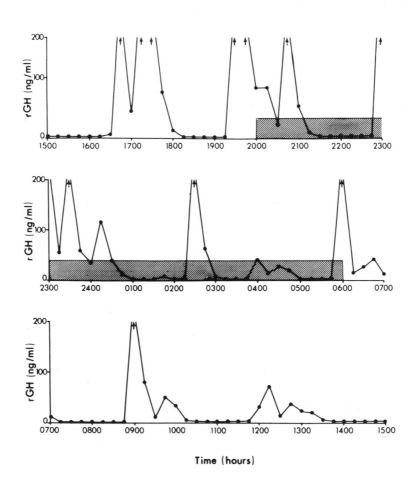

Time (hours)

Figure 1 : A 24 hour r-GH profile obtained from one chronically
cannulated rat aged 4-5 months utilising a 15 minute
sampling frequency. In this and subsequent figures,
the shaded area indicates the period of darkness, and
values over 200 ng/ml are indicated by arrows, the
maximum sensitivity of the assay, unless plasma was
available for further determinations.

In the present experiments, segments of this basic ultradian
rhythm have been examined, usually for 5 or 6 hour periods. From
time to time, criticism has been made that animals in this experimental situation are stressed, and that the long duration of trough
periods (when r-GH is unmeasurable) might thus be explained. Although the reproducability and persistence of the rhythm suggest
that stress plays no part in the maintenance of trough values,
further evidence in support of this view was sought. Concurrent
corticosterone and GH profiles were obtained in 6 chronically cannulated rats, sampled from 1500 to 2015 hours, so that the time of
the normal diurnal rise in corticosterone would be encompassed.

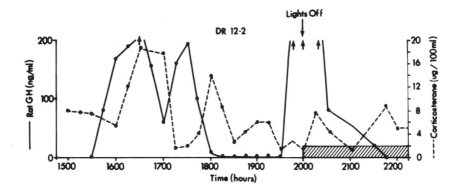

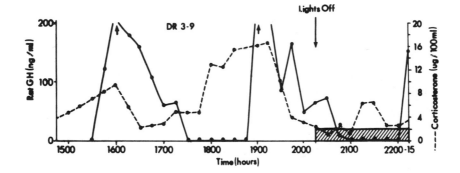

Figure 2 (a) & (b) : Concurrent r-GH and corticosterone profiles
           from 2 animals covering late afternoon and commencement
           of the dark period. Characteristic GH secretory pro-
           files are evident, together with bursts of corticoster-
           one secretion tending to be most prominent in the late
           afternoon.

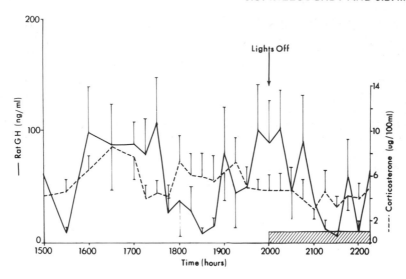

Figure 2 (c) : Concurrent mean r-GH and corticosterone values in 6
        rats sampled from 1500 - 2015 hours. The standard error
        of each mean is indicated by a vertical bar. Mean r-GH
        values fluctuate with approximately a 3 hour periodicity
        and a peak occurs at "lights off". Corticosterone mean
        values rise in the late afternoon, compatible with the
        normal diurnal rise.

Results from 2 animals are shown in Figure 2a and 2b, and the
group data in 2c. Individual and average r-GH profiles show a
periodicity of r-GH secretion of approximately 3 hours and the
occurrence of a peak at "lights off" as previously reported by
Tannenbaum and Martin,(1975b). Corticosterone levels show a
tendency to continuous pulsatile secretion, an afternoon rise and
an absence of sustained high levels normally associated with
stress. Moreover, r-GH trough values and corticosterone secretory episodes appear to be independent.

    In further experiments, the precise relationship of r-GH pro-
files to the commencement of the light period was examined. Figure 3a shows 7 r-GH secretory profiles from a group of 9 rats in
which a definite fall of r-GH from peak values is evident, com-
mencing just before "lights on". The other two rats had slightly
different profiles; only one rat which had unmeasurable values at
0600 hours failed to demonstrate a "lights on" effect. Mean r-GH
values obtained from this group are shown in Figure 3b; again the
effect of the commencement of the light period is seen together
with a recurrence of peak or trough levels approximately every 3
hours.

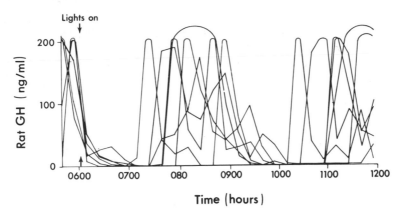

Figure 3 (a) : R-GH secretory profiles from 7 rats, sampled from
before the commencement of the light period. One of 2
other rats with slightly different profiles failed to
demonstrate a fall in r-GH levels preceding "lights on"
(see text). Peaks exceeding 200 ng/ml are indicated by
arcs.

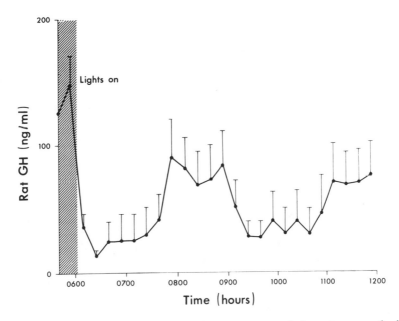

Figure 3 (b) : Mean r-GH values in a group of 9 rats sampled from
0540 to 1155 hours. A crisp depression of mean r-GH
values precedes the occurrence of "lights on" demonstrating entrainment the ultradian r-GH rhythm to the light
dark cycle; a variation of mean values with a periodicity
of approximately 3 hours is also demonstrated.

Because the occurrence of a peak followed by an abrupt decline
of r-GH levels preceded the commencement of the light period in all
but one rat, the effect of blinding on this secretory pattern was
determined. Rats blinded by orbital enucleation for six weeks were
sampled from 0540 to 1155 hours. While all rats demonstrated r-GH
secretory episodes usually exceeding 200 ng/ml, and with a periodicity of about 3 hours, only 2 of 8 rats retained an apparent
"lights on" effect. The profile of mean r-GH values in this group
of 8 rats is shown in Figure 4. The mean values are similar to
those in normal rats and the commencement of the light period no
longer is preceded by a definite decline of GH values. Some suggestion of a 3 hourly variation in mean r-GH values persists and
may have resulted from the entraining effect of the normal daily
activity patterns of intact rats which were housed in the same
room as the blind animals.

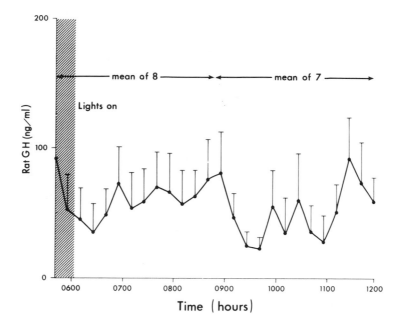

Figure 4 : Mean r-GH values from blinded rats sampled from 0540 to
           1155 hours. The definite decline in mean r-GH values
           preceding "lights on" in normal rats is no longer evi-
           dent; instead an attenuated 3 hourly periodicity of
           mean r-GH values persists.

To determine other factors that might influence r-GH secretion, studies were performed in mature, young and aged rats, seek-
ing evidence for an age related alteration in r-GH secretion.
R-GH profiles in these animals suggest that basically similar

secretory patterns occur, as judged by inspection of 5 hour r-GH
profiles.   Figures 5a and 5b show secretory profiles from 150 and
750 g rats, respectively 44 days and 1.5 years of age.   Figure 1
shows a 24 hour r-GH secretory profiles from a 4.5 months old rat.
Although the complexity and duration of secretory episodes vary in
these animals, trough values are unmeasurable, r-GH secretory episodes occur 3 hourly, and peaks generally exceed 200 ng/ml.   A
careful analysis of 24 hour profiles would be necessary to defin-
itively indicate ontogenic changes.

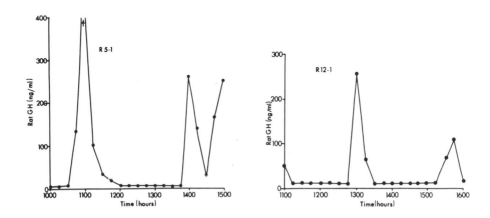

Figure 5 (a) & (b) : 5 hour r-GH secretory profiles from 44 day
          old and 1.5 year old rats, respectively, demonstrating
          the similar frequency of secretory profiles from rats of
          very different ages.   See also Figure 1.

As there is sleep augmentation of GH secretion in humans and
some laboratory primates, the possibility that sleep periods in
the rat might influence r-GH values was examined in chronically
cannulated rats implanted with EEG, EMG, and electro-oculographic
electrodes (Willoughby et al., 1975).   R-GH values during secretory episodes and troughs were found to be unrelated either to
sleep cycles, wakefulness, or preceding slow wave sleep duration.
Like GH secretion in the rhesus monkey, r-GH secretion seems independent of sleep/wake activity.

Dietary and metabolic factors such as hypoglycemia, hyperglycemia, and fasting up to 24 hours also have little effect on r-GH
secretory profiles (Tannenbaum and Martin, 1975c).

It appeared likely from the regularity of the r-GH ultradian
rhythm, its entrainment to the light dark cycle, and the lack of a

significant non-stressful influence upon it, that the phenomenon
was subserved by a neural mechanism. Further investigation has
therefore attempted to locate such a neural substrate.

    As originally described (Martin et al., 1974), hypothalamic
lesions abolish or impair r-GH secretory episodes. Subsequently,
more detailed studies have shown that large lesions in the ventro-
medial nucleus of the hypothalamus (VMH) which extend outside the
limits of this nucleus are required to abolish pulsatile r-GH
secretion completely; animals with lesions restricted to the VMH
demonstrate only impaired pulsatile GH secretion.

    Because there was a dramatic effect of large VMH lesions on
pulsatile r-GH secretion, recent experiments have investigated the
effects of Halász hypothalamic cuts on the secretory pattern.
Preliminary data confirms the original view of Halász et
al.,(1971) that isolation of the medial basal hypothalamus per-
mits continued secretion of r-GH. Five hour r-GH profiles from
rats with complete hypothalamic islands are shown in Figures 6a,
6b, and 6c. Secretory episodes persist despite the severe hydro-
cephalus present and small extent of the functional island remaining (Figure 7). However, some disturbance in r-GH control is apparent in these animals; secretory episodes appear briefer, and
although a 3 hour periodicity may be approximated for major secretory episodes, more frequent pulses of altered amplitude have also
been demonstrated. Elevated trough levels have been observed occasionally, but not consistently, even in the same animal.

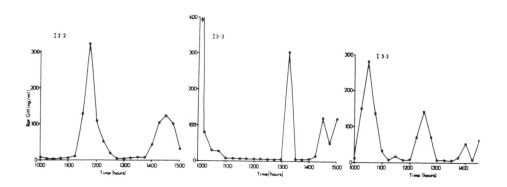

Figure 6 (a), (b), & (c) : Three r-GH secretory profiles from rats
         with complete hypothalamic deafferentation. More fre-
         quent secretory episodes appear in (b) & (c) than are
         normally seen, although the profile in (a) appears
         nearly normal.

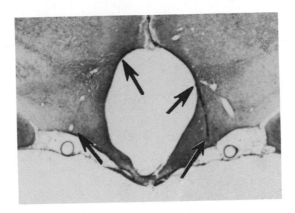

Figure 7 : Photo-micrograph of a coronal section through the hypothalamus of rat I3, whose GH profile appears in 6 (b).
There is severe dilatation of the III ventricle, and
the knife cuts are indicated by arrows (age of knife
cut - 8 weeks).

The literature on pharmacological studies of r-GH secretion
is extensive and often contradictory, and there have been no
studies on the pharmacology of physiological r-GH secretion. In
the following experiments, chronically cannulated animals were pretreated with alpha-methyl-para-tyrosine (αMT), para-chlorophenyla-
lanine (PCPA) or normal saline (Saline) and r-GH profiles obtained.
Dosages, timings, and routes of administration of the drugs are
shown in Table I.

TABLE I

Treatment	Dosage	Route	Pretreatment Interval
None	–	–	–
Saline	0.5 ml	I.P.[1]	60-90 mins
αMT	250 mg/kg	I.P.	60-120 mins
PCPA	350 mg/kg	I.P.	18 hours

[1] Intraperitoneal

TABLE II

Treatment	No. of rats	Mean GH level±SEM[1]	p value[2]
None	10	54.2±4.1	N.S.
Saline	10	58.8±6	–
αMT	10	21.8±7.5	p<.01
PCPA	10	27.8±6.9	p<.01

[1] Standard error of the mean
[2] Significance of difference compared to saline-treated group, determined by t-test.

Animals tolerated saline and αMT treatments well, and appeared in good health; however, most animals became drowsy, inactive and lost weight following PCPA administration, and some died 2 or 3 days after sampling. Both drug-treated groups contained animals with unmeasurable r-GH levels throughout the entire sampling period and also some animals with apparently normal r-GH secretory profiles. So that the effects of these treatments on r-GH secretion could be assessed, the largest area measured by planimetry under a 3-hour segment of each 5 hour r-GH profile was used, and the mean r-GH levels thus obtained for each group were compared by t-test. A 3 hour segment was chosen because normal r-GH secretory episodes have a 3 hour periodicity and therefore it provides a guide to total 24 hour r-GH secretion. As shown in Table II, both drug treated groups demonstrated significantly lower mean r-GH values than the saline treated group. Thus, αMT, and possibly PCPA, significantly impair pulsatile GH secretion.

CONCLUSIONS

Physiological r-GH secretion in the male rat is characterized by periodic secretory episodes containing 1 to 3 peaks which commence abruptly, usually exceed 200 ng/ml in magnitude, and are separated by troughs lasting 1 to 2 hours when r-GH is unmeasurable. It has been established by Tannenbaum and Martin (1975b) that episodes occur with a 3.3 hour periodicity. Because r-GH secretory episodes vary in size, 24 hour r-GH profiles would be required to compare groups of experimental animals reliably. However, 24 hour sampling is impractical, and animals have been considered to secrete r-GH normally if a 5 to 6 hour sampling period shows r-GH peaks exceeding 200 ng/ml, trough levels that are unmeasurable, and when 2 secretory episodes are obtained,

evidence of a 3 hour periodicity. Using these criteria, the same
r-GH secretory pattern is present in young mature (44-day old) as
well as old mature (1.5-year old) male rats, and it would therefore appear to be the fundamental secretory pattern in these
animals. Previous attempts to define circadian, nyctohemeral or
ultradian patterns have used decapitated rat data obtained at
widely spaced intervals, usually 3 to 4 hours, and consequently
conclusions have only occasionally been relevant to normal r-GH
secretory physiology. Previous workers have defined periodic
fluctuations of mean r-GH levels (Dunn et al., 1973); relatively
constant random mean r-GH levels in rats older than 20 days have
also been documented (Blázquez et al., 1974).

Tannenbaum and Martin (1975b) have demonstrated randomisation
of 3 hour secretory episodes between rats maintained in isolation
in constant light, and the present results in blinded animals also
confirm that the ultradian rhythm is entrained to the light-dark
cycle.

The findings of normal r-GH secretory profiles and similar
mean plasma r-GH levels in blinded and normal mature male rats is
in substantial agreement with the findings of Sorrentino et al.
(1971) in their study on the effects of blinding, and other sensory
deprivations on growth in rats. They found only a slight reduction
in the rate of body weight increase, and no change in mean r-GH
levels (approx. 45 ng/ml), although pituitary GH contents were reduced. While the reduced growth rate and plasma and pituitary
r-GH levels produced a blinding or constant darkness in young rats
is reversed by pinealectomy (Sorrentino et al., 1971; Relkin,
1972), a role for the pineal gland in the reduction of light-onset
r-GH levels seems unlikely. Firstly, r-GH levels usually decline
from peak levels before the occurrence of "lights on", and in any
case, pineal gland function is usually inhibited by the light period. Entrainment of the r-GH ultradian rhythm to the light-dark
cycle is suggested therefore, rather than light triggered suppression of r-GH secretion.

Earlier work implicating the VMH in the initiation of secretory episodes is supported by the persistence of episodic secretion of r-GH in animals with hypothalamic islands. Taken in conjunction with the pharmacological studies, strong evidence emerges
for a facilitatory dopaminergic mechansim for r-GH release in the
rat. Specifically, αMT (which depletes central norepinephrine and
dopamine) impaired pulsatile r-GH secretion. Hypothalamic deafferentation as reported by Weiner (1973) results in unmeasurable
hypothalamic norepinephrine levels and normal dopamine levels.
Such islands permitted persistent episodic r-GH secretion, thus
strongly implicating the dopaminergic neurons remaining in the
medial basal hypothalamus in the episodic secretory mechanism.

The possibility that deafferentation of the medial basal hypothalamus removes inhibitory neural influences (Mitchell et al., 1973)
is lent some support by the finding of an increase in frequency of
secretory episodes in some rats, although correlation of r-GH profiles with growth rates has not yet been obtained.

Interpretation of the results of PCPA administration needs to
be cautious. Unhealthy animals generally secrete r-GH abnormally,
viz secretory episodes tend to be lower and more frequent and occasionally r-GH levels remain unmeasurable throughout. Thus, the
non-specific or "stress" effects of PCPA injection may explain the
reduced r-GH mean values in this group. However, a facilitatory
serotoninergic mechanism for r-GH secretion in the rat is not excluded by the present data, and they would support the findings of
other workers (Collu et al., 1972; Smythe et al., 1975). Because
episodic r-GH secretion persists in rats with hypothalamic islands
where hypothalamic serotonin levels are significantly reduced
(Weiner, 1973) any role that extrahypothalamic serotoninergic afferents have in pulsatile r-GH secretion is likely to be only
modulatory. Further experiments using lower dosages of PCPA and
examination of brain serotonin levels will be necessary to resolve
its role more accurately.

Although stress-sensitive, the generally unvarying nature of
pulsatile r-GH secretion in the male rat is indicative of its
fundamental nature. While hypothalamic islands maintain pituitary
function and responsiveness to some stimuli in rat (Halász and
Pupp, 1965) and rhesus monkey (Krey et al., 1975a; Krey et al.,
1975b; Butler et al., 1975a; Butler et al., 1975b), pulsatile release of FSH and LH has also been demonstrated in ovariectomised
monkeys (Krey et al., 1975a) and rats (Blake and Sawyer, 1974)
with hypothalamic islands. These observations together with the
present findings on pulsatile r-GH release, indicate that neural
mechanisms in the medial basal hypothalamus are sufficient for
episodic AP hormone release. However, AP hormone fluctuations occurring as a result of longer endogenous rhythms (diurnal, oestrus
cycle, etc.) usually depend on extrahypothalamic inputs for their
maintenance (Halász and Pupp, 1965; Krey et al., 1975b; Halász et
al., 1967).

It is evident from the studies of Blake and Sawyer (1974)
that the periodicity of LH surges in ovariectomised rats bearing
hypothalamic islands is 20 - 30 minutes. In the present studies,
episodic GH secretion occurred no more often than 1 hourly,
usually 2 - 3 hourly. Concurrent PRL measurements in our rats
(unpublished observations) indicate that episodic r-PRL secretion persists, independent of r-GH. Thus, the isolated medial
basal hypothalamus supports intermittent secretion of r-LH,
r-GH and r-PRL and with different inherent rhythms. It can there-

fore be hypothesised that this small area of neural tissue contains a number of independent hypothalamic pacemakers.

Pulsatile GH secretion is present in many species and supportive evidence is accumulating for such a phenomenon for other AP hormones. Further electrophysiological and pharmacological investigation of the medial basal hypothalamus will be valuable in understanding the neural mechanisms that subserve these intrinsic biological rhythms.

ACKNOWLEDGEMENTS

The authors wish to thank Adah Saunders and Judy Audet for technical assistance and Gail Hannaford for secretarial help. The Hormone Distribution Officer, NIAMD, Bethesda, Maryland, generously supplied radioimmunoassay materials. John O. Willoughby is a Medical Research Council of Canada Fellow and Joseph B. Martin is an M.R.C. Associate. Supported by grant MA 3967 from the Medical Research Council of Canada.

REFERENCES

1. Blake, C.A. and Sawyer, C.H. (1974) Endocrinology 94, 730-736.

2. Blázquez, E., Simon, F.A., Blázquez, M. and Foà, P.P. (1974) Proc. Soc. Exp. Biol. Med. 147, 780-783.

3. Boyar, R.M., Finkelstein, J.W., Roffwarg, H., Kapen, S., Weitzman, E.D. and Hellman, H. (1972a) New Engl. J. Med. 287, 582-586.

4. Boyar, R., Perlow, M., Hellman, L., Kapen, S. and Weitzman, E. (1972b) J. Clin. Endocrinol. Metab. 35, 73-81.

5. Brown, M.R. and Hedge, G.A. (1972) Neuroendocrinology 9, 158-174.

6. Butler, W.R., Krey, L.C., Espinosa-Campos, J. and Knobil, E. (1975a) Endocrinology 96, 1094-1098.

7. Butler, W.R., Krey, L.C., Lu, K.H., Peckham, W.D. and Knobil, E. (1975b) Endocrinology 96, 1099-1105.

8. Collu, R., Fraschini, F., Visconti, P. and Martini, L. (1972) Endocrinology 90, 1231-1237.

9. Dierschke, D.J., Battacharya, A.N., Atkinson, L.E. and Knobil, E. (1970) Endocrinology 87, 850-853.

10. Dunn, J.D., Schindler, W.J., Hutchins, M.D., Scheving, L.E. and Turpen, C. (1973) Neuroendocrinology 13, 69-78.

11. Finkelstein, J.W., Roffwarg, H.P., Boyar, R.M., Kream, J. and Hellman, L. (1972) J. Clin. Endocrinol. Metab. 35, 665-670.

12. Frohman, L.A. and Bernardis, L.L. (1970) Endocrinology 86, 305-312.

13. Gallagher, T.F., Yoshida, K., Roffwarg, H.D., Fukushima, D.K., Weitzman, E.D. and Hellman, L. (1973) J. Clin. Endocrinol. Metab. 36, 1058-1073.

14. Gay, V.L. and Sheth, N.A. (1972) Endocrinology 90, 158-162.

15. Glick, S.M. and Goldsmith, S. (1968) In: Growth Hormone (A. Pecile and E.E. Müller, eds.) I.C.S. 158, Excerpta Medica, Amsterdam, pp 84-88.

16. Halász, B. and Pupp, L. (1965) Endocrinology 77, 553-562.

17. Halász, B., Slusher, M.A. and Gorski, R.A. (1967) Neuro-endocrinology 2, 43-55.

18. Halász, B., Schalch, D.S., and Gorski, R.A. (1971) Endo-crinology 89, 198-203.

19. Hellman, L., Nakada, F., Curti, J., Weitzman, E.D., Kream, J., Roffwarg, H., Ellman, S., Fukushima, D.K. and Gallagher, T.F. (1970) J. Clin. Endocrinol. Metab. 30, 411-422.

20. Honda, Y., Takahashi, K., Takahashi, S., Azumi, K., Irie, M., Sakuma, M., Tsushima, T. and Shizumi, K. (1969) J. Clin. Endocrinol. Metab. 29, 20-29.

21. Krey, L.C., Butler, W.R. and Knobil, E. (1975a) Endocrinology 96, 1073-1087.

22. Krey, L.C., Lu, K-H., Butler, W.R., Hotchkiss, J., Piva, F. and Knobil, E. (1975b) Endocrinology 96, 1088-1093.

23. Krieger, D.T., Ossowski, R., Fogel, M. and Allen, W. (1972) J. Clin. Endocrinol. Metab. 35, 619-623.

24. MacIntyre, H.B. and Odell, W.D. (1974) Neuroendocrinology 16, 8-21.

25. Martin, J.B., Renaud, L.P. and Brazeau, P. (1974) Science 186, 538-540.

26. Mitchell, J.A., Hutchins, M., Schindler, W.J. and Critchlow, V. (1973) Neuroendocrinology 12, 161-173.

27. Neill, J.D. (1972) Endocrinology 90, 568-572.

28. Nett, T.M., Akbar, A.M. and Niswender, G.D. (1974) Endocrinology 94, 713-718.

29. Parker, D.C., Sassin, J.F., Mace, J.W., Gotlin, R.W. and Rossman, L.G. (1969) J. Clin. Endocrinol. Metab. 29, 871-874.

30. Parker, D.C., Morishima, M., Koerker, D.J., Gale, C.C. and Goodner, C.J. (1972) Endocrinology 91, 1462-1467.

31. Parker, D.C., Rossman, L.G. and Vanderlaan, E.F. (1973) J. Clin. Endocrinol. Metab. 38, 646-651.

32. Quabbé, H-J., Schilling, E. and Helge, H. (1966) J. Clin. Endocrinol. Metab. 26, 1173-1177.

33. Relkin, R. (1972) J. Endocrinol. 53, 289-293.

34. Rubin, R.T., Kales, A., Adler, R., Fagan, T. and Odell, W. (1972) Science 175, 196-198.

35. Sassin, J., Jacoby, J.H., Finkelstein, J., Fukushima, D. and Weitzman, E. (1971) Neurology 21, 431-432.

36. Sassin, J.F., Frantz, A.G., Weitzman, E.D. and Kapen, S. (1972) Science 177, 1205-1207.

37. Schindler, W.J., Hutchins, M.O. and Septimus, E.J. (1972) Endocrinology 91, 483-490.

38. Smythe, G.A., Brandstater, J.F. and Lazarus, L. (1975) Neuroendocrinology 17, 245-257.

39. Sorrentino, S., Schalch, D.S. and Reiter, R.J. (1971) In: Growth and Growth Hormone (A. Pecile and E.E. Müller, eds) I.C.S. 244, Excerpta Medica, Amsterdam, pp 330-348.

40. Takahashi, Y., Kipnis, D.M. and Daughaday, W.H. (1968) J. Clin. Invest. 47, 2079-2090.

41. Tannenbaum, G. (1975) Ph.D. Thesis, Dept. of Psychology, McGill University.

42. Tannenbaum, G. and Martin, J.B. (1975a) Fed. Proc. <u>34</u>, 273.

43. Tannenbaum, G. and Martin, J.B. (1975b) Endocrinology (submitted for publication).

44. Tannenbaum, G. and Martin, J.B. (1975c) Endocrinology (submitted for publication).

45. Vanhaelst, L., Golstein, J., Van Cauter, E., L'Hermite, M. and Robyn, C. (1973) Compt. Rend. Acad. Sci. <u>276</u>, 1875-1877.

46. Weiner, R.I. (1973) In: <u>Drug Effects on Neuroendocrine Regulation</u> (E. Zimmerman, W.H. Gispen, B.H. Marks and D. de Weid, eds.) <u>Prog. Brain Res. 39</u>, Excerpta Medica, Amsterdam, pp 165-170.

47. Willoughby, J.O., Martin, J.B., Renaud, L.P. and Brazeau, P. (1975) Endocrinology (submitted for publication).

HORMONAL CONTROL OF LIVER PROLACTIN RECEPTORS

Paul A. Kelly, Louise Ferland, Fernand Labrie
and Andre De Lean

Medical Research Council Group in Molecular
Endocrinology, Centre Hospitalier de l'Université Laval, Quebec G1V 4G2, Canada

Binding of polypeptide hormones to specific receptors located
on the cell plasma membrane is the first event in the action of
these hormones in their target tissues. In agreement with this
concept of peptide hormone action, identification of a number of
specific hormone receptors has recently been accomplished (Roth,
1974).

This presentation will be restricted to hormone receptors for
prolactin or lactogenic hormones. It will include a discussion of
prolactin receptors in general followed by a more detailed description of the liver prolactin receptor chosen as a model for studies
of hormonal control of peptide receptor levels.

Radioreceptor Assays

The presence of very high binding of iodinated prolactin in
membrane fractions of rabbit mammary glands made easier the development of the prolactin radioreceptor assay (RRA) (Shiu et al.
1973) which had a number of advantages over the existing bioassays
for prolactin. These bioassays were in fact rather insensitive and
difficult to carry out. The prolactin RRA, on the other hand, is
simple and gives potency estimates of a number of prolactin preparations identical to results obtained by bioassay. Another major
advantage of receptor assays is that they are not species specific,
as are most radioimmunoassays, since presumably the biologically
active part of the molecule binds to the receptor. This assay
could then be used to screen potentially active fragments of the
prolactin molecule in the search for smaller active peptides.

Radioreceptor assays for growth hormone (GH) were also developed. One uses pregnant rabbit livers as a source of receptors (Tsushima and Friesen, 1973) while the other uses circulating monocytes (Gordon et al., 1974). Using the prolactin radioreceptor assay, we were in fact able to quantitate levels of a rat placental lactogen which had been predicted on the basis of biological data (Kelly et al., 1975). We have also applied both the prolactin and GH RRA to the identification of prolactin- or growth hormone-like activities in serum or placental extracts of a number of species, including the hamster, mouse, guinea pig, sheep, goat and cow (Kelly et al., 1975; Tsushima et al, 1974) in addition to the monkey and human for which placental lactogens had already been described.

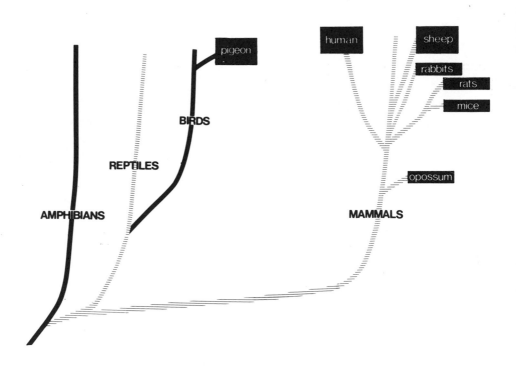

Figure 1: Species distribution of liver prolactin or growth hormone binding sites.

Distribution of prolactin receptors

Specific binding sites for human growth hormone and prolactin have been identified in plasma membrane fractions of a large number of tissues including liver, lactating mammary gland, mammary tumor, kidney, adrenal, ovary and uterus (Posner et al., 1974; Kelly et al., 1974; Frantz et al., 1974; Kelly et al., 1974b; Turkington, 1974; Costlow et al., 1974).

Appreciable binding of either human growth hormone or ovine prolactin has also been observed in liver membrane fractions of a number of species. Fig. 1 summarizes those species in which greater than 3% of the added radioactivity was specifically bound to the membranes. A number of lower orders were examined, but phylogenetically, significant binding was first observed in membrane fractions from pigeon liver. A number of mammalian species had marked binding of PRL or GH, and in most cases, the level of binding was highest in liver.

Modulation of prolactin receptors

The concept that hormone receptors are not static systems, but rather change according to the physiological state of the animal has many interesting implications in term of control of cellular activity. We chose as a model system for our study the prolactin receptor in rat liver. These binding sites have been shown to be specific for lactogenic hormones, i.e. prolactin, primate growth hormones or placental lactogens (Posner et al., 1974). The first interesting observation was that the level of these binding sites is very low in male rats and quite high in female animals. Furthermore, when these binding sites were studied as a function of the developmental state of the rat, we observed a marked increase of the receptors levels following puberty and during pregnancy (Kelly et al., 1974c). More recently, we have demonstrated a fluctuation in the concentration of these binding sites during the estrous cycle as well as a rapid decline following hypophysectomy (Kelly et al., 1975c).

Prolactin has been reported to have at least 46 actions in the various species in which it is secreted (Bein and Nicoll, 1968). In rats, prolactin has specifically been reported to affect hepatic free fatty acid synthesis (MacLeod et al., 1968) and RNA synthesis (Chen et al., 1972). Although a coupling of prolactin binding to one of these events has not yet been established, prolactin binding sites in rat liver do conform to the other requirements which define a hormone receptor, namely, there are specific for only prolactin or prolactin-related hormones and they have an affinity constant of a magniture sufficient to bind circulating levels of hormones ($Ka = 1.5 \times 10^9 M^{-1}$). We have conclusively shown, however, that these sites are not sites associated with the degradation of the prolactin

or growth hormone molecule (Posner <u>et al</u>., 1974a; Kelly <u>et al</u>.,
1974b).

Assay of prolactin receptor

    For the studies described in this report, crude plasma membra-
ne fractions were prepared by differential centrifugation. Prolactin (oPRL) was iodinated with lactoperoxidase to approximately 80
µCi/µg. For the assay of PRL binding, 200 µg membrane protein was
combined with approximately 100,000 cpm ^{125}I-oPRL. The data are
expressed as the percent specific binding calculated as the difference between the cpm bound in the absence (total binding) and presence (non-specific binding) of excess oPRL divided by the total
cpm added to the assay tube times 100.

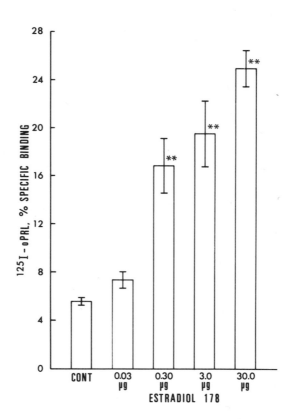

Figure 2: Specific binding of ^{125}I-oPRL to liver membranes of female rats ovariectomized 6 weeks previously and injected daily for
7 days with vehicle alone or the indicated doses of estradiol-17β.

Double antibody radioimmunoassays for rat prolactin were carried out on plasma samples using the materials supplied by NIAMDD. Results are expressed as equivalents Rat PRL-RP-1 (ng/ml plasma).

Stimulatory effect of estrogens

Since prolactin binding sites were increased following puberty and during pregnancy (Kelly et al., 1974b, c) and these periods are normally associated with increased production of ovarian steroids, the effect of estrogens and progesterone on prolactin binding sites was examined. The male, which has very low prolactin binding was as a model. The administration of 50 µg estrone or estradiol (E_2) per day for 8 days induced levels of prolactin binding normally observed in female rats whereas progesterone was without effect (Posner et al., 1974b). A single injection of 1 or 2 mg of estradiol valerate, a long-acting preparation, resulted in similar increased in binding (Kelly et al., 1974c).

Fig. 2 shows that much smaller amounts of estradiol-17β (E_2) can also be effective in inducing prolactin binding. Female rats ovariectomized for 6 weeks were injected daily for 7 days with the vehicle alone or 0.03, 0.30, 3.0 or 30 µg E_2. For this and the subsequent studies, steroids were dissolved in a small amount of ethanol and then suspended in a solution of 1% gelatin in 0.9% NaCl. Control rats had PRL binding values of 5.6 ± 0.3%. Binding was significantly increased to 16.9 ± 2.3% in rats injected with 0.3 µg/ E_2 per day. Maximal binding was observed in rats treated with 30 µg E_2 (25.0 ± 1.5%). These data confirm the fact that physiological as well as pharmacological doses of E_2 can stimulate prolactin receptor levels.

Stimularoty effect of prolactin

The loss of prolactin binding in rat liver following hypophysectomy implied the importance of a pituitary factor in the maintaince of these binding sites (Kelly et al., 1975c). A direct effect of prolactin on its own receptor was first implied when we demonstrated that prolactin binding to rat liver in hypophysectomized rats given a pituitary implant under the kidney capsule began to increase approximately 3 days following the increase in serum prolactin levels (Posner et al., 1975). Costlow et al. (1975) have also shown that direct administration of 2 mg prolactin to hypophysectomized female rats increased prolactin binding in rat liver.

Another method of demonstrating a direct effect of prolactin on its own receptor is to study prolactin receptor levels in animals bearing prolactin-secreting tumors. The tumor chosen in this case was MtTF4, a prolactin-growth hormone-, and ACTH-secreting tumor (Lis et al., 1975). Six weeks after transplantation, at a time when tumors were well-developed, the animals were sacrified

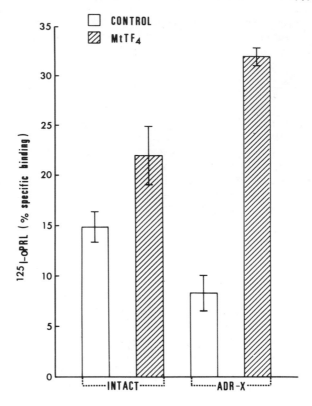

Figure 3: Specific binding of ^{125}I-oPRL to liver membranes of normal rats and rats bearing a prolactin-secreting tumor (MtTF4).

and livers removed. The specific binding of PRL to intact and adrenalectomized (ADR-X) control or tumor-bearing rats is shown in Figure 3. For both intact and ADR-X rats, presence of the PRL-secreting tumor was associated with significant stimulation of PRL binding ($p < 0.01$). These results are similar to these reported by Posner (1975b) for MtT/F4, MtT/F45 and MtT/W5 tumors.

Although prolactin is capable of increasing prolactin binding in hypophysectomized animals, it is not able to increase binding to levels found in intact female animals. Costoff et al (1975) found that even with replacement of a number of other anterior pituitary hormones binding was never greater than 30% of intact levels.

Inhibitory effect of anti-estrogens

Since prolactin binding could be stimulated by estrogens, fluctuated with the estrous cycle, and was reduced by ovariectomy, it was felt of interest to study the effect of anti-estrogenic compounds on prolactin binding. At doses of 15 mg/kg, the anti-estrogens clomiphene, ICI 46474 and nafoxidine were capable of significantly reducing E_2-stimulated prolactin binding in male rats (Kelly et al., 1975c). In female animals, we have recently found that a highly potent anti-estrogen, RU-16117 (11α-methoxy ethinyl-estradiol), a product of Roussel, Paris, is capable of reducing E_2-stimulated binding by 30-70% at doses 1000 times less than those required for the other anti-estrogens (Kelly et al., 1975d).

Inhibitory effect of androgens

In view of the fact that prolactin binding is higher in female than male animals, the effect of androgen administration on prolactin binding and plasma prolactin was next examined, looking at both basal as well as estrogen-stimulated levels. Fig. 4 illustrates changes in prolactin binding (A) and plasma prolactin (B) in rats injected with E_2 (0.25 µg/day), testosterone (T, 500 µg/day) or a combination of E_2 and T. Rats were ovariectomized (OVX) 3 weeks previously, and were treated for 8 days. E_2-treatment causes a 4.1-fold increase in PRL binding while T alone had no effect. Addition of T to E_2 treatment caused a 76% reduction in PRL binding. E_2-treatment had no significant effect on plasma prolactin while T alone or in combination with E_2 reduced PRL levels (p < 0.05).

The androgen-estrogen antagonism on prolactin binding observed in females was also apparent in male rats. Male animals (intact and castrated for 1 month) were treated once daily with estradiol benzoate (EB, 10 µg/100 g B.W.) or testosterone propionate (TP, 100 µg/100 g B.W.) for 8 days. The level of prolactin binding in liver membranes of these rats is shown in the upper panel of Fig. 5. EB treatment in intact and castrated rats increased PRL binding from a control level of 0.1 ± 1% to 10.2 ± 1.4% and 2.9 ± 0.3 to 14.6 ± 1.2%, respectively. Addition of TP to E_2 treatment caused a 62 to 73% decrease in the E_2-induced PRL binding. Plasma prolactin levels in these animals are shown in the lower panel of Fig. 5. A strong stimulation of plasma prolactin by EB was observed in both intact and castrated rats. Contrary to the effect on PRL binding, addition of TP to EB treatment did not reduce the EB-stimulated plasma prolactin levels. In these experiments, where testosterone was utilized, we failed to observe a stimulation of plasma prolactin levels by androgen treatment as has previously been reported (Meites and Clemens, 1972; Kalra et al., 1973). We thus decided to rule out the possible conversion of androgen to estrogen by utilizing 5α-dihydrotestosterone (DHT).

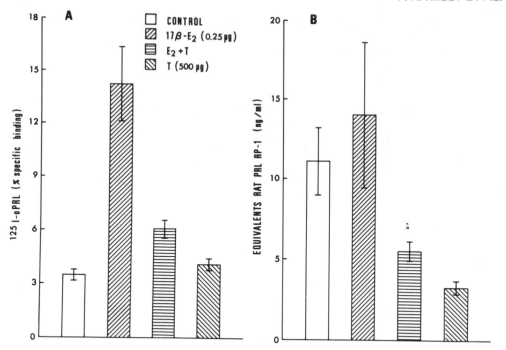

Figure 4: Specific binding of ^{125}I-oPRL to liver membranes (A) and plasma prolactin (B) of female rats ovariectomized 3 weeks previously and injected daily for 8 days with E$_2$, testosterone (T) or a combination of E$_2$ and T.

    The dose-response of T and (DHT) on prolactin binding is shown in Fig. 6. Female rats ovariectomized for 2 weeks were treated twice a day for 8 days with either E$_2$ (0.05 µg/100 g,B.W.), T or DHT (2.5, 10, 40 µg/100 g,B.W.) or a combination of the two. DHT, at a dose of 10 µg/100 g B.W. or greater significantly reduced the basal level of PRL binding (Pannel A). The lower panel (B) shows that DHT also led to a marked inhibition of E$_2$-stimulated increased PRL binding from 11.2 ± 1.0% to 9.5 ± 0.7, 5.2 ± 0.4 and 1.6 ± 0.2% for the three doses of DHT, respectively. T was less effective than DHT, causing a significant reduction only at 40 µg/100 g, B.W. Plasma prolactin levels (not shown) in these animals were not significantly stimulated by E$_2$-treatment nor inhibited T or DHT treatment.

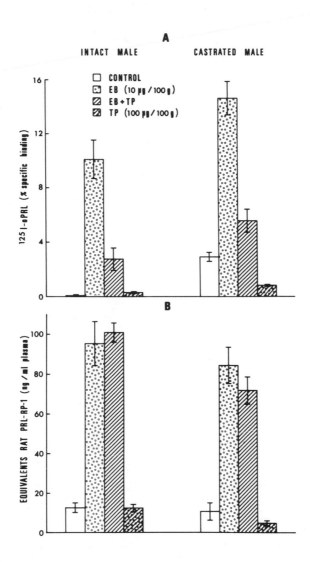

Figure 5: Specific binding of ^{125}I-oPRL to liver membranes (A) and plasma prolactin (B) in intact and castrated male rats treated with estradiol benzoate, testosterone propionate or a combination of the two steroids.

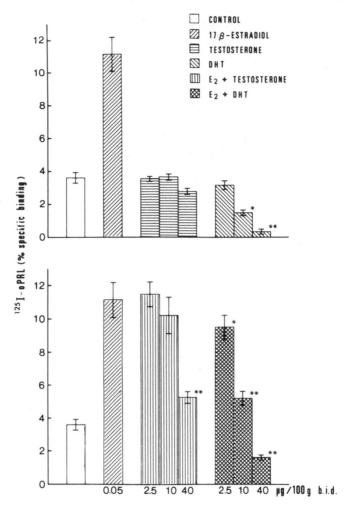

Figure 6: Specific binding of ^{125}I-oPRL to liver membranes of female rats ovariectomized for 2 weeks and treated twice a day for 8 days with E_2, T, DHT or a combination of E_2 and androgen. The upper panel (A) illustrates the effect of androgens alone and the lower panel (B) the combination of E_2 plus androgen.

Dissociation between estradiol stimulatory effect on prolactin receptor and plasma prolactin levels

In an attempt to get a further indication whether estradiol stimulates prolactin binding via an increase of plasma prolactin levels or by a direct effect of E_2 on liver binding sites, a dose-response was carried out on both the level of prolactin binding as well as on plasma prolactin (Fig. 7). Rats ovariectomized for 2

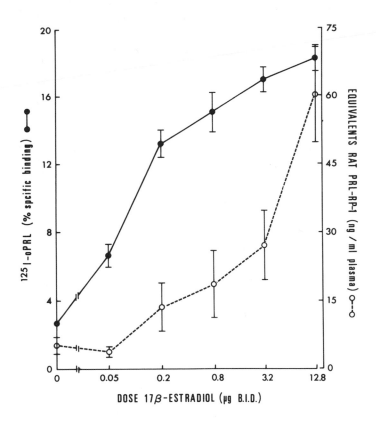

Figure 7: Dose response of estradiol-17β on prolactin binding and plasma prolactin in female rats ovariectomized 2 weeks previously and injected twice a day for 8 days with the indicated amounts of E_2.

weeks were treated twice a day (b.i.d.) for 8 days with 0.05, 0.2 0.8, 3.2 or 12.8 µG E_2. As little as 0.05 µg E_2 increased prolactin binding from 2.7 ± 0.7% to 6.7 ± 0.7% (p < 0.01) with maximal binding observed with 12.8 µg (18.2 ± 0.8%). The plasma prolactin concentration, on the other hand, began to increase significantly in rats receiving 3.2 µg E_2 (27.1 ± 7.6 ng/ml vs 5.1 ± 1.9 ng/ml in control rats), with highest PRL levels observed in rats receiving 12.8 µg E_2.

With such a large difference of the sensitivity (approximately 60-fold) between the dose-response-curves for prolactin binding and plasma prolactin levels, it seems unlikely that the increase in prolactin binding following E_2 treatment is only mediated by an increase in circulating prolactin levels. It should however be noticed that animals were killed between 9:00 and 11:00 hours and that estrogen effects on plasma PRL levels could be more apparent at other times of the day.

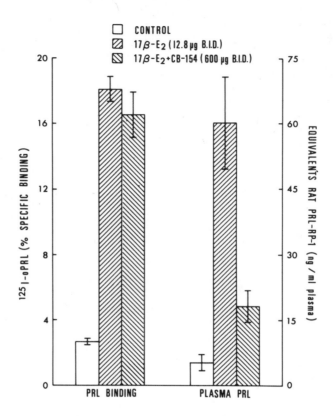

Figure 8: Specific binding of ^{125}I-oPRL and plasma prolactin levels in OVX female rats injected twice a day for 8 days with E$_2$ or E$_2$ plus CB-154 (600 μg, b.i.d.)

The concept that E$_2$ stimulates the PRL receptor directly is strengthened by the results of the following study in which a prolactin-lowering drug, CB-154 was injected (600 μg, b.i.d.) together with 12.8 μg E$_2$. Fig. 8 shows that prolactin binding (on the left) was not significantly changed in rats receiving E$_2$ and CB-154, whereas plasma prolactin levels were reduced from 60.2 ± 10.5 to 18.2 ± 3.7 ng/ml (p < 0.01).

The various factors affecting prolactin receptor levels in
the rat liver are schematically presented in Fig. 9. Both estradiol and prolactin have been shown to have a positive effect on the
development of prolactin binding sites. Hypophysectomy and prolactin replacement experiments of Costoff et al. (1975) indicate that
prolactin is necessary for the maintainance of prolactin binding
sites, but at best only a partial restoration of receptors can be
obtained with prolactin alone, thus indicating that other factors
are likely to be involved in this process.

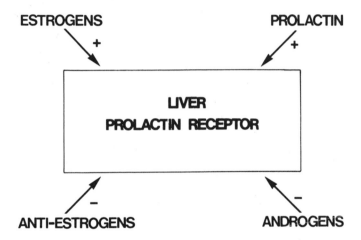

Figure   9: Factors affecting the prolactin receptor in rat liver.

Antiestrogens reduce estradiol-stimulated prolactin binding,
probably as a result of their competition with the estradiol receptor. Androgens are capable of reducing both basal as well as estradiol-stimulated prolactin binding, regardless of their effect
on plasma prolactin, thus indicating a possible direct influence
of steroid hormones on the modulation of prolactin binding sites.

REFERENCES

Bern, H.A. and C.S. Nicoll (1968) Recent Prog. Horm. Res. 24, 681.

Chen, H.A., D.H. Hamer, H.J. Neiniger and H. Meier (1972) Biochim. Biophys. Acta 287, 90.

Costlow, M.E., R.A. Buschow and W.L. McGuire (1974) Science 184, 85.

Costlow, M.E., R.A. Buschow, G.C. Chamrass and W.L. McGuire (1975) The 57th Meeting of the Endocrine Society, New York, p. 79.

Frantz, W.L., J.H. MacIndoe and R.W. Turkington (1974) J. Endocrinol. 60, 485.

Gordon, P., M.A. Lesniak, C.M. Hendricks and J. Roth (1974) In S. Raiti (ed.) Advances in Human Growth Hormone Research, Government Printing Office, Washington, D.C., p. 545.

Kalra, P.S., C.P. Fawcett, L. Krulich and S.M. McCann (1973) Endocrinology 92, 1256.

Kelly, P.A., C. Bradley, R.P.C. Shiu, J. Meites and H.G. Friesen (1974a) Proc. Soc. Exp. Biol. Med. 146, 816.

Kelly, P.A., B.I. Posner, T. Tsushima, R.P.C. Shiu, and H.G. Friesen (1974b) In S. Raiti (ed.) Advances in Human Growth Hormone Research, Government Printing Office, Washington, D.C., p. 567.

Kelly, P.A., B.I. Posner, H.G. Friesen (1974c) Endocrinology 95, 532.

Kelly, P.A., R.P.C. Shiu, M.C. Robertson and H.G. Friesen (1975a) Endocrinology 96, 1187.

Kelly, P.A., R.P. C. Shiu, T. Tsushima and H.G. Friesen (1975b) Submitted to Endocrinology

Kelly, P.A., B.I. Posner, and H.G. Friesen (1975c) Endocrinology, in press.

Kelly, P.A., L. Ferland, F. Labrie and J.P. Raynaud (1975d) Manuscript in preparation.

Lis, M., M.C. Guerinot and M. Chretien (1975) Endocrinology 96, 739.

MacLeod, R.M., M.B. Boss, S.C. Huang and M.C. Smith (1968) Endocrinology 82, 253.

Meites, J. and J.A. Clemens (1972) Vitam. Horm. 30, 165.

Nolin, J.M., G.T. Campell, D.D. Nansel and E.M. Bogdanov (1975) Fed. Proc. 34, 251.

Posner, B.I., P.A. Kelly and H.G. Friesen (1974a) Endocrinology 95, 521.

Posner, B.I., P.A. Kelly and H.G. Friesen (1974b) Proc. Nat. Acad. Sci. (USA) 71, 2407.

Posner, B.I., P.A. Kelly, H.G. Friesen (1975a) Science 187, 57.

Posner, B.I. (1975b) The 57th Meeting of the Endocrine Society, New York, p. 84.

Roth, J. (1973) Metabolism 22, 1059.

Shiu, R.P.C., P.A. Kelly, H.G. Friesen (1973) Science 180, 968.

Tsushima, T. and H.G. Friesen (1973) J. Clin. Endocrinol. Metab. 37, 334.

Tsushima, T., R.P.C. Shiu, P.A. Kelly and H.G. Friesen (1974) In S. Raiti (ed.) Advances in Human Growth Hormone Research, Government Printing Office, Washington, D.C., p. 372.

Turkington, R.W. (1974) Cancer Res. 34, 758.

Chemistry and Assay of Hypothalamic Hormones

SUPPRESSION OF GONADOTROPIN RELEASE AND OVULATION IN ANIMALS BY

INHIBITORY ANALOGS OF LUTEINIZING HORMONE-RELEASING HORMONE

David H. Coy, Esther J. Coy, Jesus A. Vilchez-Martinez, Antonio de la Cruz, Akira Arimura and Andrew V. Schally

Department of Medicine, Tulane Univ. School of Medicine and Veterans Administration Hospital, New Orleans, Louisiana USA 70112

INITIAL APPROACHES

The basic assumption in developing competitive inhibitors of luteinizing hormone/follicle stimulating hormone-releasing hormone (LH/FSH-RH), the structure of which is shown in Figure 1, was that analogs could be designed which could retain the ability to bind to pituitary receptor sites whilst being devoid of gonadotropin-releasing activity. The first indication that this approach was valid came out of work by Vale et al. (1972) who found that removal of histidine from the peptide chain gave a nonapeptide of very low LH-RH activity which was capable of inhibiting the action of LH-RH on cultures of anterior pituitary cells. This inhibition was, however, weak and subsequently could not be demonstrated in vivo in rats (Vilchez-Martinez et al., 1974a). Other inhibitors based on the original decapeptide sequence were shown (Vilchez-Martinez et al., 1974a) to be active in vivo ; however, these were also too weak to be of practical value. It became obvious, therefore, that ways must be found to substantially raise the binding affinity of an inhibitor, again without increasing agonistic activity to any great extent.

SUPER-ACTIVE ANALOGS OF LH-RH AND THEIR USE IN THE DESIGN OF COMPETITIVE INHIBITORS

When Fujino and co-workers (1972) discovered that [desGly-NH$_2^{10}$] -LH-RH ethylamide (pGlu-His-Trp-Ser-Tyr-Gly-Leu-Arg-Pro-NHCH$_2$CH$_3$) was about four times more active than LH-RH, it seemed probable to us that this was a result of increased binding efficiency, and that advantage could be taken of this property by

339

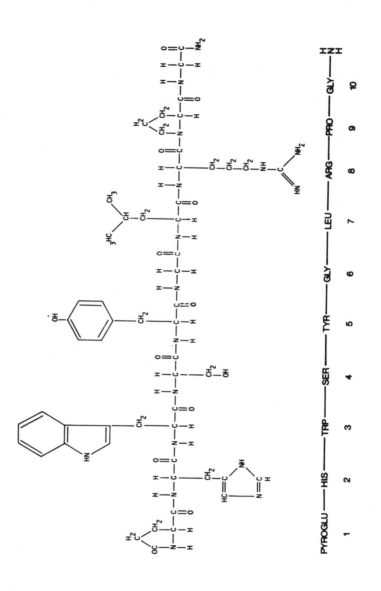

FIGURE 1: Structure of LH/FSH-Releasing Hormone

incorporating the C-terminal modification into some of the inhibitory peptides already developed. Thus, [deHis^2,desGly-NH$_2$^{10}] -LH-
RH ethylamide was prepared (Coy et al., 1974a) which, as expected,
was a significantly better inhibitor of administered LH-RH than
[desHis^2] -LH-RH in several animal models (Vilchez-Martinez et al.,
1974a,b;1975).

    [DesGly-NH$_2$^{10}] -LH-RH trifluoroethylamide (Coy et al., 1975)
was subsequently found to be twice as active as the ethylamide
analog; however, the corresponding [desHis^2]-peptide did not appear
to be a better in vivo inhibitor of LH-RH (Vilchez-Martinez et al.,
1976). At about the same time, another modification of LH-RH was
reported (Monahan et al., 1973) which also resulted in a peptide of
increased gonadotropin-releasing activity and which has subsequently
turned out to be of even greater significance from the point of view
of design of inhibitors. The analog, [D-Ala^6] -LH-RH, was found to
be approximately 7 times more active than LH-RH (Coy et al., 1974b;
Arimura et al., 1974) and its [desHis^2] -derivative (Monahan et al.,
1973) was more effective as an in vitro inhibitor than [desHis^2] -
LH-RH. Furthermore, we found this peptide to be a better antagonist
than [desHis^2,desGly-NH$_2$^{10}] -LH-RH ethylamide in several of our in
vivo assay systems.

    The third class of highly active agonists which have been
developed contain a D-amino acid in position 6 in conjunction with
a C-terminal alkylamide modification. Several of these peptides
display very high gonadotropin-releasing activity. For instance,
[D-Ala^6,desGly-NH$_2$^{10}] -LH-RH ethylamide (Coy et al., 1974; Fujino
et al., 1974a; Arimura et al., 1974) and[D-Leu^6,desGly^{10}] -LH-RH
ethylamide (Vilchez-Martinez et al., 1974c; Fujino et al., 1974b)
promote prolonged release of LH and FSH when compared with LH-RH
in immature male rats (Figure 2). In terms of total amounts of LH
and FSH released, these analogs are 20-30 times more active than
LH-RH and it was anticipated that they would offer ideal structures
from which to develop inhibitors with the same excellent receptor
site-binding characteristics. Unfortunately, in practice this has
not turned out to be the case. For instance, [desHis^2,D-Ala^6,
desGly-NH$_2$^{10}] -LH-RH ethylamide, an obvious choice for direct comparison with other [desHis^2] -peptides, did exhibit somewhat greater
inhibitory activity than [desHis^2,D-Ala^6] -LH-RH, but by no means in
proportion to the agonistic activities of the parent peptides. It
was also discouraging to find that inhibitors of this type also
tended to have higher inherent gonadotropin-releasing activities at
the doses necessary to give high blockade of LH-RH (Vilchez-Martinez
et al., 1975a).

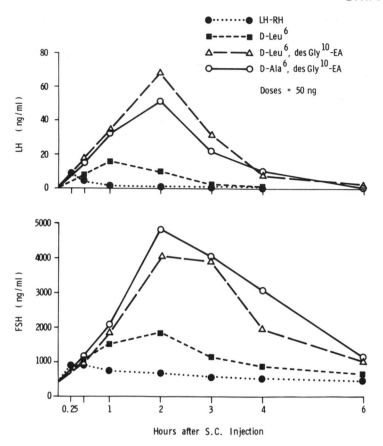

FIGURE 2: Serum LH and FSH levels after s.c. injection of saline, LH-RH, [D-Leu⁶]-LH-RH, [D-Ala⁶desGly¹⁰]-LH-RH ethylamide, and [D-Leu⁶,desGly¹⁰]-LH-RH ethylamide.

NEW INHIBITORS DERIVED FROM D-AMINO ACID-6-LH-RH ANALOGS -- ASSAY METHODS

An analysis of the information already described indicated to us and other groups that the main emphasis in searching for improved antagonists should center around super-active precursor peptides with D-amino acids in the six position. Investigation of the structure-activity relationships of this position revealed to us that [D-Leu⁶]-LH-RH was more active than [D-Ala⁶]-LH-RH (Vilchez-Martinez et al., 1974c) and this seemed to indicate that it might be possible to increase the LH-RH activity even more by the selection of appropriate side-chains for the D-amino acid. A series of analogs was, therefore, synthesized in which an increase in the lypophylic character of the side-chain was found to coincide with an increase in biological activity in immature male rats (Coy et al.,1976): D-Glu[6], 1.8; D-Ala[6], 7.0; D-Leu[6], 9.0; D-Phe[6], 10; D-Trp[6], 13 times the activity of LH-RH.

The two most potent peptides of the series, [D-Phe[6]] - and [D-Trp[6]] -LH-RH, have <u>in vivo</u> gonadotropin-releasing activities not far short of [D-Ala[6],desGly-NH$_2$[10]] -LH-RH ethylamide and induce similar patterns of LH and FSH release (Figure 3).

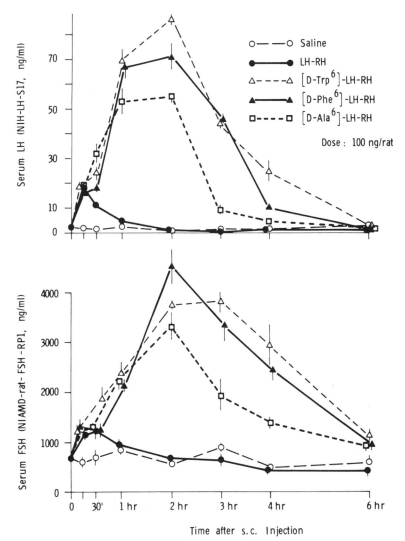

FIGURE 3: Serum LH and FSH levels after s.c. injection of saline, 100 ng of LH-RH, [D-Ala[6]] -LH-RH, [D-Phe[6]] -LH-RH, and [D-Trp[6]] -LH-RH.

Interestingly, Labrie et al., (unpublished observations) have found that [D-Phe⁶] - and [D-Trp⁶] -LH-RH are far more active than [D-Ala⁶, desGly-NH₂¹⁰] -LH-RH ethylamide in vitro - the reverse of the in vivo situation. Surprisingly, the ethylamide derivatives of the [D-Phe⁶]- and [D-Trp⁶] - analogs were less active both in vivo and in vitro in contrast to the results with [D-Ala⁶]- and [D-Leu⁶]- -LH-RH.

We have prepared many inhibitory analogs with D-Leu, D-Phe, or D-Trp in position 6. The greatest amount of work has been carried out on the first two types, owing to the decreased yields obtained when synthesizing peptides with more than one residue of Trp. In evaluating analogs for their relative inhibitory activities and potential effectiveness for inhibiting natural gonadotropin surges and ovulation, we felt it necessary to observe the time courses of their activities, particularly when the prolonged and displaced peak activities of the parent peptides are considered.

In the assay method devised (Vilchez-Martinez et al., 1976), 25-day-old male rats are injected s.c. with either 500 µg of an LH-RH antagonist or with vehicle as control. LH-RH (200 ng) or saline is then injected s.c. at the same time and, in separate groups, at 30 minute intervals after injection of the inhibitor. Blood is collected 30 minutes after each LH-RH and saline administration and analyzed for gonadotropin levels by radioimmunoassay. Thus, this method allows us to measure the percentage inhibition of both the LH and FSH release after administration of a dose of LH-RH at anytime and also to determine the agonistic activity, if any, of the inhibitor. For example, the results of this method as applied to [desHis², D-Phe⁶] -LH-RH are shown in Figure 4. Maximal inhibition of LH-RH takes place when it is injected simultaneously with the analog (zero time on the graph). At 240 minutes, the ability of the peptide to inhibit has disappeared and at no time is there significant release of LH by the analog alone. The pattern of inhibition of FSH-release (not shown) is similar.

At this point, the most effective inhibitors which we have found contain a [D-Phe²] -modification, which has proved to be superior for the production of inhibitors than deletion of the histidine residue. Rees et al. (1974) discovered that D-Phe²-LH-RH was considerably more active than [desHis²] -LH-RH in preventing the action of LH-RH on cultures of anterior pituitary cells. We have found this also to be the situation in vivo (Vilchez-Martinez, et al., 1976) and have incorporated this new alteration into our super-active agonist peptides with excellent results. Most of these peptides are rather insoluble in physiological saline solution and for bioassay are dissolved in 20% propylene glycol/ 0.9% saline solution. A direct comparison of [D-Phe²,D-Leu⁶] -LH-RH and [desHis²,D-Leu⁶]-LH-RH shows (Figure 5) that the peak inhibitory activities of the two peptides

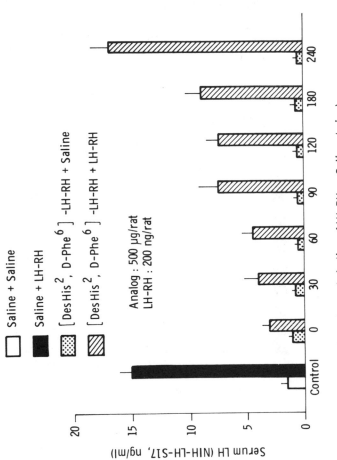

FIGURE 4: Time course of anti-LH-RH activity of [desHis^2,D-Phe^6]-LH-RH in immature male rats. Inhibitor was injected s.c. at 0 time and the rats decapitated 30 minutes after LH-RH or saline administration.

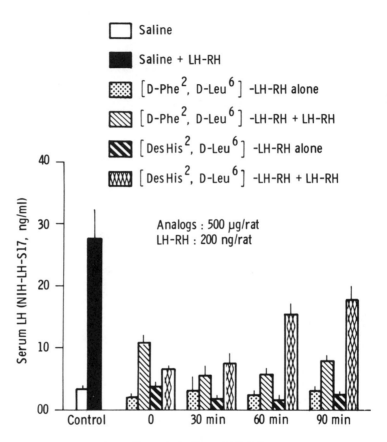

FIGURE 5: Time course of anti–LH–RH activities of [D-Phe[2],D-Leu[6]] – LH-RH and [desHis[2],D-Leu[6]] -LH-RH in immature male rats. Inhibitors were injected s.c. at 0 time and the rats decapitated 30 minutes after LH-RH or saline administration.

are different, 30-60 minutes for the former and 0 minute for the latter. At each time interval, other than 0 minute, the [D-Phe^2] - peptide is more active than the [desHis^2]-peptide. This is in fact the case with every pair of [D-Phe^2]- and [desHis^2]-analogs which we have examined to date. In vitro experiments (Labrie et al., unpublished results) give similar results, the 50% inhibition doses being about 3 times less for the [D-Phe^2] -analogs.

Direct comparisons were also made between the inhibitory activities of [D-Phe^2]-peptides with D-Ala, D-Leu, or D-Phe in position 6, and it was found that their effectiveness increased progressively in that order (Figures 6 and 7). Again the same trend is observed in vitro (Labrie et al., unpublished observations). The first peptide of the series, [D-Phe^2,D-Ala^6] -LH-RH, has also been made by Foell and Yardley (1974) and extensively tested in ovulation blockade experiments by Corbin and Beattie (1975). The most potent of the three peptides, [D-Phe^2, D-Phe^6]-LH-RH, produced significant inhibition of LH-RH for up to 8 hours after its injection into immature male rats (Figure 8), which is 2-3 hours longer than with the [D-Ala^6]- and [D-Leu^6]- analogs.

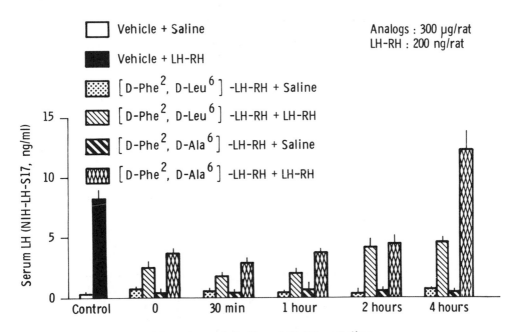

FIGURE 6: Comparison of anti-LH-RH activities of [D-Phe^2,D-Ala^6] - LH-RH and [D-Phe^2,D-Leu^6]-LH-RH in immature male rats. Inhibitors were injected s.c. at 0 time and the rats were decapitated 30 minutes after LH-RH or saline administration.

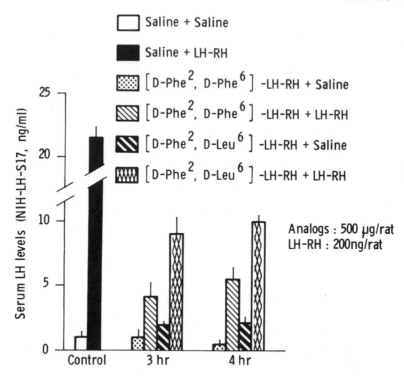

FIGURE 7: Comparison of anti-LH-RH activities of [D-Phe^2,D-Phe^6]-LH-RH and [D-Phe^2,D-Leu^6]-LH-RH in immature male rats. Inhibitors were injected s.c. at 0 time and the rats were decapitated 30 minutes after LH-RH or saline administration.

Thus, several of the peptides which were developed appeared suitable for attempts to block endogenous LH-RH in animals. Initial experiments were carried out with [D-Phe^2,D-Leu^6]-LH-RH in naturally cycling hamsters and, after some exploratory work, 750 μg doses of the analog injected s.c. at 3, 4, 5 and 6 p.m. on the afternoon of proestrus led to an 83% lowering of the LH surge (de la Cruz et al., 1975). Disappointingly, this was accompanied by only 30% suppression of ovulation when animals were examined the following morning. The reason for this was discovered later (de la Cruz et al., 1976a) when it was shown that hamsters were able to ovulate fully with approximately only 10% of the gonadotropins normally released during proestrus

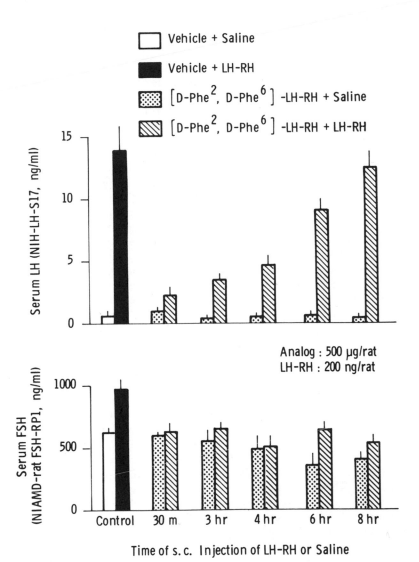

FIGURE 8: Time course of anti LH/FSH-releasing activities of [D-Phe2,D-Phe6]-LH-RH in immature male rats. Inhibitor was injected s.c. at 0 time and rats decapitated 30 minutes after LH-RH or saline administration.

Later experiments using 4-day-cycling rats according to a similar protocol gave 83% blockade of ovulation (Table I).

As we stated above, [D-Phe^2,D-Ala^6] -LH-RH, which is less active than [D-Phe^2,D-Leu^6] -LH-RH, has been rigorously tested by Corbin and Beattie (1975). They found that this peptide could also inhibit ovulation in rats, induced ovulation in the rabbit, and prevent pregnancy when administered pre-coitally to rats.

The best results with the [D-Ala^6] - and [D-Leu^6]- peptides are obtained when multiple doses of quite large amounts are given, in other words their length of action is not sufficient to produce complete inhibition of the LH surge which takes place over an 8-hour period in the rat. [D-Phe^2,D-Phe^6]-LH-RH is active, however, for about this period of time (Figure 8) and it seemed possible that single injections of this analog at lower dose levels would give comparable results. When this was tried, the results were not good and we subsequently found that the gonadotropin-releasing activity of this peptide, although not detectable in immature male rats, proved to be very significant in female proestrus animals and too high to enable complete blockade of ovulation to take place. Attempts were immediately made to synthesize peptides with lower LH-RH activity which retained the desirable properties of [D-Phe^2, D-Phe^6] -LH-RH. Among these, two peptides have been found which meet these requirements, [D-Phe^2,Phe^3,D-Phe^6] -LH-RH, and [D-Phe^2,Phe^5, D-Phe^6] -LH-RH which, respectively, have Phe in place of Trp and Tyr. These modifications were chosen on the basis that [Phe^3] -LH-RH and [Phe^5] -LH-RH have LH releasing activities of 0.1% and 50%-60%, respectively, of LH-RH itself. It appeared probable that these changes could be incorporated into [D-Phe^2,D-Phe^6]-LH-RH without drastically lowering its binding affinity whilst decreasing its gonadotropin-releasing activity.

A comparison of the inhibitory activities of all three analogs in the immature male rat system at 30 minutes and 4 hours after injection is shown in Figure 9. The two derivatives were only slightly inferior inhibitors to [D-Phe^2,D-Phe^6] -LH-RH and yet were later found to have lower LH/FSH-releasing properties, particularly in the case of the [Phe^3]-peptide.

A single s.c. injection of 1.5 mg (6 mg/kg) of [D-Phe^2,Phe^3, D-Phe^6] -LH-RH given at noon on the proestrous day resulted in a 95% reduction of total LH released and 84% reduction of the FSH released (de la Cruz et al., 1976b). This was accompanied by an 86% suppression of ovulation. Only one animal out of five ovulated, producing a reduced number of ova when examined the following morning (Table I). No rebound of gonadotropin levels occurred up until 6 a.m. on the following estrous day. Elevation of FSH levels in control animals continued well into the estrous morning, long

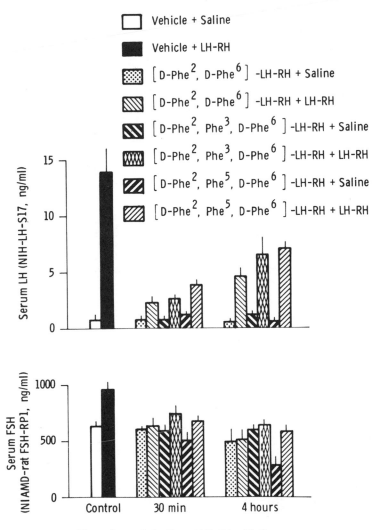

FIGURE 9: Comparison of the anti-LH-RH activities of [D-Phe^2,D-Phe^6]-LH-RH, [D-Phe^2,Phe^3,D-Phe^6]-LH-RH, and [D-Phe^2,Phe^5,D-Phe^6]-LH-RH. Inhibitors (500 µg) were injected s.c. at 0 time and rats decapitated 30 minutes after LH-RH (200 ng) or saline administration.

TABLE I: SUPPRESSION OF OVULATION · IN RATS* BY INHIBITORY ANALOGUES OF LH-RH

TREATMENT	DOSE**	NUMBER OF ANIMALS	NUMBER OF ANIMALS OVULATING	NUMBER OF OVA (mean ± S.E.)	PERCENTAGE OF SUPPRESSION	P
DILUENT $\underline{a}$	x 3	6	6	13.3 ± 0.8		
[D-Phe^2-Phe^3-D-Phe^6]-LH-RH	1 mg x 3	5	0	0.	100.0	0.001
[D-Phe^2-D-Leu^6]-LH-RH	2 mg x 3	5	1	2.4 ± 2.4	82.8	0.01
[Des-His^2-D-Leu^6]-LH-RH	4 mg x 3	5	5	11.8 ± 0.9	11.3	NS
DILUENT $\underline{a}$	x 1	5	5	13.1 ± 0.5		
[D-Phe^2-Phe^3-D-Phe^6]-LH-RH	1.0 mg x 1	5	1	2.2 ± 2.2	82.0	0.01
" "	1.5 mg x 1	5	1	1.8 ± 1.8	86.4	0.01

* 4-day estrous cycle. Body weight: 202.6 ± 1.6 g

** Three s.c. injections were administered at 12:00, 14:30, and 17:00 hrs or single s.c. injection at 12:00 of the proestrous day (C.S.T.).

$\underline{a}$ 20% propylene glycol/saline

N.S. = not significant

after the LH peak had disappeared and increased pituitary sensitivity
to LH-RH had returned to normal. This phenomenon has been observed
by many groups and no fully satisfactory explanation appears to have
been formulated. The results, which we obtained, where blockade of
both early and late FSH release took place, seem to rule out two
explanations that have been recently suggested by Zeballos and McCann
(1975). One, that the late release of FSH is caused by a separate
releasing factor, unless it has receptor sites virtually identical
to those for LH-RH, and the other that it is produced directly by
steroid hormones which should be unaffected by an LH-RH antagonist.
It seems to us that a more likely explanation is that LH-RH, in
addition to releasing stored FSH, also promotes the synthesis of
fresh hormone which, in turn, is also released by LH-RH with some
delay. [D-Phe^2,Phe^5,Phe^6]-LH-RH which has been tested by Labrie's
group in a similar fashion behaves quite similarly to the [Phe^3]-
peptide.

We have done some preliminary work on the effects of injections
of [D-Phe^2,Phe^3,D-Phe^6] -LH-RH at other times of the estrus cycle
of rats. As might be expected from its time course of action, its
ability to block ovulation drops off rapidly if injections are given
earlier than 12:00 noon on proestrus. Injection of a dose of
6 mg/kg at 12:00 noon on diestrous day 2 did give slight suppression
of ovulation, but administration at the same time on diestrous day 1
produced no effect on ovulation. These results tend to conflict
with a report by Corbin and Beattie (1975), who found that injections
of [D-Phe^2,D-Ala^6]-LH-RH at "appropriate times" on any day prior to
the gonadotropin surge result in high degrees of blockade of ovulation.
However, no details were given concerning their experimental designs.

We are now beginning a program to test the most potent inhibitory
analogs in primates and are hopeful that similarly positive results
can be obtained. In addition, new peptides are being developed which
should be effective at lower dose levels for even longer periods of
time.

REFERENCES

Arimura, A., Vilchez-Martinez, J.A., Coy, D.H., Coy, E.J., Hirotsu,
    Y., and Schally, A.V. (1974) Endocrinology 95, 1174-1177.
Corbin, A., and Beattie, C.W. (1975) Endocrine Res. Commun. 2, 1-23.
Coy, D.H., Coy, E.J., Schally, A.V., Vilchez-Martinez, J.A., Debeljuk,
    L., Carter, W.H., and Arimura, A. (1974a) Biochemistry 13,
    323-326.
Coy, D.H., Coy, E.J., Schally, A.V., Vilchez-Martinez, J.A., Hirotsu,
    Y., and Arimura, A (1974b) Biochem. Biophys. Res. Commun. 57,
    335-340.

Coy, D.H., Vilchez-Martinez, J.A., Coy, E.J., Arimura, A., and Schally, A.V. (1976), J. Med. Chem., in press.

Coy, D.H., Vilchez-Martinez, J.A., Coy, E.J., Nishi, N., Arimura, A., and Schally, A.V. (1975) Biochemistry 14, 1848-1851.

de la Cruz, A., Arimura, A., and Schally, A.V. (1976a) Endocrinology, in press.

de la Cruz, A., Coy, D.H., Schally, A.V., Coy, E.J., de la Cruz, K.G., and Arimura, A. (1975) Proc.Soc.Exp.Biol.Med. 149, 576-579.

de la Cruz, A., Coy, D.H., Vilchez-Martinez, A.J., Arimura, A., and Schally, A.V. (1976), Science, in press.

Foell, T.J. and Yardley, J.P. (1974) U.S. Patent 3,855,199.

Fujino, M., Fukuda, T., Shinagawa, S., Kobayashi, S., Yamakazi, I., Nakagama, R., Seely, J.H., White, W.F., Rippel, R.H. (1974a) Biochem.Biophys. Res.Commun. 60, 406-413.

Fujino, M., Kobayashi, S., Obayashi, M., Shinagawa, S., Fukuda, T., Kitada, C., Nakagawa, R., Yamakazi, I., White, W.F., and Rippel, R.H. (1972) Biochem.Biophys.Res.Commun. 49, 863-869.

Fujino, M., Yamakazi, S., Kobayashi, S., Fukuda, T., Shinagawa, S., Nakayama, R., White, W.F., and Rippel, R.H. (1974) Biochem.Biophys.Res.Commun. 57, 1248-1256.

Monahan, M., Amoss, M.S., Anderson, H.A., and Vale, W. (1973), Biochemistry 12, 4616-4620.

Rees, R.W.A., Foell, T.J., Chai, S.Y., and Grant, N. (1974) J.Med. Chem. 17, 1016-1019.

Vale, W., Grant, G., Rivier, J., Monahan, M., Amoss, M., Blackwell, R., Burgus, R., and Guillemin, R. (1972). Science 176, 933-934.

Vilchez-Martinez, J.A., Coy, D.H., Arimura, A., Coy, E.J., Hirtosu, Y., and Schally, A.V. (1974c) Biochem.Biophys.Res.Commun. 59, 1226-1232.

Vilchez-Martinez, J.A., Coy, D.H., Coy, E.J., Arimura, A., and Schally, A.V. (1976) Endocrinology, in press.

Vilchez-Martinez, J.A., Coy, D.H., Coy, E.J., Schally, A.V., and Arimura, A. (1975) Fert.Ster. 26, 554-559.

Vilchez-Martinez, J.A., Schally, A.V., Coy, D.H., Coy, E.J., Debeljuk, L., and Arimura, A. (1974b) Endocrinology 95, 213-218.

Vilchez-Martinez, J.A., Schally, A.V., Debeljuk, L., Coy, D.H., Coy, E.J., Arimura, A., and Yanaihara, N. (1974a) Neuroendocrinol. 14, 121-128.

Zeballos, G. and McCann, S.M. (1975) Endocrinology 96, 1377-1385.

ISOLATION AND CHARACTERIZATION OF HYPOTHALAMIC PEPTIDE HORMONES

R. Burgus, M. Amoss[†], P. Brazeau[*], M. Brown,
N. Ling, C. Rivier, J. Rivier, W. Vale, and J. Villarreal

Salk Institute for Biological Studies, La Jolla, Cal. 92037
[*]McGill University, Montreal, Quebec
[†]Texas A & M University, College Station, Texas

The existence of peptides in the hypothalamus which are involved in the control of release of pituitary hormones is now well
established; several have been isolated and chemically characterized and much is being learned about the physiological and chemical properties of their synthetic replicates and analogs.

Although most of these substances (with the exception of substance P) were first isolated from hypothalamic tissue, there is
now evidence for the presence of some of these peptides throughout
the central nervous system (CNS) (Oliver et al., 1974; Jackson
and Reichlin, 1974; Winokur and Utiger, 1974; Barry, Pelletier,
Vale et al., this meeting) and also for the presence of substance
P (Von Euler and Gaddum, 1931) and somatostatin in gastrointestinal
tissue (Dubois, 1975; Arimura et al., 1975). Extrapituitary effects of the hypothalamic peptides have been reported in the central nervous system (Plotnikoff et al., 1971, 1973; Prange et al.,
1975; Brown and Vale, 1975) and in the gastrointestinal system
(Ruch et al., 1973; Besser, Gerich, this meeting); thus the significance of these substances is now known to be much broader than
was once supposed.

It is the purpose of this communication to describe the status
of the isolation and characterization of hypothalamic peptide hormones.

For the purposes of this discussion, the nomenclature and abbre-
viations used will be those listed in Table 1. For the most recently proposed nomenclature, see recommendations of the IUPAC-IUB
Commission on Biochemical Nomenclature (1975). Table 1 lists some

TABLE 1

Putative Hypothalamic Hormones Stimulating or Inhibiting The
Release of Pituitary Hormones

A. Stimulators of Release

Factor (Hormone)	Target Hormones
TRF (TRH)	Thyrotropin (TSH)
LRF (LHRH)	Luteinizing Hormone (LH)
FRF (FSHRH)	Follicle Stimulating Hormone (FSH)
SRF (GRF, GHRH)	Somatotropin (Growth Hormone) (GH)
PRF	Prolactin (Prl)
CRF	Corticotropin (ACTH)
MRF?	Melanotropin (MSH)

B. Inhibitors of Release

Factor (Hormone)	Target Hormones
MIF	MSH
SRIF (GIF) Somatostatin	GH
TIF	TSH
PIF	Prl
LIF?	LH
FIF?	FSH
CIF?	ACTH

of the pituitary hormones and Table 2 lists peptides for which
biological significance has been proposed and which have been isolated from hypothalamic tissue.

TRF was the first of the hypothalamic releasing hormones to
be isolated and characterized, initially from ovine (Burgus et
al., 1970) and then porcine (Nair et al., 1970) tissue. The structure of porcine LRF decapeptide was then established (Matsuo et
al., 1971) and ovine LRF was shortly thereafter shown to have the
same structure (Burgus et al., 1972). Both TRF and LRF have dual
effects on the pituitary gland; TRF stimulates not only TSH release but also PRL release (Tashjian, et al., 1971) and LRF decapeptide stimulates the release of FSH as well as that of LH (Matsuo
et al., 1971; Burgus et al., 1972). It is therefore possible
that the putative hormones PRF and FRF have been identified. The
existence of an as yet uncharacterized separate FRF as reported
by Folkers and coworkers (Johansson et al., 1973) has not been

TABLE 2.

Peptides Isolated From Brain Tissue

TRF	PGlu–His–Pro–NH$_2$
LRF/FRF	PGlu–His–Trp–Ser–Tyr–Gly–Leu–Arg–Pro–Gly–NH$_2$
Substance P	H–Arg–Pro–Lys–Pro–Gln–Gln–Phe–Phe–Gly–Leu–Met–NH$_2$
"GHRH"	H–Val–His–Leu–Ser–Ala–Glu–Lys–Glu–Ala–OH
MIF–I	H–Pro–Leu–Gly–NH$_2$
MIF–II	H–Pro–His–Phe–Arg–Gly–NH$_2$
Somatostatin	H–Ala–Gly–Cys–Lys–Asn–Phe–Phe–Trp–Lys–Thr–Phe–Thr–Ser–Cys–OH
Neurotensin	PGlu–Leu–Tyr–Glu–Asn–Lys–Pro–Arg–Arg–Pro–Tyr–Ile–Leu–OH
[Arg^8]–Vasopressin	H–Cys–Tyr–Phe–Gln–Asn–Cys–Pro–Arg–Gly–NH$_2$
α–MSH	Ac–Ser–Tyr–Ser–Met–Glu–His–Phe–Arg–Trp–Gly–Lys–Pro–Val–NH$_2$

confirmed by other laboratories (including our own) searching for
it. A pentapeptide fragment (H-Cys-Tyr-Ile-Gln-Asn-OH) arising
from incubation of oxytocin with hypothalamic tissue has been proposed as an MRF (Taleisnik and Orias, 1965; Celis et al., 1971a),
but its physiological significance remains to be established.   It
is now generally accepted (Schally et al., 1973) that the physiological significance of a "GHRH" isolated by Schally and co-
workers (Schally et al., 1971) (structure as shown in Table 2) is
highly questionable.   CRF, the first of the hypothalamic releasing factors to be studied (Guillemin and Rosenberg, 1955) has not
yet been isolated and characterized.

Two peptides, "MIF-I and "MIF-II" have been isolated from porcine
hypothalami and have been reported to have MSH-release inhibiting
activity in vitro (Nair et al., 1971, 1972). MIF-I was first observed by Celis et al. (1971b) following incubation of oxytocin with
hypothalamic tissue. This peptide, irrespective of the significance of its action on the pituitary gland has received wide
attention as a result of its proposed CNS effects (Plotnikoff et
al., 1971). The tetradecapeptide somatostatin, isolated from ovine
hypothalami (Brazeau et al, 1973; Burgus et al., 1973a) on the
basis of its ability to inhibit growth hormone release, also inhibits the release of TSH and under some conditions the release of
prolactin (Vale et al., 1974). Somatostatin might well have been
isolated as a "TIF" on the basis of its inhibition of TSH release,
since no other factor specific for inhibition of TSH release has
been observed. One of the most striking observations regarding
somatostatin has been its effect on the pancreas to inhibit the
release of insulin and glucagon (Ruch et al., 1973); it also has
other gastrointestinal effects, for example the inhibition of gastrin secretion (Bloom et al., 1974). Although the inhibition of
release of prolactin has long been known to involve hypothalamic
substances (Blackwell and Guillemin, 1973), the identification of
hypothalamic substances reported to be distinct from catecholamines
and somatostatin (Dupont et al., this meeting) remains to be accomplished. Similarly, substances corresponding to LIF/FIF (preliminary reports by Griebrokk et al. 1974 notwithstanding) or an
inhibitor of ACTH release has not been achieved; indeed, unlike
PIF, little if any physiological evidence exists for these factors.

Other substances which have now been isolated from hypothalamic
tissue preparations (Table 2) include substance P (Chang and Leeman,
1970; Chang et al., 1971), neurotensin (Carraway and Leeman, 1975),
[Arg^8]-vasopressin and α-MSH. Substance P and neurotensin, both
vasoactive substances, have no well established effect on the
pituitary gland; these peptides are of interest because substance
P is the first   brain substance also to be found in the gut
and neurotensin has some possible structural similarities to LRF
(Carraway and Leeman, 1975). The presence of vasopressin

(Guillemin and Rosenberg, 1975) and MSH (Guillemin et al., 1957)
biological activities in hypothalamic tissue has been known for
some time. We have structurally characterized in our laboratory
(unpublished results) [Arg^8]- vasopressin and α-MSH from side
fractions of ovine hypothalami. It is not surprising to find these
hormones in the hypothalamic tissue we processed, since these fragments contained some pituitary stalk tissue, but it is of interest
that the fraction of vasopressin we isolated on the basis of pres-
sor activity (Guillemin et al., 1957) had the same structure as
the ovine pituitary hormone (Acher et al., 1959). The α-MSH was
not routinely followed by biological activity, but the structure
of the peptide isolated from the ovine hypothalamic tissue preparation was not different from that of ovine pituitary origin (Lee
et al., 1963).

   Status of characterization of ovine hypothalamic hormones.
The purification and ovine hypothalamic fractions with which we
are currently working are summarized in Figures 1 and 2. The work-
-up of the alcohol-chloroform extract (fractions 2-6, Figure 1)
yielded LRF decapeptide (Ling et al., 1973), LRF B (Burgus et al.,
1973b) somatostatin (Burgus et al., 1973a) and α-MSH (unpublished
results). [Arg^8]-vasopressin was obtained from side fractions of
a previous isolation scheme for LRF (Amoss et al., 1971).
   The organic phase (fraction 5, figure 1) contains as yet uncharacterized substance(s) with CRF biological activity (measurement of radioimmunoassayable ACTH from pituitary cell culture);
at this stage CRF behaves chemically as a high molecular weight,
nonpolar acidic substance.

   In addition to the screening for substances controlling gonadotropin secretion (see below), one of the major efforts in our laboratory has been the search for a GRF. Preliminary screening of
all side fractions from the scheme in Fig. 1 and 2 by the in vitro
pituitary cell culture assay (Vale et al., 1972) for substances
releasing radioimmunoassayable GH showed the most activity in 2N
acetic acid extracts of the residue from the ethanol-chloroform
extraction (fraction 2, Fig. 2); further purification of this
fraction by gradient elution on carboxymethyl cellulose (CMC) and
gel filtration on Sephadex G-25 gave 182 g of a basic polypeptide
fraction that was active to release GH in vitro at levels of > 1
μM . Subsequent unsuccessful attempts to purify this material to
higher specific in vitro biological activity, to observe separa-
tions of fractions in a large variety of separation systems, or
to observe in vivo biological activity in rat led us to consider
that the material was an essentially pure nonspecific basic protein. Gel filtration and sodium dodecyl sulfate polyacrylamide
gel electrophoresis indicated a molecular weight of about 20,000.
Comparison of this material with other reported brain proteins by
mobilities in chromatographic and electrophoretic systems, amino

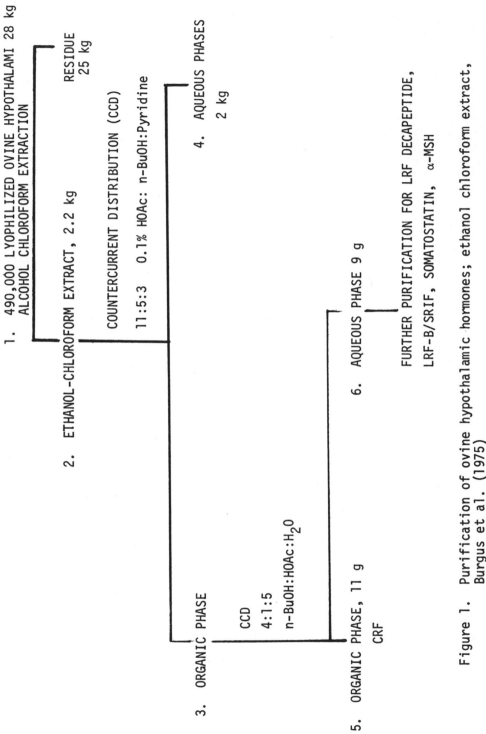

Figure 1. Purification of ovine hypothalamic hormones; ethanol chloroform extract, Burgus et al. (1975)

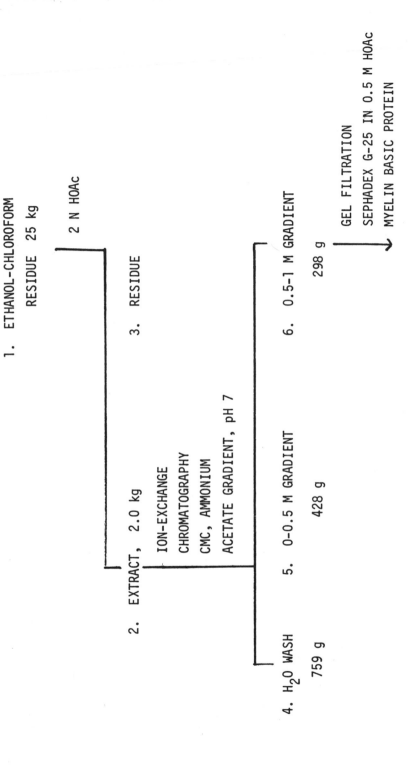

Figure 2. Purification of ovine hypothalamic hormones; extraction of ethanol chloroform residue (Villarreal et al., submitted for publication).

acid analysis of the intact protein, two-dimensional chromatograph-
ic-electrophoretic maps of tryptic digests and amino acid analysis
of fractions from tryptic digests led us to the conclusion that
the ovine brain fraction is similar or identical to bovine or porcine myelin basic protein, a structural component of myelin having
a molecular weight of ca. 18,000. As we have already reported
(Villarreal et al. submitted for publication) we have never proposed this ovine basic protein as having physiological significance
in terms of GH release (in contrast to the "GHRH" originally described by Schally et al., 1971, which is now considered by its
authors to be an artifact), but rather its presence in hypothalamic
fragments makes it an interfering substance in the in vitro cell
culture assays. A hypothalamic GRF thus remains to be characterized.

A small amount of activity to inhibit the release in vitro of
radioimmunoassayable prolactin is found in the CMC fraction 5 (Fig.
2) and appears to be distinguishable from catecholamines; this
fraction, however, contains some high molecular weight SRIF biological activity as described in the next section.

Multiple factors. Multiple factors in hypophysial portal blood
having LH releasing activity were reported by Fink (1967); one
fraction behaved as a low molecular weight material and the other
was of higher molecular weight based on gelfiltration. Shin and
Fawcett (1971) and more recently Fawcett et al. (1975) have also
described multiple LRF fractions.

We reported (Burgus and Guillemin, 1970) as part of the purification scheme of TRF that ultrafiltration of crude ovine TRF
extracts resulted in about 80% retention of TRF biological activity by a membrane with a nominal molecular weight cutoff of 500
daltons; subsequent ultrafiltration of the unretarded fraction
resulted in little retention of TRF biological activity. These
data led us to conclude that TRF biological activity was bound to
a higher molecular weight substance(s) in the crude extract; such
binding to other components of the extract might also explain why
Tsuji et al. (1968) found TRF fractions bound to anion exchange
when it is now known that the TRF molecule itself has no anionic
group.

In our program of characterization of factors controlling
gonadotropin release, we subjected 9 g. of stage 6 (Fig. 1) product
to ion-exchange chromatography on CMC (Fig. 3). Two zones of LRF
biological activity were observed. From one, which we labelled
"LRF-A", was isolated by partition chromatography and gel filtration (Amoss et al., 1971) 4.5 mg of LRF decapeptide, the structure
of which was confirmed as LRF-decapeptide (pGlu-His-Trp-Ser-Tyr-
Gly-Leu-Arg-Pro-Gly-NH$_2$) by mass spectrometry (Ling et al., 1973).

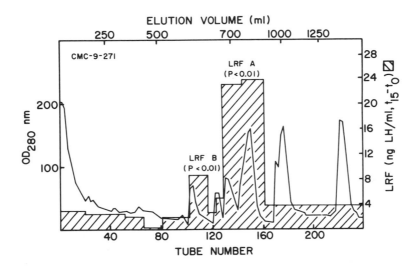

Figure 3. Ion exchange chromatography of a CMC of aqueous phase
stage 6, Figure 1. A column of Whatman CM-32 (21 x 2.7
cm.) was equilibrated in 1 M NH_4OAc (pH 4.5) and then
washed with 250 ml of H_2O. The sample, 8.3 g, was
applied in 325 ml H_2O and then a linear gradient to 0.4
M NH_4OAc (pH 7.2) was applied through a 1,330 ml mixing
volume of H_2O. The first 508 ml of eluant was collected
in bulk and then fractions of 4-8 ml were collected.

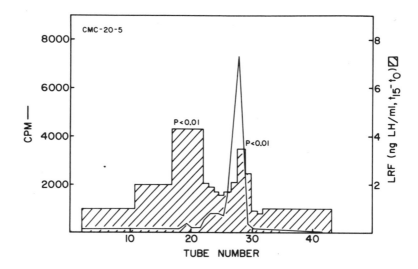

Figure 4. Ion exchange chromatography on CMC of LRF-B incubated
with tritium-labelled LRF decapeptide. Column: 9.5 x
0.7 cm. CMC equilibrated with 1 M NH4OAc (pH 4.5) and
washed with H2O. Sample was applied in 1 ml H2O and
washed on to the column in 1 ml H2O. Fractions of 0.9 m
ml were collected. A linear gradient to 0.4 M NH4OAc
was applied through a 25 ml mixing volume of water
beginning with tube no. 17.

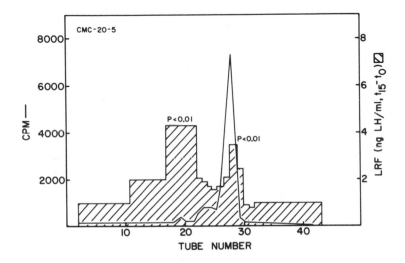

Figure 5. Partition chromatography of LRF-B incubated with tritium labelled LRF decapeptide. Column: 58.5 X 0.5 cm Sephadex G-25 equilibrated with lower phase, then upper phase of 4:1:5 nBuOH:HOAc:H$_2$O. Sample was applied in 300 µl upper phase. Fractions of 0.25 ml were collected.

The other zone, labelled "LRF-B", contained 531 mg of material.
All of the radioactivity from a marker of tritium labelled LRF
(prepared from tritium labelled proline at a specific activity of
36 Ci/mmole was found in the LRF-A zone; thus it seemed unlikely
that LRF-B simply represented LRF decapeptide bound to other substances in the extract. We further tested this possibility by
incubating 2% or 24 mg of LRF-B from the CMC columns with 2 µCi
of tritium labelled LRF decapeptide for three hours at room temperature in 200 µl aqueous solution. Half of the incubation mixture
was applied to an analytical CMC column (Fig. 4) and the other
half was applied to a partition column (Fig. 5). In both systems
the bulk of biological activity was separated from the radioactivity; some LRF biological activity found in the LRF decapeptide
zone can be accounted for by some remaining decapeptide from the
previous purification stage and by the biological activity of the
trace of tritium labelled LRF. From these observations we concluded (Burgus et al., 1973b) that LRF decapeptide is not readily
bound to substances in the LRF-B zone; moreover, if such binding
were to occur it would have to involve low molecular weight substances, since LRF-B biological activity is retarded upon gelfiltration on Sephadex G-25.

Subsequent purification of LRF-B (summarized in Table 3) yielded too little peptide (less than 10 µg) to characterize. The in
vitro cell culture assay (Vale et al. 1972) showed that LRF-B
stimulated the release of immunoassayable FSH in proportions
similar or identical to that of LRF decapeptide (Table 4); LRF-B
therefore differs from the possible "FSH-RH" reported by Johansson
et al. (1973). It may, however, be similar to the low molecular
weight species observed by Fawcett et al. (1975).

Multiple forms of other hypothalamic hormones have been observed. Currie et al. (1974) and Johansson et al. (1974), reported
two growth hormone releasing substances in porcine hypothalamic
extracts; at least one of these, however, "A-GHRH", appears to
have properties similar to myelin basic protein. Schally et al.
(1975) have reported on three types of immunoreactive SRIF's with
different molecular weights and Arimura et al (1975) has found
two materials, one large and one smaller molecular weight in rat
stomach and pancreas which are active in the somatostatin radioimmunoassay. We have also observed larger molecular weight immunoreactive somatostatin(s) in ovine brain extracts. We also find
SRIF biological in vitro activity in all purification stages of
LRF-B. None of these substances has been fully characterized.
The reports of two different MIF peptides have already been cited.

The physiological significance of all of these multiple factors
remains to be established. Some of these (as in the case of TRF)
may represent binding of presently characterized hormones to other

TABLE 3

Purification of Ovine "LRF-B"

	Stage	Weight	Units[†]LRF X 10^5
1.	Ion-exchange CMC	531 mg	0.6 - 3.0
2.	Partition on Sephadex G-25 4:1:5 n-BuOH:HOAc:H_2O (BAW)	95 mg	0.1
3.	Gel Filtration, Sephadex G-25	29 mg	0.1
4.	Partition on Sephadex G-25 (BAW)	5 mg	0.1
5.	Electrophoresis, pH 6	10 µg	0.1

[†] Estimated from single dose _in_ vivo (Amoss _et al._, 1971) for stages 2-5.

TABLE 4

Cell Culture Assay of Secretion of LH and FSH by "LRF-B"

Treatment	LRF Activity in pg/Fragment	
	LH Release	FSH Release
LRF-B Stage 4 (Table 3) partition BAW	1.3	1.3
LRF-B Stage 5 (Table 3) Electrophoresis	3.9	3.3

substances; the specificity of any such binding substance is as
yet unknown. In other cases, such as the LRF's and some of the
SRIF's, there may be separate chemical entities involved. The
possibility cannot be excluded that some or all of the multiple
factors are simply nonspecific artifacts of the hormones arising
from the isolation procedures; but these substances may represent
naturally occuring structural analogs or biological precursors to
known hormones and therefore be of considerable interest in
defining the metabolism and mechanisms of action of these peptides.

In conclusion, several of the hypothalamic hypophysiotropic
hormones have now been characterized, making it possible to prepare
their synthetic replicates and analogs for a wide variety of
physiological and clinical applications. Several more of the putative hormones for which physiological and chemical evidence exists,
such as GRF, CRF, PIF, and the multiple forms of known hormones
remain to be isolated and characterized. The increasing biological
significance of the known brain hormones, especially with regard
to extrapituitary effects and their occurrence in tissues other
than hypothalamus now being observed leads us to eagerly anticipate
the discovery of other physiologically important brain substances.

ACKNOWLEDGMENTS

The authors are grateful for the excellent technical assistance
of M. Butcher, L. Chan, L. Clark, S. Garcia, M. Mercado, L. Osaki,
R. Schroder and R. Wolbers. Research supported by AID (Contract
No. csd-2785), NIH (AM 16707; AM 18811; and HD 09690), National
Foundation (1-411), the Rockefeller Foundation, the Ford Foundation,
and the Edna McConnell Clark Foundation.

REFERENCES

Acher, R., Chauvet, J. and Lenci, M.T. (1959) C. R. Acad. Sci. (Paris) 248, 1435-1438.

Amoss, M., Burgus, R., Blackwell, R., Vale, W., Fellows, R.E. and Guillemin, R. (1971) Biochem. Biophys. Res. Commun. 44, 205-210.

Arimura, A., Sato, H., Dupont, A., Nishi, N. and Schally, A.V. (1975) Science 189, 1007-1009.

Blackwell, R. and Guillemin, R. (1973) Ann. Rev. of Physiol. 35. 357-390.

Bloom, S.R., Mortimer, C.H., Thorner, M.O., Besser, G.M., Hall, R., Gomez-Pan, A., Roy, V.M., Russell, R.C.G., Coy, D.H., Kastin, A.J. and Schally, A.V. (1974) Lancet 2, 1106-1109.

Brazeau, P., Vale, W., Burgus, R., Ling, N., Butcher, M., Rivier, J. and Guillemin, R. (1973) Science 179, 77-79.

Brown, M. and Vale, W. (1975) Endocrinology 97, 1151-1156.

Burgus, R., T. Dunn, D. Desiderio, D. Ward, W. Vale and R. Guillemin. (1970) Nature 226, 321-325.

Burgus, R. and Guillemin, R. (1970) In: Hypophysiotropic Hormones of the Hypothalamus (J. Meites, ed.), Williams & Wilkins, Baltimore, Md., pp. 227-241.

Burgus, R., Butcher, M., Amoss, M., Ling, N., Monahan, M., Rivier, J., Fellows, R., Blackwell, R., Vale, W. and Guillemin, R. (1972) Proc. Nat. Acad. Sci. (USA) 69, 278-282.

Burgus, R., Ling, N., Butcher, M. and Guillemin, R. (1973a) Proc. Nat. Acad. Sci. (USA) 70, 684-688.

Burgus, R., Rivier, J. and Amoss, M. (1973b) The Endocrine Society, June 20-22 (Abstract).

Carraway, R. and Leeman, S.E. (1975) J. Biol. Chem. 250, 1907-1911.

Celis, M.E., Taleisnik, S. and Walter, R. (1971a) Proc. Nat. Acad. Sci. (USA) 68, 1428-1433.

Celis, M.E., Taleisnik, S., Schwartz, I.L. and Walter, R. (1971b) Biophysical J. 11, 98a.

Chang, M.M. and Leeman, S.E. (1970) J. Biol. Chem. 245, 4784-4790.

Chang, M.M., Leeman, S.E. and Niall, H.D. (1971) Nature New Biol. 232, 86-87.

Currie, B.L., Johansson, K.N.G., Greibrokk, T., Folkers,K. and Bowers, C.Y. (1974) Biochem. Biophys. Res. Commun. 60, 605-609.

Dubois, M.P. (1975) Proc. Nat. Acad. Sci. (USA) 72, 1340-1343.

Fawcett, C.P., Beezley, A.E. and Wheaton, J.E. (1975) Endocrinology 96, 1311-1314.

Fink, G. (1967) Nature 215, 159-161.

Greibrokk, T., Currie, B.L., Johansson, K.N.G., Hansen, J.J., Folkers, K. and Bowers, C.Y. (1974) Biochem. Biophys. Res. Commun. 59, 704-709.

Guillemin, R. and Rosenberg, B. (1955) Endocrinology 57, 599-607.

Guillemin, R., Hearn, W.R., Cheek, W.R. and Housholder, D.E. (1957) Endocrinology 60, 488-506.

IUPAC-IUB Commission on Biochemical Nomenclature (1975) Biochem. 14, 2559-2560.

Jackson, I.M.D. and Reichlin, S. (1974) Endocrinology 95, 854-862.

Johansson, K.N.G., Currie, B.L., Folkers, K. and Bowers, C.Y. (1973) Biochem. Biophys. Res. Commun. 50, 8-13.

Johansson, K.N.G., Currie, B.L., Folkers, K. and Bowers, C.Y. (1974) Biochem. Biophys. Res. Commun. 60, 610-615.

Lee, T.H., Lerner, A.B. and Buettner-Janusch, V. (1963) Biochem. Biophys. Acta 71, 706-709.

Ling, N., Rivier, J., Burgus, R. and Guillemin, R. (1973) Biochemistry 12:26, 5305-5310.

Matsuo, H., Baba, Y., Nair, R.M.G., Arimura, A. and Schally, A.V. (1971) Biochem. Biophys. Res. Commun. 43, 1334-1339.

Nair, R.M.G., Barrett, J.F., Bowers, C.Y. and Schally, A.V. (1970) Biochemistry 9, 1103-1106.

Nair, R.M.G., Kastin, A.J. and Schally, A.V. (1971) Biochem. Biophys. Res. Commun. 43, 1376-1381.

Nair, R.M.G., Kastin, A.J. and Schally, A.V. (1972) Biochem. Biophys. Res. Commun. 47, 1420-1425.

Oliver, C.R., Eskay, L., Ben-Johnathan, N. and Porter, J.C. (1974) Endocrinology 95, 540-546.

Plotnikoff, N.P., Kastin, A.J., Anderson, M.S. and Schally, A.V. (1971) Life Sci. 10, 1279-1283.

Plotnikoff, N.P., Prange, A.J. Jr., Breese, G.R., Anderson, M.S. and Wilson, I.C. (1973) Science 178, 417-418.

Prange, A.J. Jr., Breese, G.R., Jahnke, G.D., Martin, B.R., Cooper, B.R., Catt, J.M., Wilson, I.C., Alltop, L.B., Lipton, M.A., Bissetti, G., Nemeroff, C.B. and Loosen, P.T. (1975) Life Sci. 16, 1907-1914.

Ruch, W., Koerker, D.J., Carino, M., Johnsen, S.D., Webster, B.R., Ensinck, J.W., Goodner, C.J. and Gale, C.C. (1973) In: Advances in Human Growth Hormone Research (S. Raiti, ed.), U. S. Gov't. Printing Ofc., DHEW, Publ. No. (N.I.H.) 74-612, pp 271-289.

Schally, A.V., Baba, Y., Nair, R.M.G. and Bennett, C.D. (1971) J. Biol. Chem. 246, 6647-6650.

Schally, A.V., Arimura, A. and Kastin, A.J. (1973). Science 179, 341-350.

Schally, A.V., Dupont, A., Arimura, A., Redding, T.W. and Linthicum, G.L. (1975) Fed. Proc. 34, 584.

Shin, S. and Fawcett, C.P. (1971) Endocrinology 88, 70A.

Taleisnik, S. and Orias, R. (1965) Am. J. Physiol. 208, 293-296.

Tashjian, A.H. Jr., Barowsky, N.J. and Jensen, D.K. (1971) Biochem. Biophys. Res. Commun. 43, 516-523.

Tsuji, S., Sakoda, M. and Asami, M. (1968) In: Integrative Mechanisms of Neuroendocrine System (S. Itoh, ed.), Hokkaido Univ. School of Med., Hokkaido, Japan, pp. 63-85.

Vale, W., Grant, G., Amoss, M., Blackwell, R. and Guillemin, R. (1972) Endocrinology 91, 562-572.

Vale, W., Rivier, C., Brazeau, P. and Guillemin, R. (1974) Endocrinology 95, 968-977.

VonEuler, U.S. and Gaddum, J.H. (1931) J. Physiol. 72, 74-87.

Winokur, A. and Utiger, R.D. (1974) Science 185, 265-267.

ANALOGS OF SOMATOSTATIN PART A.   CHEMISTRY AND IN VITRO RESULTS

H. Immer*, N.A. Abraham*, V. Nelson*, K. Sestanj*,
M. Götz*, P. Brazeau** and J.B. Martin**

*Ayerst Research Laboratories, St. Laurent, Quebec
**Research Institute, Montreal General Hospital, Montreal,
Quebec

Recently, we reported on the synthesis of Somatostatin by a
classical fragment approach (Immer et al., 1974). This method avoids
the problematic cyclization of dihydrosomatostatin (Rivier, J.E.F.,
1974, Fujii, N. and Yajima, H., 1975) and leads to the desired
product in high yield. Essentially, the same synthetic scheme was
employed for the preparation of three groups of somatostatin analogs
discussed here:

1) Shortened Analogs of Somatostatin.
2) Elongated Analogs of Somatostatin
3) Retroenantio Analogs of Somatostatin Derivatives.

To allow rapid understanding of the structural changes, the
following notation has been introduced:

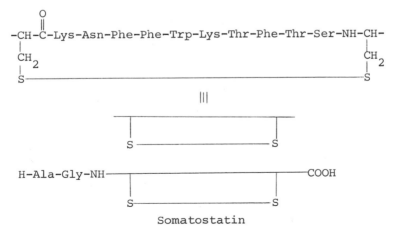

Somatostatin

373

The <u>in vitro</u> data discussed were obtained essentially according to the method published (Vale <u>et al</u>., 1972) using cultures of enzymatically dispersed anterior pituitary cells and measuring the RGH by radioimmunoassay.

1) SHORTENED ANALOGS OF SOMATOSTATIN.

Figures 1-3 show the dose-response curves of [desamino[1]]-, [descarboxy[14]]-and [desamino[1]][descarboxy[14]]-somatostatin. The results demonstrate that the peptide terminal functions are unessential for growth hormone release inhibiting activity. This finding induced us to prepare des[Ala[1]Gly[2]][acetyl[3]][descarboxy[14]] somatostatin, which differs from a reported long-acting analog (Brazeau <u>et al</u>., 1974) only by the absence of the terminal carboxy function. The compound retained high activity (Fig. 4) without prolongation of <u>in vivo</u> action (see Part B).

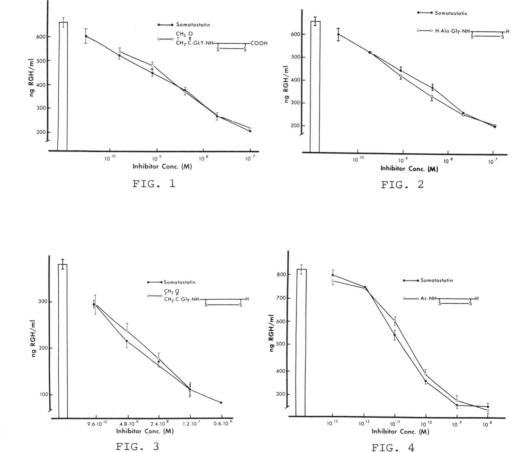

FIG. 1   FIG. 2

FIG. 3   FIG. 4

A further simplification of the somatostatin molecule led to the substance of Figure 5, which still retains high activity and at the same time is synthetically more easily accessible than somatostatin.

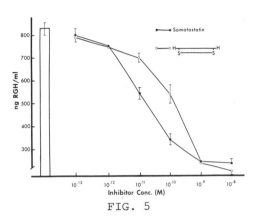

FIG. 5

2) ELONGATED ANALOGS OF SOMATOSTATIN.

Chain elongation of oxytocin and vasopressin has led to analogs termed hormonogens. These are characterized by considerably reduced in vitro activity and relatively high and protracted activity in vivo due to the delayed formation of the parent compound through enzymatic removal of the elongating groups (Rudinger, J., 1971).

Somatostatin was elongated at the amine terminal by di-Gly, (Fig. 6), tri-Gly (Fig. 7) and Leu-di-Gly (Fig. 8). It was shown above that the terminal carboxy is unessential for activity. The carboxy group was therefor omitted in the last example (Fig. 9). All of these compounds are in vitro highly active inhibitors of GH-secretion. The heptadecapeptide tri-Gly-somatostatin shows the highest potency of all analogs discussed. Since the choice of the elongating groups is very restricted and arbitrary, it is foreseeable that empirical screening of other elongating groups would lead to the detection of even more active derivatives.

In summary, the elongation of the somatostatin molecule has created compounds of increased in vitro potency. Unless one assumes high enzymatic activity in the pituitary cell preparations, these results cannot be accommodated by the hormonogen theory.

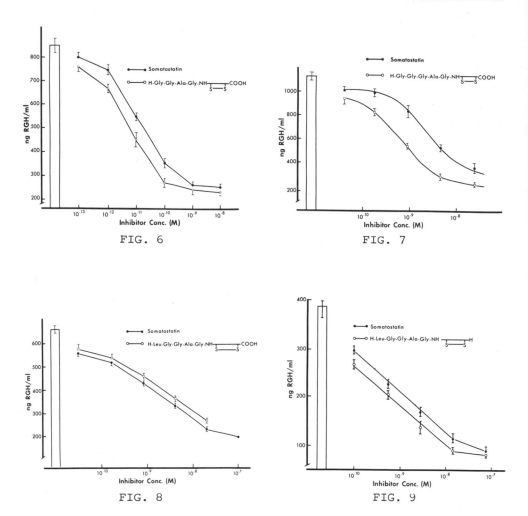

FIG. 6   FIG. 7

FIG. 8   FIG. 9

3) RETROENANTIO ANALOGS OF SOMATOSTATIN DERIVATIVES.

Retroenantio isomers are obtained by reversal of the direction of the peptide bond and inversion of all asymmetric centers of a given peptide. This manipulation should not affect the topology of the side chains. The synthesis of retroenantio analogs is only attractive if the terminal functions are either absent- as in the case of homodetic cyclic peptides- or of no importance for activity in the parent molecule (Shemyakin, M.M., et al., 1969). This prerequisite is not realized in the case of all retroenantio hormones reported up to this date (Rudinger, J., 1971, Hechter, O., et al., 1975).

[Desamino[1]] [descarboxy[14]]-somatostatin and des[Ala[1]Gly[2]]
[desamino[3]] [descarboxy[14]]-somatostatin are devoid of terminal
functional groups and still exhibit high GH release inhibiting
activity (Fig. 3 and 5). Thus their retroenantio isomers are
ideal candidates for a synthetic effort. Experimental details of
the preparation of 1 and 2 will be reported in a forthcoming paper.

$$
\begin{array}{l}
\quad\quad O \\
\quad\quad || \\
CH_2C-ser-thr-phe-thr-lys-trp-phe-phe-asn-lys-cys-gly-NH-Et \\
| \\
CH_3 \\
| \\
S
\end{array}
$$

Structure 1

$$
\begin{array}{l}
\quad\quad O \\
\quad\quad || \\
CH_2C-ser-thr-phe-thr-lys-trp-phe-phe-asn-lys-NHCH_2 \\
| \quad\quad\quad\quad\quad\quad\quad\quad\quad\quad\quad\quad\quad\quad\quad\quad\quad | \\
CH_2 \quad\quad\quad\quad\quad\quad\quad\quad\quad\quad\quad\quad\quad\quad\quad CH_2 \\
| \quad\quad\quad\quad\quad\quad\quad\quad\quad\quad\quad\quad\quad\quad\quad\quad\quad | \\
S\quad\quad\quad\quad\quad\quad\quad\quad\quad\quad\quad\quad\quad\quad\quad\quad\quad\quad S
\end{array}
$$

Structure 2

(small letters indicate D-configuration of amino acids)

    Figure 10 clearly demonstrates that the retroenantio isomer 2
shows significant GH release inhibition, whereas isomer 1 is
practically inactive. This is in contrast to the parent compounds,
both of which are highly active. The activity of substance 2
indicates that the cyclic backbone is not of crucial importance
for hormonal action. Consequently, the lack of activity of 1 must
be related to the presence of the side chain. The following
hypothesis could accommodate these results. A prerequisite for
GH release inhibition is the enzymatic cleavage of a peptide bond
of the side chain. Obviously this cannot be achieved in the all
D-form 1, which is expected to be stable towards proteolytic enzymes.
This hypothesis is schematically expressed in Fig. 11.

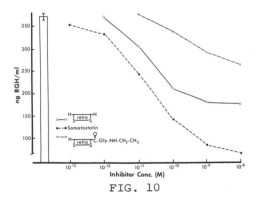

FIG. 10

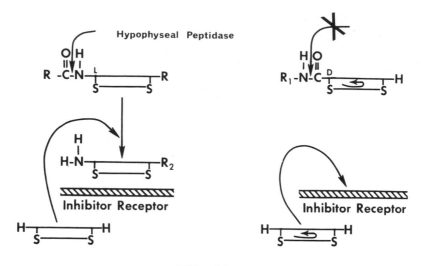

FIG. 11

In conclusion, structure 2 represents the first retroenantio compound with pronounced hormonal activity.

REFERENCES

Brazeau, P., Vale, W., Rivier, J. and Guillemin, R.
(1974) Biochem. Biophys. Res. Commun. 60, 1202-1207.

Fujii, N. and Yajimo, H. (1975) Chem. Pharm. Bull. 23, 1596-1603.

Hechter, O., Kato, T., Nakagawa, S.H., Yong, F. and Flouret, G.
(1975) Proc. Nat. Sci. USA 72, 563-566.

Immer, H.U., Sestanj, K., Nelson, V.R. and Götz, M.
(1974) Helv. Chim. Acta. 57, 730-734.

Rivier, J.E.F. (1974) J. Amer. Chem. Soc. 96, 2986-2991.

Rudinger, J. (1971) In: Drug Design (E.J. Ariëns ed.) vol. 2,
Academic Press New York and London, pp 394-397 and 368-369.

Shemyakin, M.M., Ovchinnikov Yu. A. and Yvanov, V.T.
(1969) Angew. Chem. Internat. Edit. 8, 492-499.

Vale, W., Grant, G., Amoss, M., Blackwell, R. and Guillemin, R.
(1972) Endocrinology 91, 562-5.

PART B. IN VIVO ACTIVITIES: PROLONGATION OF ACTION WITH PROTA-

MINE ZINC

P. Brazeau
Research Institute, Montreal General Hospital
Montreal, Quebec
and
J.B. Martin
Division of Neurology, Department of Medicine
Montreal General Hospital, McGill University
Montreal, Quebec

INTRODUCTION

The elucidation of the structure of somatostatin (GH release-inhibiting factor - SRIF) (Brazeau et al., 1973) and the demonstration that it is effective in inhibiting insulin and glucagon release by direct effects on the pancreas (Koerker et al., 1974) has resulted in a number of attempts to develop a long-acting preparation for potential clinical use. The duration of action of SRIF is limited to 5-10 minutes after intravenous administration (Brazeau et al., 1973) and to a maximum of 20-30 minutes after subcutaneous injection (Brazeau et al., 1974a; Martin, 1974) in the rat. Similar findings are reported in primates, including man.

A combination of SRIF with protamine zinc (PZ) was reported to suppress the GH response to pentobarbital for up to 16 hours in the rat (Brazeau et al., 1974a) and to inhibit physiologic pulsatile GH secretion in the rat (Martin et al., 1974). Subsequent reports indicated that this combination was not effective in the dog and monkey (unpublished reports). However, Besser et al. (1974) have recently shown that PZ combined with cyclic or linear SRIF is effective in suppressing GH in man for up to 5 hours.

Analogues of SRIF have also been tested for GH-inhibiting effects. Acylated-cys[3] analogues initially showed promise of long action when tested in the rat (Brazeau et al., 1974b), but subsequent findings and our own recent experience has indicated that their effect is inconsistent in different bioassays.

379

In the present experiments, a number of additional analogues of SRIF have been synthesized as described in Part A and their effects tested in vivo. The results indicate that the short-term activity of SRIF can be enhanced several fold by minor structural modifications and that these effects can be demonstrated in vivo. However, prolonged activity was not evident unless the agents were administered in combination with an acidic suspension of PZ. These results provide promise of an effective long-acting preparation of SRIF which may be of use in clinical studies.

METHODS

Animals: Male Sprague Dawley rats weighing 175–200 g were used except for the animals that were implanted with intracardiac cannulae. The latter weighed 350–450 g.

In vivo bioassays: A number of critical factors were taken into consideration in the development of an in vivo bioassay for SRIF. Several reports have shown that morphine is a potent stimulant of GH release in the rat (Kokka et al., 1972; Brazeau et al., 1974c; Martin et al., 1975); its effects are several fold greater than pentobarbital and evidence indicates that its site of action is at a hypothalamic level (Martin et al., 1975). Morphine has no effect when directly applied to hemi-pituitaries (Martin et al., 1975) or monolayer cultures in vitro (Brazeau et al., 1974c). The rapid effects of morphine are consistent with an effect mediated by release of endogenous GH-releasing factor (GRF).

Physiologic secretion of GH in the rat has been shown to be characterized by episodic or pulsatile release (Martin et al., 1974). Detailed studies by Tannenbaum, Willoughby and Martin (see paper by Willoughby and Martin, page 303) have shown a consistent timing of the secretory bursts in relation to clocktime. In colonies where lights are turned on at 6:00 hr, there are prominent bursts of GH release at 7:30 to 9:00 hrs, at 10:00 to 12:00 hrs and at 13:30 to 14:30 hrs. Between these rather discrete bursts of GH release, plasma GH levels are undetectable (<5 ng/ml). We have found that administration of morphine during the trough period at 12:15 to 12:30 hrs results in a highly homogeneous response in GH. Consequently, all animals were tested with morphine starting at 12:20 and sacrificed by decapitation 20–25 minutes later. Individually tested analogs were administered s.c. at various intervals up to 12 hrs before morphine. Control injections consisted of the vehicle alone.

In a few preliminary studies, SRIF and several analogues were also administered to animals bearing chronic intracardiac cannulae to test for suppression of physiologic episodic GH release using techniques which have been previously reported (Martin et al., 1974).

PZ-SRIF was prepared as previously described (Brazeau et al., 1974a) except that pH of the final suspension was reduced to 5.2-5.6.

RESULTS

a) Acute effects: The acute effects of cyclic SRIF and several analogues when tested in vivo against the GH stimulating effects of morphine were comparable to those observed in vitro (Figure 1). The des [Ala^{1}Gly^2] [acetyl^3] [descarboxyl^{14}] analogue had a potency similar to native SRIF. Tri-Gly-SRIF and Leu-di-Gly-SRIF were approximately 3.0-5.0 times more potent than SRIF. The [desamino^1] [descarboxy^{14}] analogue was slightly more potent than cyclic SRIF, a finding in variance with the in vitro results (see Part A).

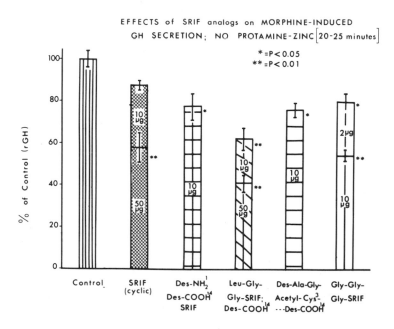

Figure 1

b) Prolonged effects (morphine model): None of the analogues showed any inhibitory effects on GH responses to morphine at 3, 6 or 12 hrs when administered in saline. The results at 3 hrs are illustrated in Figure 2. Combination of SRIF and several analogues in suspension with PZ was effective in suppressing the GH response

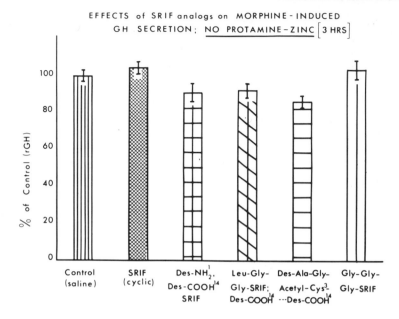

Figure 2

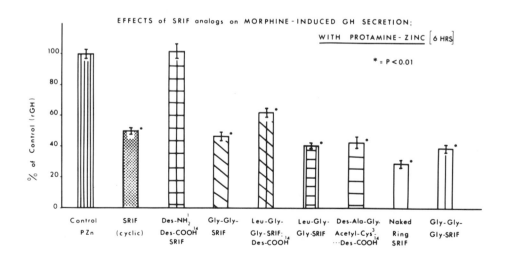

Figure 3

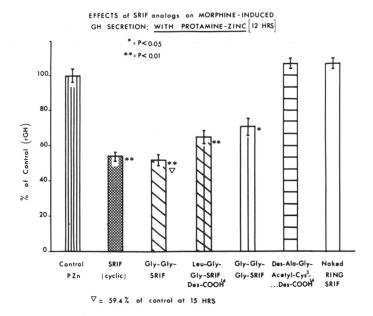

Figure 4

to morphine and the inhibitory effect persisted in some cases for
as long as 12 hrs (Figures 3 and 4).

All of the analogues with the exception of the [desamino[1]]
[descarboxy[14]]-SRIF compound were highly effective in inhibiting
GH responses at 6 hrs (Figure 3).

c) Prolonged activity on pulsatile GH secretion: In preliminary studies, two of the compounds have been tested for effects
on suppression of physiologic GH release in the rat. PZ-SRIF is
effective in suppressing pulsatile GH for at least 6 hrs in the
rat (Martin et al., 1974) (Figure 5). The acetyl derivative was
also effective when combined with PZ (Figure 6). A reduction in
the amplitude of GH surges was observed in 6 of 8 animals.

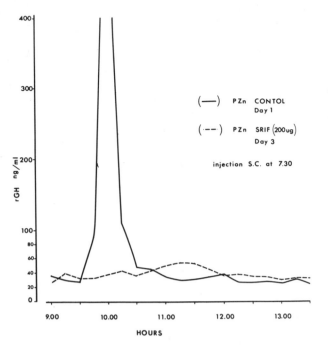

Figure 5

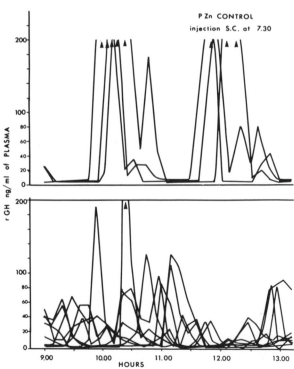

Figure 6

DISCUSSION

These results indicate that several elongations of somatostatin can significantly enhance the GH inhibitory effects of SRIF
in vivo. The elongation did not, however, result in any demonstr-
able prolongation of action except in combination with PZ. Although several analogues in combination with PZ were slightly more
effective that SRIF itself, the differences were not great.

We believe that the effective suppression of GH for more than
6 hrs by SRIF and various analogues administered in combination
with PZ is a significant effect and that, to date, this affords
the most promising method for prolongation of SRIF action. Preliminary studies on suppression of pulsatile secretion in the rat
and the demonstration of glucose and glucagon lowering effects in
diabetic dogs (P. Brazeau and R. Unger, unpublished results) leads
us to believe that further studies with this vehicle are warranted.

ACKNOWLEDGEMENTS

The authors wish to thank Judy Audet and Diane Duperré for
technical assistance and Gail Hannaford for secretarial help.
Supported by grants No. MA-5298 and MA-3967 from the Medical
Research Council of Canada.

REFERENCES

1. Brazeau, P., Vale, W., Burgus, R., Ling, N., Burcher, M.,
    Rivier, J. and Guillemin, R. (1973) Science 179, 77-79.

2. Brazeau, P., Rivier, J., Vale, W. and Guillemin, R. (1974a)
    Endocrinology 94, 184-187.

3. Brazeau, P., Vale, W. and Guillemin, R. (1974b) B.B.R.C. 60,
    1202-1207.

4. Brazeau, P., Vale, W. and Guillemin, R. (1974c) In: Narcotics
    and the Hypothalamus (E. Zimmerman and R. George, eds.) Raven
    Press, New York, pp 109-119.

5. Koerker, D.J., Ruch, W., Chideckel, E., Palmer, J., Goodner,
    C.J., Ensinck, J. and Gale, C.C. (1974) Science 184, 482-484.

6. Kokka, N., Garcia, J.F., George, R. and Ellioh, H.W. (1972a)
    Endocrinology 90, 735-743.

7.   Martin, J.B. (1974) Endocrinology 94, 497–503.

8.   Martin, J.B., Renaud, L.P. and Brazeau, P. (1974) Science 186, 538–540.

9.   Martin, J.B., Audet, J. and Saunders, A. (1975) Endocrinology 96, 881–889.

IN VIVO METHODS FOR STUDYING THE ACTION OF HYPOTHALAMIC HORMONES

WITH SPECIAL REFERENCE TO THEIR ANTISERA AS TOOLS FOR INVESTIGATION

Akira Arimura

Tulane University School of Medicine and Veterans

Administration Hospital, New Orleans, Louisiana, U.S.A.

INTRODUCTION

Physiological actions of the hypothalamic hypophysiotropic hormones were extensively studied before these hormones were isolated. Experiments were performed using crude extracts of hypothalamic tissue in order to understand the action of a hypothalamic hormone. The physiological role of a hypothalamic hormone was indirectly studied by suppressing or stimulating production or release of the hormone by making a lesion or stimulating a certain area in the brain. To learn its biokinetics, the content of the hypothalamic hormone under various conditions was measured by using bioassays. The enormous amount of data thus accumulated by many investigators has greatly contributed to our knowledge of neuroendocrinology.

However, the major advancement in this field of study may be the isolation, characterization and synthesis of TRH, LHRH and somatostatin. The availability of synthetic preparations of these hormones has made possible the study of their actions in vivo and in vitro without considering interference by substances which are possibly contained in the crude or semipurified natural hormone preparations. Furthermore, these synthetic hormones were used as antigens to generate specific antisera which could be used to establish a specific radioimmunoassay for the hormone. It is also possible to block the action of the endogenous hormone through neutralization by the antiserum, thus revealing its physiological role and action. Such basic studies have indeed provided very useful information for understanding the physiology of the hypothalamic hormones. At this meeting, I would like to talk about some of our in vivo studies on LHRH and somatostatin using synthetic preparations of these hormones as well as their antisera.

LHRH

The most sensitive and convenient in vivo method for determining
LHRH activity may be the one originally reported by Ramirez and
McCann (1963) using ovariectomized progesterone- estrogen treated
rats.   In our experiments, the injection of as small a dose as 0.2
ng synthetic LHRH into these animals increased serum LH levels significantly 30 min after injection.   The magnitude of the rise in LH
is dose-related in a range of up to 2.5 ng.   Because of its great
sensitivity and easiness, this assay for LHRH has been used during
our effort in purification, isolation and structure studies of LHRH.
LHRH, either natural or synthetic, as well as crude extracts of hypothalamic tissue, stimulate the release of both LH and FSH from
the pituitary in vitro in a dose-related manner, whereas these materials do not consistently stimulate the release of FSH in ovariectomized steroids-treated rats.   Since during in vitro stimulation,
the pituitary gonadotrophs may be continuously exposed to LHRH or
FSHRH in the medium, prolonged exposure of the pituitary to the
hormone might be essential for full stimulation of FSH release.
Since a possibly brief exposure of the pituitary to LHRH in vivo,
following a single injection of the decapeptide, might be effective in stimulating LH release, but relatively ineffective in FSH
release, a prolonged iv infusion of the hormone was tested for FSH
releasing activity in immature male rats.   As expected, a considerable rise in serum FSH as well as LH levels was induced by a 2-4 hr
iv infusion of LHRH (Arimura et al., 1972a).   This prolonged infusion in immature male rats is now being used in our laboratories as
a method for in vivo assay for FSHRH activity.

These findings have cast a problem on the different response
mechanisms of LH and FSH gonadotrophs.   One of the most commonly
considered problem is whether protein or RNA synthesis is essential for the release mechanism of either LH or FSH, or both.   Samli
and Geschwind (1967) and Crighton et al. (1968) reported that release of LH was not dependent upon protein or RNA synthesis in their
in vitro studies.   Jutisz and de la Llosa (1967) and Watanabe et al.
(1968) reported that FSH release required protein synthesis.   However, since those experiments were performed under different conditions, it is difficult to draw a conclusion from them.

To investigate this problem, immature male rats were pretreated
with 100 ug Actinomycin D (Act D)/100 g.b.w. ip or saline, and they
were challenged by 150 to 300 ng LHRH through a prolonged infusion
or a quick injection (Vilchez-Martinez et al., 1975).   Other studies
using the uptake of ^{3}H-uridine indicated that this dose of Act D
administered under similar conditions suppressed by 30% the incorporation of ^{3}H-uridine into the RNA of the pituitary gland.   The
blockade of RNA synthesis became apparent as early as 45 min after
injection and lasted for at least 4 hr thereafter (Bowers et al.,

1967). The increase in serum LH and FSH levels after quick iv injection of LHRH was unaffected by pretreatment with Act D regardless of whether the antibiotic was injected 1 or 2 hr before LHRH.
When the animals were infused with LHRH for 4 hrs, the elevation of
serum LH at 1 hr after the initiation of the infusion was not affected by Act D which was injected 1 hr before LHRH, but the responses at 2, 3 and 4 hr were significantly suppressed. A similar
suppression by Act D was also observed for FSH response.

One might argue that the delayed suppression may be due to the
non-specific toxic effect of Act D. However, this may not be the
case, since the same results were obtained when Act D was injected
2 hr before LHRH. LH response at 1 hr, which was 3 hr after Act D,
was not impaired in this study, being in contrast to the suppression
of LH response at 2 hr after infusion started in the preceeding study which was also 3 hr after Act D (Vilchez-Martinez et al., 1975).

The results suggest that the initial phase of both LH and FSH
responses to LHRH does not require DNA-dependent RNA synthesis,
whereas the later phase does. RNA or protein synthesis may be necessary for maintenance of the increased secretion of both LH and
FSH during the later period of continuous infusion with LHRH.

Influence of endogenous LHRH can be eliminated through its neutralization by the antiserum. Injection of rabbit antiserum to LHRH
to the proestrus rats before the critical period prevented the pre-
ovulatory surge of LH and FSH and blocked ovulation (Arimura et al.,
1974). The results suggested that either LHRH regulates the secretion of both LH and FSH, or that FSHRH is immunologically indistin-
guishable from LHRH decapeptide. Similar results were reported by
Koch and his colleagues (1973).

de la Cruz (1975), in our laboratories, extended the study on the
effect of anti-LHRH serum on the pituitary-gonadal function in cycling golden hamsters. In this study, sheep antiserum to LHRH was
utilized. In the first experiment, hamsters received 0.5 ml of the
antiserum iv at 9 a.m. of any stage of the estrous cycle. None of
these hamsters ovulated on the morning of the presumptive estrus,
while control animals receiving 0.5 ml normal sheep serum fully
ovulated. The characteristic vaginal discharge occurring on the
morning of estrus was present in the hamsters treated with the antiserum on P_1 but absent in those treated with the antiserum on E, D_1
or D_2. The duration of anti-ovulatory activity of 0.5 ml of the
antiserum which was injected on D_1 lasted 13.2 days and 12.5 days
after iv and sc administration, respectively. The minimum iv dose
of the antiserum to block ovulation was 0.2 ml when administered at
noon on P. At least 50 ng LHRH was needed to overcome the anti-
ovulatory activity of 0.2 ml antiserum.

In normal hamsters, LH surge was observed between 3 and 7 p.m. on

proestrus.   Injection of 0.2 ml of the antiserum at noon completely
suppressed LH surge.   IV injection of 50 ng LHRH at 4 p.m. on proestrus induced full ovulation in the   antiserum-treated animals;
however, the integrated levels of serum LH after injection of 50
ng LHRH in these hamsters were approximately 10% of those in the intact animals.   In other words, only 10% of LH which is normally secreted in the afternoon of proestrus appears to be sufficient to
induce full ovulation.   Any antagonist or reagent which will be prepared in an attempt to block ovulation by suppressing LH secretion
must suppress normal LH release by 90% or more, if the ovarian responsiveness to LH remains unaltered.

Phenobarbital injection at 1 p.m. on P as well as the antiserum
injected at 9 a.m. at any stage of estrous cycle suppressed preovulatory LH surge.   200 ng LHRH at 4 p.m. on P induced
LH release of a similar magnitude in both phenobarbital-blocked and
antiserum-blocked hamsters; however, only 1 out of 5 rats receiving
the antiserum on D_1 ovulated, whereas all of the phenobarbital-
blocked hamsters fully ovulated.   Treatment with estradiol on D_2
augmented LH response but did not improve the ovarian respnse to
LH.   The failure of ovulation may be most probably interpreted by
suppression by the antiserum of follicular maturation.   These findings suggest that anti-LHRH serum blocked ovulation through different mechanisms, first, by suppressing follicular maturation, second, by suppressing estrogen secretion which otherwise triggers LH
release and third, by blocking preovulatory LH surge.   A similar
mode of action was reported for antiserum to LH by Ely and Schwarz
(1971).   They suggested that a lower dose of the antiserum to LH
than is required to prevent ovulation at proestrus would prevent
estrogen secretion and the ensuing ovulation when injected at diestrus in rats.

When 0.5 ml of the antiserum was injected on D_1, serum estradiol levels remained at the same levels during the cycle but never
felt below the levels in ovariectomized- adrenolectomized hamsters.
In the hamsters receiving normal sheep serum, estradiol levels increased, reaching a peak in the afternoon of proestrus.   The LH response to LHRH in the afternoon of proestrus was the same for both
of these groups of animals.   The results indicated that a gradual
increase in estrogen secretion during the estrous cycle is regulated by the hypothalamus, by means of LHRH and thus LH and FSH,
but this increase does not appear to contribute to the greater LH
response which is normally observed in the afternoon of P.

The fact that treatment with antiserum to LHRH suppressed tonic
secretion of gonadotropin was supported by other experiments in
which the sheep antiserum was given to male rats every 2 days beginning the day after castration (Arimura et al., 1975a). Both serum
LH and FSH levels were already elevated on the day after castration.
Treatment with 1 ml of the antiserum to LHRH once every 2 days

resulted in a parallel reduction of serum LH and FSH levels, which remained suppressed throughout the study. In the control castrated rats injected with normal sheep serum, serum LH and FSH levels remained elevated or increased further. These animals were sacrificed 3 weeks later, and it was found that there were numerous castration cells in the pituitaries from control rats, whereas castration cells were absent in the antiserum-treated rats.

Zambrano et al. (1974) reported that the incubation of pituitary glands with LHRH in the culture medium for 3 to 6 hrs led to formation of typical "signet ring" castration cells. They interpreted the finding to indicate that castration cells are formed by increased secretion of LHRH into the hypophysial portal vessels. The complete absence of castration cells in the castrated rats which received the anti-LHRH serum starting on the day after castration can be accounted for as the result of the neutralization of endogenous LHRH by the antiserum.

The requirement of the pituitary for the maintenance of early pregnancy is well established (Pencharz and Long, 1933; Selye et al., 1933). Laurence and Hassouna (1973) reported that administration of antiserum to LH in rats delayed implantation or terminated pregnancy, thus suggesting the importance of LH during early gestation. To what extent is the LH secretion during early pregnancy dependent on LHRH? We have recently completed a series of studies on this problem (Nishi et al., 1975; Arimura et al., 1975b). γ-globulin was isolated from sheep anti-LHRH serum and dissolved in saline in the same concentration as that in the original serum. Proestrous rats were caged with 2 male rats which had been proved fertile and the vagina was examined for the presence of spermatozoa the next morning. The day that spermatozoa were found present was designated as pregnancy day 1.

In the first series of experiments, the effect of the administration of anti-LHRH γ-globulin on implantation was investigated. The animals received 1 ml anti-LHRH γ-globulin or normal sheep γ-globulin (NSG) iv once daily from day 1 through day 7 of pregnancy. On day 8, laparotomy was performed to examine viable sites in the uterus. The operation wound was closed and the second laparotomy was performed on day 14. Some of the rats were allowed to survive until they delivered pups. The rats who received normal γ-globulin daily from days 1 through 7 or from days 3 through 5 had 14 and 13 viable sites on the average on day 8, respectively. A similar number of viable sites but of greater size were observed on day 14. They delivered pups on term. However, in the rats which revieved 1 ml anti-LHRH γ-globulin daily from day 1 through day 7 or from days 3 to 5, the viable sites on day 8 were hardly distinguishable, although the uteri were hypertrophied. Viable sites became distinguishable on day 14 in 3 out of 8 rats treated with anti-LHRH Υ -globulin from day 1 through day 7, and in 9 out of 12 rats treated from day 3 to day 5. But these viable sites were considerably smaller in size than those in NSG-treated control rats. Some of these animals delivered pups but the parturition was delayed by 4 to 6 days. Implantation failed to occur in other females.

To pinpoint the critical period when hypothalamic LHRH is most needed for normal implantation, 1 ml of anti-LHRH Γ -globulin was injected into rats on day 3,4 or 5 of pregnancy, and viable sites were inspected on days 8 and 14. The number of viable sites on day 8 were drastically reduced when anti-LHRH Υ -globulin was injected on day 4, but not on day 3 or 5. This finding was rather surprising. Our aforementioned study on the effect of anti-LHRH serum on the estrous cycle in hamsters indicated that suppression of ovulation as well as estrogen secretion by anti-LHRH serum lasted about 12 days. The fact that implantation was suppressed only when anti-LHRH was injected on day 4 shows that the action of anti-LHRH ʃ -globulin did not appear to last longer than one day. One possible explanation could be that the immunogamma globulin injected into pregnant rats is metabolized more rapidly than in normal animals.

If the rats were treated with anti-LHRH ʃ -globulin and 1 ug LH RH in 16% gelatin twice on day 4 of pregnancy, the suppressive effect of anti-LHRH on implantation was no longer present. Treatment with 1 ug estradiol on day 4 also resulted in a nearly complete restoration of implantation. Number and size of viable fetuses on days 8 and 14 were nearly normal in these animals. On the other hand, 0.01 ug estrogen on day 4 had little effect, and 0.02 ug estrogen improved implantation, but the size of viable fetuses on day 14 was smaller than in the control animals.

The effect of anti-LHRH ʃ -globulin on the gestation after implantation was also investigated. After pregnancy was confirmed by a laparotomy on day 7, these pregnant rats were given 1 ml anti-LHRH ʃ -globulin or NSG iv daily from day 7 through day 11. On day 14 of pregnancy, the second laparotomy was performed for inspecting viable sites. In NSG-treated rats, 9 to 12 well-developed viable fetuses were observed, whereas in the anti-LHRH treated rats, resorption of fetuses occurred. In none of the cases has bleeding been observed prior to the termination of gestation by anti-LHRH. This is quite a contrast to the findings on the termination of gestation by treatment with antiserum to LH, which often causes profuse bleeding, (Loewit and Laurence, 1969; Loewit et al., 1969; Madwa Raj and Moudgal, 1970).

To examine the critical time for the requirement of LHRH, 1 ml anti-LHRH ʃ -globulin was injected in the morning of day 7, 8, 9, 10, 11, or 12 and the viable sites were examined on day 14. Injection on day 7 did not affect viable fetuses on day 14, but injection on day 9 or 10 caused complete resorption of fetuses in all of

the rats treated. Injection on day 8 or 11 was partially effective
and on day 12 caused fetal resorption in only 1 out of 5 rats treated.
The results indicate that the critical days are days 9 and 10 where
LHRH is essential for the maintenance of viable fetuses.

A single injection of 1 ug LHRH in 16% gelatin once daily for 4
days from days 9 through 12 failed to reverse resorption of fetuses
caused by anti-LHRH Υ -globulin, but injections twice daily during
the same period of time completely overcame the effect of anti-
LHRH. Treatment with 4 mg progesterone daily from days 7 through
12 of gestation also prevented the fetus resorption by anti-LHRH
Υ -globulin.

Serum progesterone, as measured by RIA, was elevated on day 7
of gestation and reached a peak on days 13 to 14. A single injection of anti-LHRH on day 7 of gestation only slightly suppressed
serum progesterone levels thereafter. On the other hand, the injection on day 9 or 10 drastically reduced progesterone levels on
day 11 and thereafter. Suppression of progesterone was slight or
absent when the antiserum was injected on day 12. Therefore, there
is a good correlation between the termination of gestation and the
decrease in serum progesterone. These results as well as the prevention by progesterone of anti-LHRH-induced termination of gestation may well indicate that an increased secretion of progesterone
on days 11 through 14 of gestation is essential for the maintenance
of fetal growth and that the progesterone secretion during this
period is stimulated by hypothalamic LHRH probably through increased
secretion of LH.

It can be concluded from these studies that the hypothalamus
may play an important role in early gestation by means of LHRH at 2
times in rats. Firstly, on day 4, LHRH, through LH, stimulates estrogen secretion, which is essential for implantation of fertilized
ova, and secondly, on days 9 to 10, LHRH stimulates progesterone
secretion which is essential for maintenance of viable fetuses.

SOMATOSTATIN

The antiserum to somatostatin is similarly a powerful tool for
studying the physiological role of this hypothalamic hormone. It
has been established that administration of somatostatin suppresses
not only GH, but also TSH, prolactin, insulin, glucagon, gastrin,
gastric acid and other GI hormones. However, there has been no evidence which indicates that these suppressive actions of somatostatin
operate under physiological conditions as part of a regulatory mechanism of secretion of these hormones. Neutralization by the antibody of endogenous somatostatin which is present not only in the
brain, but also in the pancreas, stomach and intestine (Arimura

et al., 1975 a,b) could reveal the physiological role of endogenous somatostatin. I would like to report on some of the results recently obtained on GH secretion.

It is well known that noxious stress decreases circulating GH levels in the rat. In order to examine whether the reduction of GH secretion results from the increased secretion of hypothalamic somatostatin, we investigated the effect of administration of anti-somatostatin on stress-induced decrease in GH secretion in the rat. Based on the results of the experiments with anti-LHRH, we have assumed that administration of a sufficient amount of antiserum to somatostatin would neutralize the hormone in the median eminence and suppress its effect on the pituitary gland.

Two ml sheep anti-somatostatin serum was injected iv into a group of adult male rats once daily for 3 consecutive days, and 2 ml normal sheep serum was injected into another group in a similar manner. On the following day, these animals were bled twice from the jugular vein under ether at a 30-min interval. There was considerable variation in serum GH levels in the first specimen, ranging from non-detectable to 508 ng/ml in the normal sheep serum-treated rats. GH levels in the rats treated with anti-somatostatin fluctuated less. GH levels 30 min after the first bleeding remained low or decreased in 6 out of 9 rats, whereas those in the antiserum-treated rats increased in 7 out of 9 rats. Mean GH level in the antiserum-treated group was 76 ng/ml, whereas that in the normal serum-treated group was 16.8 ng, but the difference was insignificant due to the large variation in individual values.

In other experiments, severe stress, induced by 2 electroshocks on the paws, of 15-sec duration each, interrupted by a 15-sec interval, was employed. Thirty-min post-stress GH levels in the rats which were injected iv with 2 ml anti-somatostatin serum 3 hr before were significantly higher (34.4 ng) than those in the rats injected with 2 ml normal sheep serum (0.9 ng/ml) or non-treated rats (0.5 ng/ml) (Arimura et al., 1975d).

These results suggest that stress-induced reduction of GH secretion in rats is at least partly due to an increased release of endogenous somatostatin. However, a fairly large variation in the same treatment group suggests the involvement of other factors, such as GH releasing hormone, or "somatoliberin" in the regulatory mechanism of GH secretion.

Data on the effects of active and passive immunization with somatostatin on pancreatic or GI hormones are being accumulated.

CONCLUSION

Although the synthetic preparation of hypothalamic hormones can be used to investigate the mode of actions, in vivo and in vitro, it is difficult to conclude that the same action is exercised by the endogenous hormones under physiological or pathological conditions. A specific antiserum to a hypothalamic hormone which neutralizes the corresponding endogenous hormone can be used to reveal its physiological role. The data obtained in such studies may provide valuable information on the usefulness of synthetic antagonists to these hypothalamic hormones.

REFERENCES

Arimura, A., Debeljuk, L., and Schally, A.V. (1972a) Endocrinology 91: 529-532.

Arimura, A., Debeljuk, L., and Schally, A.V. (1972b) Proc. Soc. Exp. Bio. Med. 140: 609-612.

Arimura, A., Debeljuk, L., and Schally, A.V. (1974) Endocrinology 95: 323-324.

Arimura, A., Shiino, M., de la Cruz, K., Rennels, E.G., and Schally, A.V. (1975a) Endocrinology, submitted for publication.

Arimura, A., Nishi, N., and Schally A.V. (1975b) Endocrinology, submitted for publication.

Arimura, A., Sato, H., Dupont, A., Nishi, N., and Schally, A.V. (1975c) Science 189: 1007-1009.

Arimura, A., Smith, R., and Schally, A.V. (1975d) Endocrinology, submitted for publication.

Bowers, C.Y., Lee, K., and Schally, A.V. (1967) Endocrinology 82: 303-310.

Crighton, D.B., Watanabe, S., Dhariwal, A.P.S., and McCann, S.M. (1968) Proc. Soc. Exp. Bio. Med. 128: 537-540.

de la Cruz, A., Arimura, A., de la Cruz, K., and Schally, A.V. (1975) Endocrinology, in press.

Ely, C.A. and Schwarz, H.B. (1971) Endocrinology 89: 1103-1108.

Jutisz, M. and de la Llosa, M.P. (1967) Endocrinology 81: 1193-1202.

Koch, Y., Chobsieng, P., Zor, U., Fridkin, M., and Lindner, H.R. (1973) Biochem. Biophys. Res. Commun. 55: 623-629.

Laurence, K.A. and H. Hassouna, H. (1973) In: Handbook of Physiology (R.O. Greep, ed.) vol. 2, part 2, The Williams and Wilkins Company, Baltimore, pp. 339-348.

Loewit, K.K. and Laurence, K.A. (1969) Fertil. Steril. 20: 679-688.

Loewit, K.K., Badwy, S., and Laurence, K.A. (1969) Endocrinology 84: 244-251.

Madwa Raj, H.G. and Moudgal, N.R. (1970) Endocrinology 86: 874-889.

Nishi, N., Arimura, A., de la Cruz, K., and Schally, A.V. (1975) Endocrinology, submitted for publication.

Pencharz, R.I. and Long, J.A. (1933) Am. J. Anat. 53: 117-135.

Ramirez, V.D. and McCann, S.M. (1963) Endocrinology 73: 193-198.

Samli, M.H. and Geschwind, I.I. (1967) Endocrinology 81: 835-848.

Selye, H., Collip, J.B., and Thompson, D.L. (1933) Proc. Soc. Exp. Bio. Med. 30: 589-590.

Vilchez-Martinez, J.A., Arimura, A., and Schally, A.V. (1975) Acta Endocrinologica, in press.

Watanabe, S., Dhariwal, A.P.S., and McCann, S.M. (1968) Endocrinology 82: 674-684.

Zambrano, D., Cuerdo-Rocha, S., and Bergmann, I. (1974) Cell Tiss. Res. 150: 179-192.

APPLICATIONS OF ADENOHYPOPHYSEAL CELL CULTURES TO NEUROENDOCRINE STUDIES

Wylie Vale, Catherine Rivier, Marvin Brown, Lana Chan,
Nick Ling and Jean Rivier

Salk Institute for Biological Studies
La Jolla, California, 92037

Anterior pituitary cell function can be influenced by neural peptides (including the hypothalamic regulatory hormones, HRH), neurotransmitters and peripheral hormones. Because of the pituitary gland's close (vascular) coupling to the central nervous system, the secretory rates of its hormones are highly dynamic and easily modified by experimental circumstances. It is often difficult to determine if responses seen in vivo are due to direct effects on the pituitary or are mediated through extrapituitary mechanisms. In vitro assays of the hypophysiotropic substances offer isolation from such indirect effects. It has been the aim of biologists in this field to develop an in vitro assay that would be technically simple, sensitive, reliable, accurate and valid. With the availability of radioimmunoassays to the pituitary hormones, the preparations of pituitary tissues themselves became the limiting factor to the achievement of these goals.

The techniques involving short-term incubation or longer term culture of pituitary glands have been profitably applied to many physiological and biochemical problems of pituitary regulation. However, because of the heterogeneity of the responses of glands except when comparing "paired" halved glands from the same animal, investigators were led to search for other in vitro pituitary preparations which would behave more homogeneously (Guillemin and Vale, 1970).

One way of obtaining multiple equivalent cell populations is to dissociate pituitary glands enzymatically, and mix and divide them into as many experimental units as desired. Such cells had been reported by Portanova et al., 1970, and Bala et al., 1970, to secrete pituitary hormones in response to a variety of stimuli

within a few hours of dissociation. However, in our and others'
experiences, such acutely dissociated cells are not adequately sensitive to hypophysiotropic substances to allow their use in quantitative assays.

     Our solution to this problem was to maintain dissociated cells
for several days in culture, allowing them to recover from the enzymatic treatment (Vale et al., 1972b). Subsequently Hopkins and
Farquhar (1973) reported a variation on this method in which they
used cells within 16 hours following dissociation. The current
procedure (Vale and Grant, 1975) we routinely employ to dissociate
rat pituitary cells is shown in Table 1. Normal or neoplastic pituitaries from species other than the rat have been successfully

TABLE 1   Cell dissociation procedure

     Anterior pituitary glands obtained from $\male$ 180 GM rats are
     stirred at 37° in spinner flask with the following solution:

0.4%	Collagenase – Worthington Type I	
1.0%	BSA	
10 µg/ml	DNAse	
137 mM	NaCl	
5 mM	KCl	
0.7 mM	Na$_2$HPO$_4$	"HEPES–BUFFER"
25 mM	HEPES	pH 7.2
2 mg/ml	GLUCOSE	
	ANTIBIOTICS	

     After 1-2 hours the partially dissociated cells are centrifu-
ged, resuspended in 0.25% viokase in HEPES-buffer, and stirred for
≤ 10 minutes.

     Cells are washed by repeated centrifugation and resuspension
in culture medium (Dulbecco modified eagles medium, 15 mM HEPES,
10% fetal calf serum)

Yield: 1-1.5 x 10^6 cells/gland.

0.2-0.4 x 10^6 cells are distributed to each tissue culture dish in
3 mls culture medium.

dissociated and cultured, including the hamster, mouse, guinea pig,
cow, monkey, rabbit and human. While the two-step enzymatic treatment works best to dissociate cells in our experience, other investigators have also reported success with a variety of procedures
(Hopkins and Farquhar, 1973; Hymer et al., 1973; Tang and Spies,
1974). We have extensively studied the functions and sensitivities

to secretagogue of each of the adenohypophyseal hormone secreting
cell types in our cultures, however, such has not yet been the case
for cells prepared by other means. As can be seen from the cell
yield (1-1.5 x 10^6 cells/pituitary gland) and the number of cells
plated (0.2-0.4 x 10^6 cells/dish), each rat pituitary can be used
to make 2.5-7.5 dishes of cells. Since the number of replicates
used for in vitro and in vivo experiments are 3 and 6 respectively,
the animals required per experimental treatment in vitro can be as
little as 1/15th that required for a similar in vivo study.

Within 2-3 days following dissociation, the cultured pituitary
cells have attached to the bottom of the tissue culture dishes and
lost the spherical appearance typical of acutely dissociated cells.
At that time, the cells can be washed by repeated medium changing
without their being dislodged. We generally then add treatments to
the cultures and incubate for 3-5 hours for short-term experiments,
after which time the fluids are removed and frozen for future radioimmunoassay of pituitary hormone levels.

We have examined the effects of a variety of agents on the secretion of hormones by these cells. They were shown to behave as
would have been expected on the basis of other in vitro studies.
For example, prostaglandins, theophylline, cyclic AMP derivatives
and high medium potassium stimulate pituitary hormonal secretion;
low medium calcium and appropriate peripheral hormones inhibit secretion; hypothalamic regulatory hormones and extracts have various
effects depending on the particular hormones studied. The responsiveness of cells to the hypothalamic hormones LRF, TRF, or somatostatin are shown in Figures 6, 11 and 18. Since the addition of
any of the characterized HRH to cultured pituitary cells results in
a new but constant rate of secretion of the appropriate hormones
(Vale and Grant, 1975), we consider that changes in hormone levels
measured at one time reflect changes in equilibrium secretion rates.
Even though the cells retain their sensitivity to a variety of stimuli for ≥ one month, most assays are carried out within 5 days of
being plated because the intracellular stores of all pituitary hormones except for prolactin (which can continue to be produced for
years) decline with time in culture as does the magnitude of the secretory responses to a variety of stimuli (Vale et al., 1972b).
Although chronic exposure of cultured cells to LRF or TRF increases
the rate of synthesis of the appropriate pituitary hormones (Fig.1,
Vale et al., 1972b; Labrie et al., 1972; Tashjian et al., 1971),
this is accompanied by a severe depletion in hormone content: perhaps a combination of HRH and peripheral hormones or some other factors present in vivo can be used to maintain adequate hormone stores
and sensitivities to secretagogues for extended time in culture.

The remainder of this discussion will be concerned with the applications of cell culture assays to several neuroendocrine programs:
1) the purification of HRH; 2) physiological and pharmacological

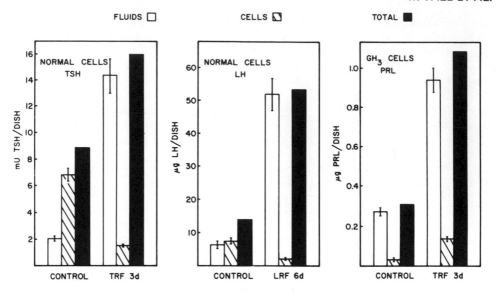

Fig. 1   Effect of TRF (3 days) or LRF (6 days) on distribu-
          tion (fluid ☐, cells ▨) and total ■ amounts of TSH
          (A) or LH (B) in normal rat pituitary cells and of
          PRL (C) in GH$_3$ rat tumor cells

studies of the interactions of various hormones, drugs and experimental conditions; and 3) the bioassay of analogs of HRH.

PURIFICATION OF HYPOTHALAMIC REGULATORY HORMONES

Somatostatin

Bioassays using cultures of anterior pituitary cells have already proven to be of value when applied to the purification of one
hormone, somatostatin (see Vale et al., 1975 for review). While
screening extracts for evidence of a growth hormone releasing factor, ethanol-acetic acid-chloroform extracts of ovine hypothalamus
were found to inhibit the secretion of growth hormone by cultured
cells. This extract was effective at doses as low as one-thousandth
of a fragment (ca. 5 μg) per ml of medium. As it has turned out,
cultured pituitary cells are far more sensitive to somatostatin responding to ≥ 0.1 nM somatostatin than are incubated hemipituitaries
which require ≥ 10 nM to observe an inhibition of GH secretion (Vale et al., 1972a). It is possible that in vivo the chronic exposure of pituitary cells to somatostatin suppresses the level of soma-

tostatin receptors thus effectively shifting the somatostatin dose
response curve to the right in a manner similar to the insulin
(Roth et al., 1975) and TRF (Hinckle and Tashjian, 1975) mediated
inhibition of the number of their cellular binding sites. Somatostatin, which was purified exclusively on the basis of the pituitary
cell culture assay, was shown, subsequent to its characterization,
to be active in vivo in a variety of species under numerous circumstances, thus validating the use of this assay for the purification
of the hormone.

     Using the culture assay, we first reported (Vale et al., 1974b)
the presence of somatostatin-like activity in extracts of the extra-
hypothalamic brain and spinal cord, an observation that was later
confirmed by radioimmunoassay (Brownstein et al., 1975; Patel et al.
1975). The presence of somatostatin in cells in the gastrointestinal tract and pancreas was demonstrated by immunohistochemical techniques (Dubois, 1975 and Hökfelt et al., 1975) and later by radioimmunoassay (Arimura et al., 1975b; Patel et al., 1975). Although
slight somatostatin-like biological activity was seen in extracts
of rat pancreas (Vale et al., 1975), extracts of frog or pigeon pancreas contain higher levels of somatostatin-like activity (Fig. 2).
We are presently using this bioassay to purify the substances

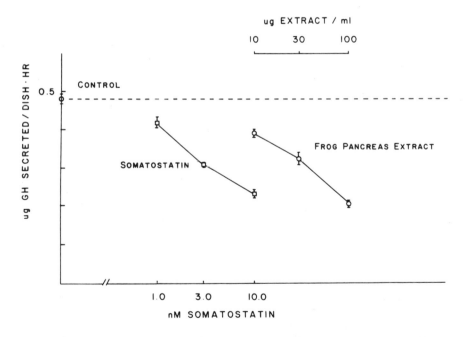

Fig. 2   Effect of somatostatin and boiled 2N HOAc extract of
          frog pancreas on GH secretion by cultured rat pitui-
          tary cells

TABLE 2   DRUGS ON PRL SECRETION BY CULTURED RAT PITUITARY CELLS

TREATMENTS	ng PRL/DISH·HR

EXPERIMENT A

Control	203 ± 4
3 µM Dopamine (DA)	86 ± 2
10 µM Pimozide (PIM)	192 ± 12
3 µM Da + 0.4 nM Pim	103 ± 3
3 µM Da + 2 nM Pim	152 ± 8
3 µM Da + 10 nM Pim	181 ± 9

EXPERIMENT B

Control	174 ± 6
0.1 nM CB 154	138 ± 8
1.0 nM CB 154	66 ± 13
10 nM CB 154	54 ± 17

EXPERIMENT C

Control	63 ± 1
3 µM DA	18 ± 1
1 µM Haloperidol (HAL)	66 ± 5
3 µM Da + 10 nM HAL	29 ± 2
3 µM Da + 100 nM HAL	53 ± 2
3 µM Da + 1 µM HAL	63 ± 1

EXPERIMENT D

Control	87 ± 3
0.1 µM Apomorphine	74 ± 2
1.0 µM Apomorphine	36 ± 2

EXPERIMENT E

Control	132 ± 3
3 µM Carbachol (CAR)	89 ± 6
1 µM Atropine (ATR)	134 ± 6
3 µM CAR + 1 nM ATR	110 ± 2
3 µM CAR + 10 nM ATR	120 ± 4
3 µM CAR + 1 µM ATR	130 ± 6

responsible for the GH release inhibiting (somatostatin-like) activities in brain and pancreas extracts. Likewise the factors responsible for TSH inhibitory activity (possibly also due to somatostatin, see below), in hypothalamic and brain extracts (Vale et al.,
1975a) are being purified.

Prolactin Release Inhibiting Factor

The pituitary cells are sensitive to a variety of agents which
can influence the rate of PRL secretion. Consistent with the results of McLeod (1969); Birge et al. (1970); Clemens et al. (1974);
McLeod and Leyhmeyer (1973) using short-term hemipituitary incubations, we find that dopaminergic agonists such as dopamine, apomorphine or CB 154 (Table 2) can inhibit the secretion of PRL by cultured pituitary cells and that the dopaminergic antagonists perphenazine, haloperidol, and pimozide can prevent the effects of dopaminergic agonists on PRL secretion. We have observed that partially
purified hypothalamic and cerebral cortical extracts contain a PRL
release inhibiting activity that is not suppressible by dopamine
antagonists (Figure 3) (Vale et al., 1974b; Vale and Rivier, 1975)

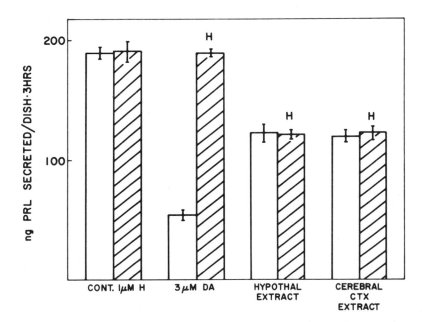

Fig. 3   Effect of haloperidol (H) on the in vitro inhibition
          of PRL secretion by dopamine (DA), hypothalamic or
          cerebral cortical extract

suggesting that there is a substance other than catecholamines in brain extracts that can behave as a PRL release inhibiting factor. This hypothesis is supported by the data of Quejada et al. (1974) using pituitary hypothalamus co-incubates and subsequently by the results of Dupont and Redding (1975) from experiments similar to ours.

The addition of cholinergic agonists such as carbachol, acetylcholine or oxotremorine also can inhibit PRL secretion by cultured pituitary cells (Vale and Rivier, 1975). The effect of carbachol is reversed by very low concentrations of atropine (Table 2) and much higher levels of D-tumocurarine indicating that the cholinergic receptors involved in this response are probably of a muscarinic type. Only very high concentrations ($\geq$ 100 μM of carbachol) inhibit PRL secretion by hemipituitary glands during short-term incubations providing perhaps another example of the sensitization of pituitary cells resulting from their removal from the in vivo environment for several days. These observations represent another example of the differences between cultured pituitary cells and incubated hemipituitary glands, although it is not obvious which method's results should be considered more physiologically significant. There are considerable difficulties involved in interpreting data obtained with incubated hemipituitary glands in view of observations that, following the several hours of preincubation required to lower spontaneous hormone secretion rates, all but the cortex of the tissue shows morphological evidence of necrosis (Hopkins and Farquhar, 1973; Guillemin and Vale, 1970). As is the case for results obtained with all in vitro experiments, they are most convincing when consistent with appropriate in vivo studies.

Cholinergic agonists and antagonists have been shown to modify PRL secretion in vivo (Grandison et al., 1974; Libertun and McCann, 1974; Gala et al., 1972), however, the level (pituitary, CNS or both) at which these effects are primarily mediated has not clearly been determined. Our in vitro results indicate that possible direct effects of these agents at the pituitary level should be considered. The PRL release inhibiting activity of our hypothalamic and cerebral cortical extracts cannot be explained by the presence of acetyl choline as neither atropine or D-tubocurarine block the effects of these extracts on PRL secretion (Fig. 4).

A variety of substances, neurotransmitters (dopamine, norepinephrine, cholinergic agonists), hypothalamic peptide hormones (somatostatin, TRF), and peripheral hormones (estrogens, thyroid hormones) can modify PRL secretion by the anterior pituitary (see Vale and Rivier, 1975, for review). The existence of such a vast array of putative regulators for a single cell type (implying the presence of multiple functional receptors), while providing an exciting model system for the study of the interactions of the various classes of hormones, certainly complicates the task of those searching for additional substances modifying PRL secretion. All of the data considered, it would appear that there exists an additional hormone (s) that is neither dopamine, acetyl choline, nor somatostatin that is found in brain extracts and is capable of inhibiting PRL secretion in vitro, the physiologic role of this substance, and, indeed, all of the hormones influencing PRL secretion remains at issue.

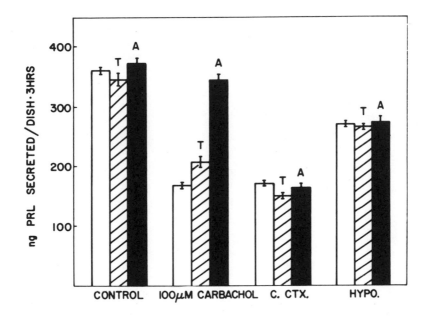

Fig. 4   Effect of atropine (A) or d-tubocurarine (T) on the in vitro inhibition of PRL secretion by carbachol (CA), hypothalamic (HYPO) or cerebral cortical (C. CTX) extract

Corticotropin Releasing Factor (CRF)

Cultured pituitary cells secrete radioimmunoassayable ACTH in response to a variety of stimuli (Table 3) including high medium potassium, theophylline, cyclic AMP derivatives, vasopressin, α-adrenergic agonists and hypothalamic extracts which presumably contain a CRF. Furthermore, dexamethasone-21-PO$_4$ pretreatment of cells inhibits the secretion of ACTH due to this CRF as would have been expected based on results with other in vitro systems (Fleis-

TABLE 3   EFFECTS OF VARIOUS SUBSTANCES AND EXPERIMENTAL CONDITIONS ON THE SECRETION OF ACTH BY RAT PITUITARY CELL CULTURES

Additions		pg ACTH secreted dish·hr	± SEM
EXP. A	to		
– 3 mM ^{8}BrcAMP		49	± 10
		1152	± 111
10 x $[K^+]_o$		184	± 18
EXP. B t_{-16} hrs	to		
–	–	274	30
2.0 nM DEX	–	207	73
20 nM DEX	–	170	10
200 nM DEX	–	139	21
2 µM DEX	–	40	20
–	500 nM DEX	69	4
–	0.1 f/ml HYP[1]	1511	172
2.0 nM DEX	HYP	1260	140
20 nM DEX	HYP	625	80
200 nM DEX	HYP	332	4
2 µM	HYP	315	55
–	500 nM DEX + HYP	477	38
–	5 mM AMN	1806	171
–	5 mM AMN + HYP	3205	98
EXP. C T_{-2} hrs	to		
–	–	192	35
–	0.05 f/ml HYP	852	108
–	3 µM Norepinephrine (NE)	785	69
–	10 µM Phentolamine (PHE)	157	40
–	Phe + HYP	889	139
–	Phe + NE	325	75
10 µM Dibenzaline	–	211	211
10 µM Dibenzaline	HYP	751	69
10 µM Dibenzaline	NE	210	65

[1] Hypothalamic fraction (HYP)

cher and Vale, 1968; Sayers and Portanova, 1974). We are presently
purifying a CRF (s) found in ovine hypothalamic extracts using this
culture assay and have been able to rule out various known ACTH secretagogues as being responsible for this activity. Consistent with
the results of Portanova and Sayers (1973) who used acutely dissociated pituitary cells the dose response curves of the CRF activity
of hypothalamic extracts can be distinguished from that of vasopressin as shown in Figure 5. Phentolamine and dibenzaline, α-adrenergic antagonists, block the release of ACTH in vitro due to norepinephrine (Table 3) while not inhibiting the response to a CRF fraction.

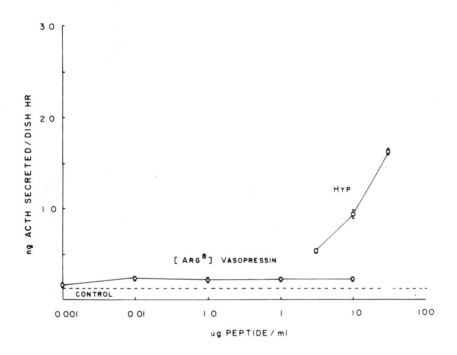

Fig. 5   Stimulation of ACTH secretion in vitro by hypothala-
          mic fraction (HYP) or [Arg^8]vasopressin

INTERACTIONS OF HYPOPHYSIOTROPIC SUBSTANCES

This section will provide additional examples of the use of pituitary cell cultures to investigate the interactions of multiple
hormones, drugs and experimental conditions.

We have used this method to reveal possible physiological actions of the hypothalamic hormones. The results (Vale <u>et al</u>.,
1973a) of the experiment shown in Figure 6 were the first indication

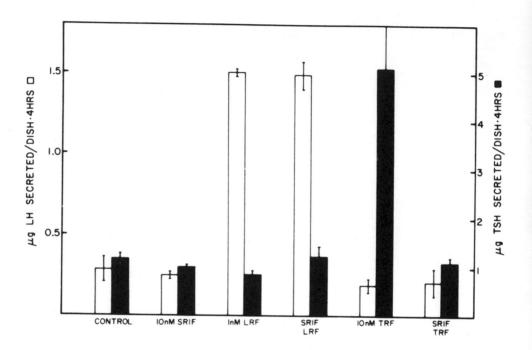

Fig. 6   Effect of somatostatin (SRIF) on TRF and LRF me-
           diated secretion of TSH (■) or LH (□) <u>in vitro</u>

that somatostatin could inhibit the secretion of TSH mediated by
TRF while not influencing the amount of LH stimulated by LRF. Evidence for an effect opposite to that of TRH on the synthesis of TSH
in pituitary cell cultures is shown in Figure 7 where somatostatin
lowers total culture TSH levels in`absence of TRF and inhibits the
TRF-induced rise in total culture TSH content. The effects (Figure
8) of the individual and simultaneous administration of the neurohormones TRF and somatostatin and the peripheral feedback inhibitor,
thyroxin, suggest that all three of these hormones can interact to
provide fine regulation of TSH secretion (Vale <u>et al</u>., 1974a).

Of course, a variety of pharmacological substances and experimental circumstances can modify the secretion of pituitary hormones
<u>in vitro</u> (see reviews, Geschwind, 1969; Boss <u>et al</u>., 1975). Agents

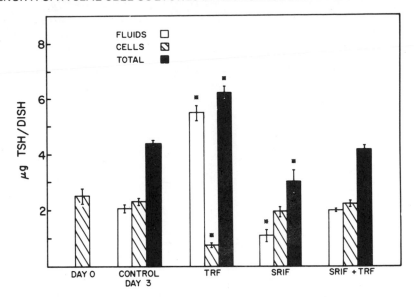

Fig. 7   Effect of 3 day exposure to somatostatin (SRIF) or
            TRH on the distribution (fluids ☐, cells ◩) or total
            amounts of TSH in pituitary cell cultures.

such as theophylline and the E series of prostaglandins which increase intracellular cyclic AMP levels, stimulate TSH secretion
only slightly when acting alone but markedly potentiate the response (TSH release) to both TRF (Table 4) and elevated medium potassium. Such results and those of others (see Labrie et al., 1976
for review) are consistent with an involvement of cyclic AMP in the
regulation of TSH secretion. However, since the amount of TSH secreted by cells treated with TRF and prostaglandins or theophylline is much greater than that secreted by cells exposed to supra-
maximal concentrations of TRF, both substances may not necessarily
act through identical mechanisms. It is thus possible that cyclic
AMP is not the sole mediator of the action of TRF but in some way
facilitates secretion in concert with other intracellular "messen-
gers".

Experiments with other in vitro preparations had shown that
extracellular calcium ion is required for the secretion of pituitary hormones mediated by hypothalamic regulatory hormones and a variety of other substances (Vale et al., 1967; Vale and Guillemin,

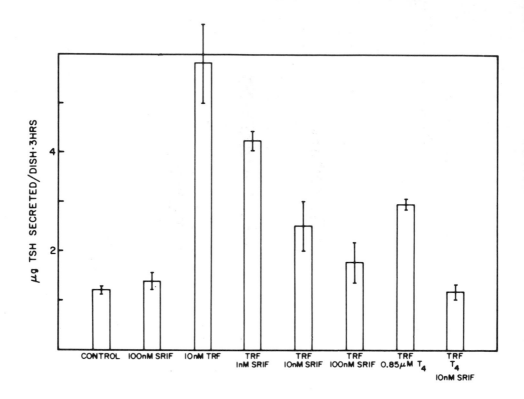

Fig. 8   Interaction of TRF, somatostatin (SRIF) and thyroxi-
            ne (T₄) on secretion of TSH <u>in vitro</u>

1967; Samli and Geschwind, 1968; Wakabayashi, 1969; for review,
Geschwind, 1969 or Boss <u>et al</u>., 1975).   The dependence on $[Ca^{++}]$o
of the LRF mediated LH secretory response of cultured pituitary
cells is shown in Figure 9a.   The stimulation (Figure 9b) of pituitary hormone secretion by the calcium ionophore A23187 which increases the permeability of membranes to divalent cations particularly
calcium (Pressman, 1973) is also consistent with a role of calcium
in this secretory mechanism.

      More direct evidence for this role is obtained from studies
using the GH_3 GH and PRL secreting rat pituitary tumor cell line.
TRF, which stimulates PRL secretion by these cells, also accelera-
tes the rate of ^{45}Ca efflux from cells previously incubated in the
isotope and subjected to washing out by periodic medium change
(Figure 10).   Concentrations of TRF as low as as 3 nM enhance ^{45}Ca
efflux while 333-fold higher levels of 2 TRF analogs which have
less than 0.1% TRF potency to stimulate hormone secretion or bind
to pituitary cells (Vale <u>et al</u>., 1973c; Hinkle <u>et al</u>., 1974) had no

TABLE 4   INTERACTION OF TRF AND ELEVATED MEDIUM
                 $[K^+]$ WITH PGE_1 OR THEOPHYLLINE

Addition	mU TSH/dish ± SEM
Experiment A	
Control	0.25 ± 0.01
3 mM TRF	2.32 ± 0.24
150 nM TRF	3.65 ± 0.05
1 µM PGE_1	0.53 ± 0.04
10 µM PGE_1	0.54 ± 0.05
1 µM PGE_1 + 3 nM TRF	4.72 ± 0.54
10 µM PGE_1 + 150 nM TRF	6.52 ± 0.08
Experiment B	
Control	0.78 ± 0.17
$[10 \times K^+]$	2.10 ± 0.05
10 mM theophylline	1.61 ± 0.14
10 µM PGE_1	1.5 ± 0.13
$[10 \times K^+]$ + 10 mM theophylline	5.55 ± 0.20
$[10 \times K^+]$ + 10 µM PGE_1	5.20 ± 0.34

effect, thereby demonstrating the specificity of this phenomenon.
The increase in ^{45}Ca efflux might reflect a TRF mediated redistri-
bution of intracellular calcium resulting in higher concentrations
of free cytoplasmic calcium which more readily equilibrates with
the extracellular fluid.

The anterior pituitary gland is a heterogeneous organ composed
of many cell types. When "non-cell type specific" parameters such
as cyclic AMP levels, ion fluxes and cell division rates are monitored in mixed cell populations, the effects on a particular cell
type cannot be determined. One approach is to use cloned cells
such as the GH_3 line as described in the calcium efflux experiments.
We have also examined the effects of TRF on mitotic rates of this
cell line. In our experiments, the addition of TRF to GH_3 cells results in a slight inhibition of cell proliferation and a suppression
of $[^3H]$ thymidine incorporation into DNA. Glucorticoids such as
dexamethasone, which stimulate GH secretion by this line, also in-

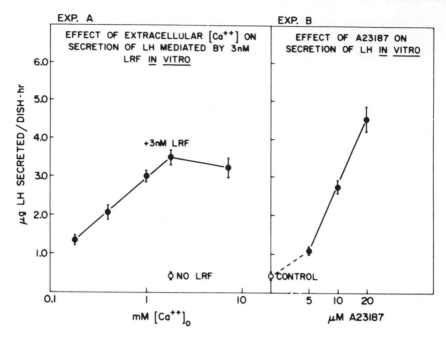

Fig. 9A   Effects of extracellular [Ca^{++}] on the LRF mediated
           secretion of LH in vitro

Fig. 9B   Stimulation of LH secretion in vitro by the calcium
           ionophore A23187

hibit cell division (Tashjian et al., 1970). TRF and dexamethasone
interact to produce pronounced inhibition of proliferation. Likewise, TRF, which only moderately inhibits GH secretion when acting
alone, has a marked effect on the GH secretion stimulated by dexamethasone (Table 5). Thyroxine has been reported to enhance the
division rate of the closely related GH$_1$ cells and to inhibit PRL
and stimulate GH secretion (Samuels et al., 1973). Thus, although
we cannot correlate effects on cell proliferation with effects on
the secretion of either PRL or GH, TRF, dexamethasone and thyroxine
can be considered as regulators not only of function but of cell
division as well in these lines.

TABLE 5   EFFECT OF TRF AND DEXAMETHASONE (DEX) ON SECRETION
           OF GH AND PROLIFERATION OF GH_3 CELLS

Experiment A

Medium: F-10 + 15% HS

cells x 10^{-3}/dish ± SEM

Additions	day 0	day 2	day 5
Control	144 ± 2	365 ± 14	708 ± 2
100 nM TRF		329 ± 3	596 ± 22
200 nM DEX		291 ± 4	485 ± 2
200 nM DEX + 100 nM TRF		220 ± 4	289 ± 3

Experiment B

Medium: F-10 + 15% HS + 2.5% FCS   ngGH/Dish·24 hrs ± SEM

Additions	ngGH/Dish·24 hrs ± SEM
Control	28 ± 3
2 nM DEX	40 ± 5
20 nM DEX	53 ± 8
200 nM DEX	72 ± 9
100 nM TRF	26 ± 3
2 nM DEX + 100 nM TRF	20 ± 2
20 nM DEX + 100 nM TRF	38 ± 5
200 nM DEX + 100 nM TRF	42 ± 6

ASSAY OF ANALOGS OF HYPOTHALAMIC REGULATORY HORMONES

Hundred of analogs of TRF, LRF and somatostatin have been synthesized and biologically tested in order to investigate the structural determinants of biological activity and to design therapeuti-
cally useful peptides for the management of a variety of endocrinopathies. In vitro assays using cultures of dissociated pituitary
cells have been powerful tools in the development of the pharmacology of HRH, providing valid, sensitive and highly quantitative assays of agonists and antagonists.

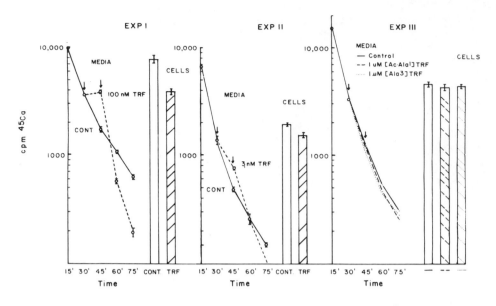

Fig. 10   Effect of TRF or TRF analogs on rate of ^{45}Ca efflux
           from GH$_3$ cells. Times of peptide additions during
           washout indicated by arrows

Luteinizing Hormone Releasing Factor (LRF)

    An example of a culture assay of LRF and two highly potent a-
gonists is shown in Figure 11 where the effects of multiple doses
of two peptides on the LH secretory rate has been used to calculate
the relative potencies shown in Table 6 and Figure 12.

    As we reported over 2 years ago (Monahan et al., 1973a, b), re-
placement of Gly found in the 6th position by D-Alanine increases
the potency almost four-fold. Subsequently, substitution by other
D-amino acids (Table 6) were found by us and others to enhance activity, (Vale et al., 1975b, c; Rivier et al., 1975; Vilchez-Martinez et al., 1974). [D-Lys^6] LRF with a free amino group can be u-
sed for coupling to molecules such as lauric acid or dextran T-2000
with maintenance of considerable biological activity. While basic
or aliphatic amino acids enhance the in vitro biological activity

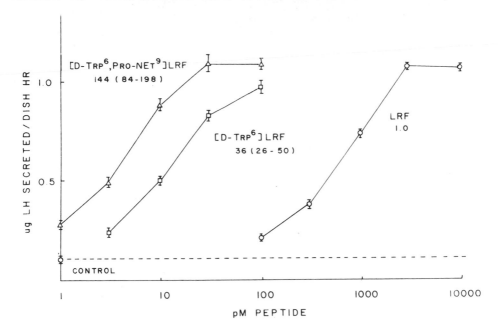

Fig. 11   Stimulation of LH secretion by LRF and 2 analogs in
vitro. Potencies with 95% confidence limits shown
under each structure

3-4 fold, the aromatic D-amino acids $_7$D-Tyr^6, D-Phe^6, or D-Trp^6 increase potency still more with [D-Trp^6]LRF having 36 times the in
vitro potency of LRF (Vale et al., 1975b).

Table 6 shows biological effects of changes in other parts of
the LRF molecule. Fujino et al. (1974) found that des-Gly^{10}-[Pro-
N-ethylamide^9] LRF, which is referred to in this paper as [Pro-N-
ethylamide^9]LRF had enhanced activity. It has been reported by us
(Vale and Rivier, 1975; Vale et al., 1975b, c) and others (Coy et
al., 1974) that combining this modification with D-Ala^6 further increases the potency. We find that [D-Ala^6, Pro-N-ethylamide^9]LRF
has an in vitro potency of 14 which is approximately the product of
the potencies of the singly modified peptides. Similar observations
(Fujino et al., 1974; Vilchez-Martinez et al., 1974; Vale et al.,
1975a, b; Rivier et al., 1975a, b) have been made with other pepti-

des having other D-amino acids at the sixth position and Pro-N-ethylamide at the ninth position with [D-Trp^6, Pro-N-ethylamide^9] LRF
having an _in vitro_ potency of 140 times that of LRF (Vale _et al._,
1975b).

TABLE 6   IN VITRO POTENCIES OF LRF ANALOGS MODIFIED
                 IN THE [GLY^6] POSITION

	Relative potency
LRF	1.0
[D-Ala^6]LRF	3.7 (2.0 - 6.5)
[D-Leu^6]LRF	3.2 (2.4 - 4.1)
[D-Lys^6]LRF	3.8 (2.8 - 5.2)
[ε-Lauryl-D-Lys^6]LRF	1.6 (1.3 - 2.1)
[ε-Dextran-D-Lys^6]LRF	0.15 (0.10 - 0.21)
[D-Arg^6]LRF	3.9 (2.9 - 5.1)
[D-Met^6]LRF	1.9 (1.1 - 3.3)
[D-Tyr^6]LRF	14.0 (8.6 - 22.0)
[D-Trp^6]LRF	36.0 (26.0 - 50.0)

Another series of LRF analogs involves the N^αMe-Leu^7 modification; [D-Ala^6, N^αMeLeu^7]LRF was synthesized (Ling and Vale, 1975)
in order to test a hypothesis (Monahan _et al._, 1973a) concerning a
possible preferred conformation (s) of LRF and was found to have a
slightly higher potency than [D-Ala^6] LRF _in vitro_. Again the composite analog involving all three modifications, [D-Ala^6, N^αMeLeu^7,
Pro-N-ethylamide^9] LRF, is more active still with a potency of 31.
Not only do these analogs show high potency _in vitro_ but _in vivo_
they have both high potency and prolonged activity (Vale _et al._,
1975b, c).

In considering possible mechanisms to explain the prolonged _in
vivo_ action of these peptides, we were led by the report of Koch
_et al._ (1974) to consider that they might be resistant to _in vivo_
enzymatic degradation. Koch showed that the Tyr^5-Gly^6-Leu^7 peptide bonds in LRF are hydrolyzed during incubation with brain extracts.
Marks and Stern (1974) then reported that the Pro^9-Gly^{10} peptide

RELATIVE POTENCY

PGLU — HIS — TRP — SER — TYR — GLY — LEU — ARG — PRO — GLY — NH$_2$ 1.0   STANDARD
  1   2   3   4   5   6   7   8   9   10

——NET   4.3   (3.5 - 5.1)

————————————————————D-ALA————— ————————————————   3.7   (2.0 - 6.5)

————————————————————D-ALA————————NET   14   (10 - 16)

————————————————————D-LEU————————NET   15   (12 - 20)

————————————————————D-LYS————————NET   17   (13 - 23)

————————————————————D-TYR————————NET   68   (48 - 95)

————————————————————D-TRP————————NET   144 (84 - 198)

————————————————D-ALA-N°ME-LEU————————————————   7.2   (4.8 - 11)

————————————————D-ALA-N°ME-LEU————————NET   31   (20 - 46)

Fig. 12   In vitro LH-releasing potencies of LRF analogs.
          Solid line represents identity with LRF. Position
          of modifications indicated by horizontal position
          on line. 95% confidence limits shown in parenthe-
          sis

bone is also cleaved, and furthermore that the D-Ala[6] and Pro-N-
ethylamide[9] modifications to LRF confer resistance to this hydroly-
sis.

    In the experiment shown in Figure 13, we incubated 4 peptides
with a homogenate of rat brain, minus hypothalamus, for 20 and 60
minutes, extracted the peptides with 90% ethanol, and then assayed
the resultant biological activities in vitro. We observed that the
relative rates of inactivation of LRF and three analogs were proportional to their potencies and durations of action in vivo, with
[D-Ala[6], N methyl-Leu[7], Pro-N-ethylamide[9]] undergoing no inactivation under the conditions of this experiment.

    We have found that LRF (monitored by radioimmunoassay specific
for the C-terminal portion of the molecule) is destroyed during in-

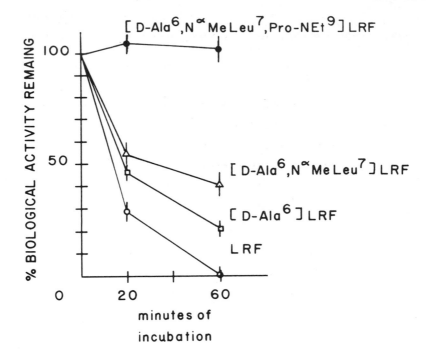

Fig. 13   Effect of incubation with brain extracts on the
           biological activities of LRF analogs. Each ana-
           log incubated at a concentration of 300 nM in an
           aqueous extract of rat brain (minus hypothalamus)
           for 20' and 60'. Biological activity assayed in
           vitro using rat pituitary cell culture assay.
           Results are expressed relative to the biological
           activity of each analog prior to incubation

cubations with extracts of many other tissues including kidney,
muscle, salivary glands, adenohypophysis, liver and testis (Vale
et al., 1975b). An LRF inactivation factor in testis (Vale et al.,
1975c) has been partially purified by 40% $(NH_4)_2SO_4$ precipitation,
dialysis and Sephadex chromatography. The physiological significance of the presence of LRF inactivation factors in several tis-

sues is not known; however, because of their ubiquity and the correlation of analogs' biological activities and relative resistances to destruction, it is tempting to suggest a role for these inactivation factors in modifying the in vivo response to LRF. Because we have also observed that cultured adenohypophyseal cells destroy LRF under the conditions of our assays, it is possible that relative resistance to degradation plays a role in determining the high specific activities of some analogs in vitro as well as in vivo.

While most active LRF analogs had in vitro dose-response curves parallel to that of LRF, we noted (Vale et al., 1972b) that the response to [Gly^2] LRF was not parallel with LRF and had a response maximal around 30% that of LRF thus behaving as a partial agonist with 30% intrinsic activity. Other modifications to the His^2 position were synthesized (Monahan et al., 1972; Rivier et al., 1972) and found (Vale et al., 1972c) to have little (<5%) intrinsic activity and to be the first reported competitive antagonists of LRF. Des-His^2-LRF is a low potency antagonist blocking the amount of LH and FSH released due to LRF by 50% at a molar excess of > 1000/1.

The ability of putative antagonists to inhibit the secretion of LH and FSH by cultured rat pituitary cells in response to a constant dose of LRF is the basis of the in vitro bioassay (Figure 14). Des-His^2 [D-Ala^6] LRF which was found to be several times more potent than des-His^2 D-Ala^6 LRF (Monahan et al., 1973c), is used as a standard in our antagonist assays and given the arbitrary potency of 1.0.

The potencies relative to des-His^2-[D-Ala^6]$_2$LRF of several LRF antagonists are shown in Figure 15. Des-His^2-[D-Ala^6, N$^\alpha$MeLeu^7] LRF has a relative potency of 2.5 while des-His^2-[D-Ala^6, Pro-N-ethylamide^9] LRF is not different from the standard. Thus the D-Ala^6 and N$^\alpha$MeLeu^7 modifications increase, while the Pro-N-ethylamide^9 alteration does not affect the potencies of the resultant histadine deleted antagonists.

We reported earlier (Monahan et al., 1973b) that [D-Ala^2]LRF was also an antagonist. Rees et al (1975) found that [D-Phe^2]LRF was several times more potent an antagonist than des-His^2-LRF. In confirmation of their results we observe [D-Phe^2]LRF to have a potency of 0.4 compared to des-His^2-LRF at 0.15. Accordingly, [D-Phe^2, D-Ala^6]LRF has a potency of over 3 and [D-Phe^2, D-Ala^6, N$^\alpha$MeLeu^7]LRF, [D-Phe^2, D-Trp^6]LRF and [D-Phe^2, D-Trp^6, N$^\alpha$MeLeu^7]LRF are 9, 30 and 50 times more potent respectively than des-His^2[D-Ala^6]LRF.

The most potent in vitro antagonists of this series, [D-Phe^2, D-Trp^6]LRF (Figure 14) and [D-Phe^2, D-Trp^6, N$^\alpha$MeLeu^7]LRF which decrease the LRF stimulated LH secretion rate by 50% at molar ratios

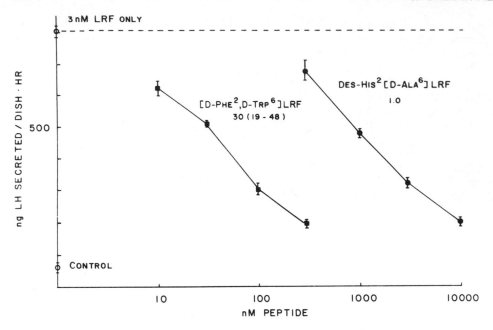

Fig. 14   Inhibition of LRF mediated LH secretion by two LRF
           antagonists.   Except for control, all dishes recei-
           ved 3 nM LRF.

of 14.1 and 9:1 (antagonist:LRF) are also the most potent in vivo.
In rats, high doses (≥ 100 μg) of [D-Phe^2, D-Trp^6] LRF given subcutaneously will block the response to LRF for more than 4 hours.
LRF analogs with the D-Phe^2 modification have been reported to be
effective inhibitors of ovulation by Corbin and Beattie (1975)
using [D-Phe^2, D-Ala^6]LRF and by Vilchez-Martinez et al. (1975) who
used [D-Phe^2, D-Phe^6]LRF which has in vitro potency of 20 in our
assays.

Somatostatin

    Somatostatin was characterized as the cyclic tetradecapeptide
shown at the top of Figure 16. Native somatostatin, synthetic somatostatin and synthetic reduced somatostatin were found (Rivier
et al., 1973; Vale et al., 1973b) to have the same potency to inhi-

UNDERLINE VITRO POTENCIES OF LRF ANTAGONISTS

Sequence	Relative Potency	
pGLU - ······- TRP - SER - TYR - GLY - LEU - ARG - PRO - GLY - NH$_2$ 1 2 3 4 5 6 7 8 9 10	0.15	(0.11 - 0.21)
——······————————————D-ALA——————————————	1.0	STANDARD
——······————————————D-ALA————————————NET	0.98	(0.58 - 1.61)
——······————————————D-ALA-N$^\alpha$ME-LEU————————————	2.5	(1.8 - 3.3)
--——D-PHE—————————————————————————	0.40	(0.29 - 0.49)
——D-PHE————————————D-ALA—————————————	3.3	(1.6 - 6.2)
——D-PHE————————————D-ALA-N$^\alpha$ME-LEU—————————	8.8	(6.5 - 12)
——D-PHE————————————D-PHE—————————————	20	(9.5 - 42)
——D-PHE————————————D-TRP—————————————	30	(19 - 48)
——D-PHE————————————D-TRP-N$^\alpha$ME-LEU—————————	52	(25 - 122)

Fig. 15   UNDERLINE In vitro antagonist potencies relative to Des-His[2]-
          [D-Ala[6]]LRF of LRF analogs. Solid line represents
          identity with sequence shown on top line. Dashed li-
          ne represents deletion.

bit GH secretion UNDERLINE in vitro. It was suggested that the oxidized, cyclic form of this peptide was the active form, and that reduced somatostatin could be rapidly oxidized during the biological assays.
The low potencies of several analogs which cannot form the disulfide bond ([Ala[3]] somatostatin, [Ala[3,14]] somatostatin and [S-Me-
Cys[3,4]]somatostatin favor this hypothesis. However, the observation that [S-MeCys[3]] somatostatin has a potency of 4% and ful intrinsic activity suggests that intramolecular associations other
than the disulfide bond maintain the molecule in a conformation
which can be recognized (although with lower affinity) by somatostatin receptors.

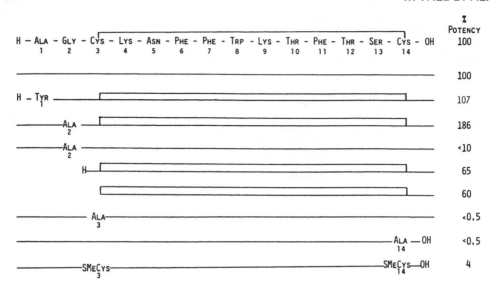

Fig. 16   *In vitro* potencies of somatostatin analogs based on
           abilities to inhibit GH secretion by rat pituitary
           cell cultures.   Identity with structure shown at top
           indicated by solid line.   Disulfide bond represented
           by 2nd solid line.

In contrast, the reduced form of $[Ala^2]$somatostatin is much
less potent than cyclic $[Ala^2]$somatostatin ($<10\%$ compared to 180%),
an observation perhaps reflecting steric hindrance of the disulfide interaction by the more rigid dipeptide side chain in the $[Ala^2]$
somatostatin.   Because of the considerable activity of analogs lacking the H-Ala-Gly side chain altogether (des-Ala[1], Gly[2]- [des-amino-
Cys[3]] somatostatin = 65%), we synthesized $[Tyr^1]$ somatostatin in
hopes of obtaining an iodinatable molecule for use in biological
and immunological studies.   Following that report (Vale *et al*.,
1973b), iodinated $[Tyr^1]$ somastostatin was used by Arimura *et al*.
(1975a) and Patel *et al*. (1975), as a trace in somatostatin radioimmunoassays.   We also prepared $[Tyr^{11}]$somatostatin, (replacing Tyr
for Phe) and found it to have 65% biological activity.

Other peptides in which alanine replaces particular amino acids in somatostatin have been synthesized and biologically tested. This series, shown in part in Figure 17, gives an appreciation of the role of the various functional groups in the presence of an intact backbone. The Asn[5] and Thr[10] functional groups in the presence of an intact backbone. The Asn[5] and Thr[10] functional groups are less critical for high biological potency than those of Phe[6], Phe[7], Trp[8], Phe[11], Thr[12], or Ser[13] which might be involved directly in the receptor-somatostatin interaction or in the maintenance of possible preferred conformations.

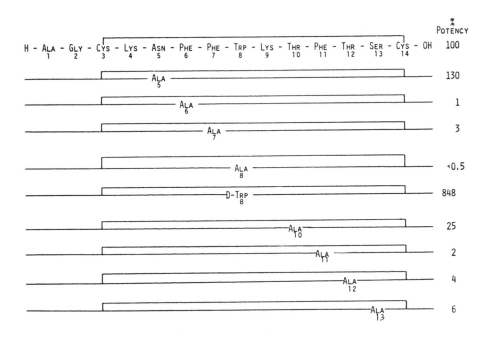

Fig. 17   In vitro potencies of somatostatin analogs

[D-Trp[8]]somatostatin was synthesized (Rivier et al., 1975a) in view of the hypothesis of Holladay and Puett (1975) that somatostatin might possess a turn in the region of the Trp[8]. This peptide is ca. 8 times more potent than somatostatin to inhibit GH in vitro (Figure 18). Recently Mars and Stern (1975) reported that brain extracts contain endopeptidases that cleave somatostatin at several sites including the Trp[8]-Lys[9] peptide bond. It is feasible that the high potency of [D-Trp[8]] somatostatin is related to a possible relative resistance to degradation.

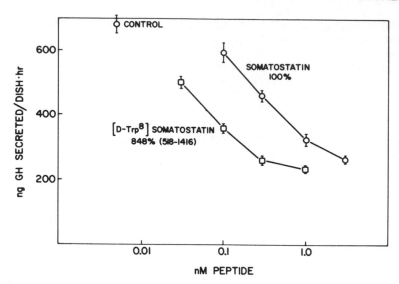

Fig. 18   Inhibition of GH secretion from culture rat pituita-
           ry cells by somatostatin (0) and [D-Trp⁸] somatosta-
           tin (□). Potency with 95% confidence limits relati-
           ve to somatostatin shown under name of peptide.

As has been emphasized before (Vale et al., 1973b, 1975a; Gerich et al., 1974; Besser et al., 1974), the lack of specificity of
somatostatin inhibiting the secretion of GH, glucagon, insulin, and
other secretory processes complicates its potential clinical appli-
cability. For example, it might be desirable to obtain an analog
with higher potency to inhibit glucagon secretion that insulin or
GH for use in juvenile onset diabetes (Gerich et al., 1974; Besser
et al., 1974; Gerich and Guillemin, 1976). Therefore, we are examining the pancreatotropic effects of our analogs by testing their
ability to inhibit the arginine stimulated release of insulin and
glucagon in vivo (Brown et al., 1976) and in vitro (Vale et al.,
1975a, b). The abilities of analogs to inhibit the secretion of
insulin and glucagon by cell cultures of neonatal rat pancreas prepared as are anterior pituitary cell cultures is the basis of our
in vitro assay for pancreatotropic hormones. The potency of [D-
Trp⁸]somatostatin to inhibit the secretion of insulin in such pan-

creas cell cultures is in agreement with its potency to inhibit GH secretion by cultured anterior pituitary cells.

ACKNOWLEDGEMENTS

The authors wish to thank Dr. R. Guillemin for advice and Dr. R. Burgus for amino acid analysis, and E. Tucker, K. Smith, L. Clark, G. Page, A. Wolf, R. Kaiser, L. Koshki, M. Mercado, R. Wolbers, R. Schroeder, R. Jacobs, A. McNeil, L. Lavie, H. Anderson, and B. Lerch for technical assistance, and Lisa Worrells and Bernice Gayer for assistance in preparing manuscript. We thank the NIAMDD rat pituitary hormone distribution program for the R/A kits used in pituitary hormone assays.

Support for research described here provided by AID/csd 2785, NIH grants AM 16787, AM18811, HD09690, Edna McConnell Clark Foundation, and the National Foundation 1-411.

REFERENCES

Arimura, A., Sato, H., Coy, D.H., and Schally, A.V. (1975a) Proc. Soc. Exp. Biol. Med. 148, 784.

Arimura, A., Sato, H., Dupont, A., Nishi, N. and Schally, A.V. (1975b) Science 189, 1007.

Bala, R.M., Burgus, R., Ferguson, K.A., Guillemin, R., Kudo, C., Olivier, C., Rodger, N.W. and Beck, J.C. (1970) In: The Hypothalamus (L. Martini, M. Motta and E. Fraschini, eds), Academic Press, New York, pp. 401-448.

Besser, G.M., Mortimer, C.H., McNeilly, A.S. and Thorner, M.O. (1974) British Medical Journal IV, 622-627.

Birge, C., Jacobs, L., Hammer, C. and Daughaday, W.H. (1970) Endocrinology 86, 120.

Boss, B., Vale, W. and Grant, G. (1975) In Biochemical Actions of Hormones (G. Litwack, ed.), Academic Press, New York, pp.

Brown, M., Rivier, J. and Vale, W. (1976) Endocrinology, in press.

Brownstein, M., Arimura, A., Sato, H., Schally, A.V. and Kizer, S. (1975) Endocrinology 96, 1456.

Corbin, A. and Beattie, B. (1975) Endocrine Research Communications 1-23.

Coy, D.H., Coy, E.J., Schally, A.V., Vilchez-Martinez, J., Hirotsu, Y. and Arimura, A. (1974) Biochem. Biophys. Res. Commun. 57, 335.

Dubois, M. (1975) Proc. Natl. Acad. Sci. (USA) 279, 1899.

Dupont, A. and Redding T.W. (1975) Endocrinology 96, 93A.

Fleischer, N. and Vale, W. (1968) Endocrinology 83, 1232.

Fujino, M., Yamazaki, I., Kobayashi, S., Fukada, T., Shinagawa, S. and Nakayama, R. (1974) Biochem. Biophys. Res. Commun. 57, 1248.

Gala, R.R., Janson, P.A. and Kuo, E.Y. (1972) Proc. Soc. Exp. Biol. Med. 140, 569.

Gerich, J.E., Lorenzi, M., Schneider, V., Karam, J., Rivier, J. and Guillemin, R. (1974) New Engl. J. of Med. 291, 544.

Gerich, J. and Guillemin, R. (1976) Somatostatin: Physiological & Clinical Significance, Ann. Rev. of Med., in press.

Geschwind, I.I. (1969) In: Frontiers in Neuroendocrinology (W. Ganong and L. Martini, eds), Oxford University Press, New York, pp. 389-431.

Grandison, E., Gelato, M. and Meites, J. (1974) Proc. Soc. Exp. Biol. Med. 145, 1236.

Guillemin, R. and Vale, W. (1970) In: Hypophysiotropic Hormones of the Hypothalamus (J. Meites, ed.), Williams & Wilkins Co., Baltimore (publ.), pp. 21-35.

Hinkle, P.M., Woroch, E.L. and Tashjian, A.H. (1974) J. Biol. Chem. 249, 3085.

Hinkle, P.M. and Tashjian, A.H. (1975) Biochemistry 14, 3845.

Hökfelt, T.S., Hellerstrom, E.C., Johansson, D., Luft, R. and Arimura, A. (1975) Acta Endocrinol. 80, 1.

Holladay, L.A. and Puett, D. (1975) Endocrinology 96, 252A.

Hopkins, C. and Farquhar, M. (1973) J. Cell Biol. 59, 276.

Hymer, W.C., Evans, W.H., Kraicer, J., Maotro, A., Davis, J. and Griswold, E. (1973) Endocrinology 92, 275.

Koch, Y., Baram, T. and Cholsieng, A.P. (1974) Biochem. Biophys. Res. Commun. 61, 95.

Labrie, F., De Léan, A., Drouin, J., Barden, N., Ferland, L., Borgeat, P., Beaulieu, M. and Morin, O. (1976) In: Hypothalamus and Endocrine Functions (F. Labrie, J. Meites and G. Pelletier, eds), Plenum Press, New York, in press.

Labrie, F., Pelletier, G., Lemay, A., Borgeat, P., Barden, N., Dupont, A., Coté, J. and Boucher, R. (1972) In: Karolinska Symposium on Research Methods in Reproductive Endocrinology (E. Diczfalusy, ed.), Geneva, pp. 301-340.

Libertun, C. and McCann, S.M. (1974) Proc. Soc. Exp. Bio. Med. 147, 498.

Ling, N. and Vale, W. (1975) Biochem. Biophys. Res. Commun. 63, 801.

McLeod, R.M. and Leymeyer, J.E. (1969) Endocrinology 92, 50A.

McLeod, R.M. (1969) Endocrinology 85, 916.

Marks, N. and Stern, F. (1974) Biochem. Biophys. Res. Commun. 61, 1458.

Marks, N. and Stern, F. (1975) FEBS Letters 55, 220.

Monahan, M., Rivier, J., Vale, W., Guillemin, R. and Burgus, R. (1972) Biochem. Biophys. Res. Commun. 47, 551.

Monahan, M., Amoss, M., Anderson, H. and Vale, W. (1973a) Biochemistry 12, 4616.

Monahan, M., Vale, W., Rivier, C., Grant, G. and Guillemin, R. (1973b) Endocrinology 93, 194A.

Patel, Y.C., Weir, G.C. and Reichlin, S. (1975) Endocrinology 96, 127A.

Patel, Y. and Reichlin, S. (1976) Endocrinology, in press.

Portanova, R., Smith, D. and Sayers, G. (1970) Proc. Soc. Exp. Biol. Med. 133, 573.

Portanova, R. and Sayers, G. (1973) Proc. Soc. Exp. Biol. Med. 143, 661.

Pressman, B.C. (1973) Fed. Proc. <u>32</u>, 1698.

Quejada, M., Illner, P., Krulich, L. and McCann, S.M. (1974) Neuro-endocrinology <u>13</u>, 151.

Rivier, J., Monahan, M., Vale, W., Grant, G., Amoss, M., Blackwell, R., Guillemin, R. and Burgus, R. (1972) Chimia <u>26</u>, 300.

Rivier, J., Brazeau, P., Vale, W., Ling, N., Burgus, R., Gilon, C., Yardley, J. and Guillemin, R. (1973) C.R. Acad. Sci. <u>276</u>, 2737.

Rivier, J., Brown, M. and Vale, W. (1975a) Biochem. Biophys. Res. Commun. <u>65</u>, 746.

Rivier, J., Ling, N., Monahan, M., Rivier, C., Brown, M. and Vale, W. (1975b) In: <u>Peptides: Chemistry, Structure and Biology</u> (Walter, R. and J. Meienhofer, eds), Ann Arbor Science (publ.), in press.

Roth, J., Kahn, R., Lesniak, M. and Gorden, P. (1975) In: <u>Recent Progress in Hormone Research</u> (R. Greep, ed.), Academic Press, New York, Vol. 31, p. 95.

Samuels, H.H., Tsai, J.S. and Cintron, R. (1973) Science <u>181</u>, 1253.

Sayers, G. and Portanova, R. (1974) Endocrinology <u>94</u>, 1723.

Shaar, C.J. and Clemens, J.A. (1974) Endocrinology <u>95</u>, 1202.

Sievertsson, H., Chang, J.K., Von Klandy, A., Rogentoft, C., Currie, B., Folkers, K. and Bowers, C. (1975) J. Biol. Chem. <u>15</u>, 222.

Tang, L.K.L. and Spies, H.G. (1974) Endocrinology <u>94</u>, 1016.

Tashjian, A.H., Bancroft, F.C. and Levine, L. (1970) J. Cell Biol. <u>47</u>, 61.

Tashjian, A., Barowsky, N. and Jensen, D. (1971) Biochem. Biophys. Res. Commun. <u>43</u>, 516.

Vale, W., Brazeau, P., Grant, G., Nussey, A., Burgus, R., Rivier, J., Ling, N. and Guillemin, R. (1972a) C.R. Acad. Sci. <u>275</u>, 2913.

Vale, W., Grant, G., Amoss, M. and Guillemin, R. (1972b) Endocrino-logy <u>91</u>, 562.

Vale, W., Grant, G., Rivier, J., Monahan, M., Amoss, M., Blackwell, R., Burgus, R. and Guillemin, R. (1972c) Science <u>176</u>, 933.

Vale, W., Brazeau, P., Rivier, C., Rivier, J. and Guillemin, R. (1973b) In: Advances in Human Growth Hormone Research (S. Raiti, ed.), U.S. Government Printing Office, DHEW, Publ. No. (NIH) 74612, Vol. I., pp. 159-182.

Vale, W., Brazeau, P., Rivier, C., Rivier, J., Grant, G., Burgus, R. and Guillemin, R. (1973a) Fed. Proc. 32, 211.

Vale, W., Grant, G., and Guillemin, R. (1973c) In: Frontiers in Neuroendocrinology (L. Martini and W. Ganong, eds), Oxford University Press, New York (publ.), pp. 375-413.

Vale, W., Rivier, C., Brazeau, P. and Guillemin, R. (1974a) Endocrinology 95, 968.

Vale, W., Rivier, C., Palkovitis, M., Saavedrna, J. and Brownstein, M. (1974b) Endocrinology 94, A-128.

Vale, W. and Grant, G. (1975) In: Methods in Enzymology, Hormones and Cyclic Nucleotides (B.W. O'Malley and J.G. Hardman, eds), Academic Press, New York, Vol. 37, chap. 15, pp. 82-93.

VALE, W. and Grant, G. (1975) In: Methods in Enzymology, Hormones and Cyclic Nucleotides (B.W. O'Malley and J.G. Hardman, eds), Academic Press, New York, Vol. 37, pp. 402-407.

Vale, W. and Rivier, C. (1975) In: Handbook of Psychopharmacology Plenum Press, New York, pp. 196-237.

Vale, W., Brazeau, P., Rivier, C., Brown, M., Boss, B., Rivier, J., Burgus, R., Ling, N. and Guillemin, R. (1975a) Rec. Prog. in Horm. Res. 31, 365.

Vale, W., Rivier, C., Brown, M., Ling, N., Leppaluoto, J., Monahan, M. and Rivier, J. (1975b) In: Clinical Endocrinology, Suppl. (I. McIntyre, ed.), Blackwell Scientific Publications (PUBL.), Oxford, England.

Vale, W., Rivier, C., Rivier, J., Ling, N., Monahan, M. and Guillemin, R. (1975c) Endocrinology 96, 99A.

Vilchez-Martinez, J.A., Coy, D.H., Arimura, A., Coy, E.J., Hirotsu, Y. and Schally, A.V. (1974) Biochem. Biophys. Res. Commun. 59, 1226.

Vilchez-Martinez, J.A., Coy, D.H., Coy, E.J., De la Cruz, A., Nishi, N. and Schally, A.V. (19) Endocrinology 96, 354A.

Localization of Hypothalamic Hormones

IMMUNOHISTOCHEMICAL LOCALIZATION OF HYPOTHALAMIC HORMONES AT THE ELECTRON MICROSCOPE LEVEL

Georges Pelletier

Medical Research Council Group in Molecular
Endocrinology, Centre Hospitalier de
l'Université Laval, Québec, G1V 4G2, Canada

Adenohypophyseal activity is under the control of neurohormones released from the hypothalamus and carried to their specific sites of action, the pituitary cells, by a portal blood system. While it was well established that hypothalamic regulatory hormones are present in high concentrations in the median eminence (Ishii, 1970; Krulich et al., 1971), it has been only recently reported that TRH and somatostatin are present in some extra-hypothalamic areas (Brownstein et al., 1974; Brownstein et al., 1975). A direct inhibitory effect of somatostatin on the secretion of insulin, glucagon (Koerker et al., 1974) and gastrin (Hayes et al., 1975) has also been reported thus suggesting that this neurohormone could be possibly produced and/or stored in the pancreas and gastrointestinal tract. In order to gain a better understanding of the mechanisms of packaging and secretion of LH-RH and somatostatin in the brain and target tissues detailed immunohistochemical studies were performed on the localization of these peptides.

LOCALIZATION OF LH-RH IN THE BRAIN

Using an immunofluorescence technique, Barry et al. (1973) have shown that LH-RH of the guinea pig was mainly concentrated in the median eminence. When the animal was previously injected with colchicine, they observed a few positive perikarya scattered in a large area extending from the preoptic area to the caudal part of the tuber. Recently, with the peroxidase-labeled antibody technique Baker et al. (1974), Setalo et al. (1974) and Kordon et al. (1974) have localized LH-RH in nerve fibers in the external zone of the median eminence of several species. None of the authors has been able to show immunostained cell bodies. Zimmerman et al.

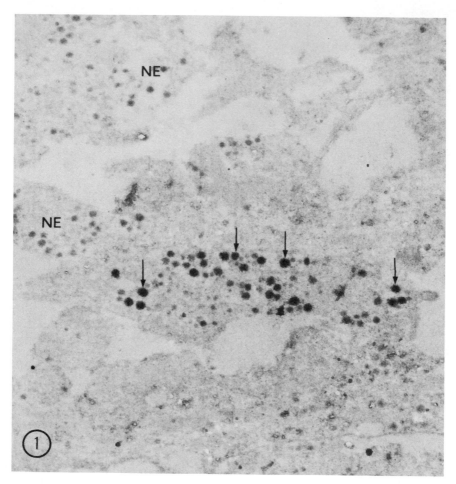

Figure 1.   Electron microscopic immunohistochemical detection of
            LH-RH in the median eminence.   The reaction secondary
            to the accumulation of the peroxidase-anti-peroxidase
            complex is found over the granules (→) of a nerve
            ending located in the external zone.   Other nerve en-
            dings (NE) are unstained.   X 33,300.

(1974) have however described, in the mouse, the presence of
LH-RH in the perikaryon of a few neurons of the arcuate nucleus
and also in tanycytes. Suprisingly, these authors did not find
any positive nerve fibers in the external zone of the median
eminence.

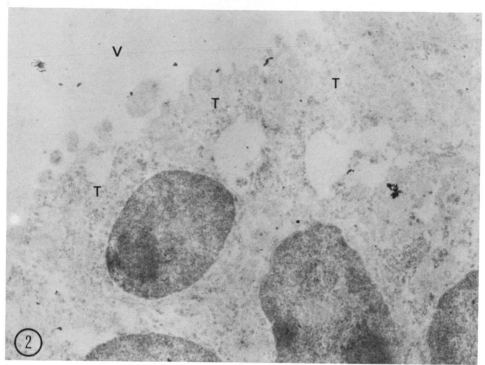

Figure 2. Immunohistochemical detection of LH-RH in the median
           eminence. Absolutely no reaction can be detected in
           the tanycytes (T). V: third ventricle. X 12,500.

        In order to explore accurately all brain areas, we have stu-
died serial paraffin sections of the whole brain in the rat and
guinea pig. With an immunohistochemical technique involving use
of the peroxidase-anti-peroxidase complex at the light microscope
level, a procedure which is much more sensitive than immunofluorescence or the peroxidase-labeled antibody technique (Sternberger,
1974), we have found a positive reaction for LH-RH in the external
zone of the lateral parts of the median eminence. This reaction
is present throughout the median eminence although more concentrated in its caudal portion. No positive perikarya were detected in
the hypothalamus. At the electron microscope level, we found that
the positive reaction was present exclusively in a few nerve endings
of the external zone of the median eminence (Pelletier et al.,
1974a). As evidenced in Fig. 1, the reaction is localized exclusively in the secretory granules of the positive nerve endings.
The diameter of the LH-RH-containing granules ranged from 750 to
950 A°. Absolutely no reaction was observed in the tanycytes of
the median eminence (Fig. 2).

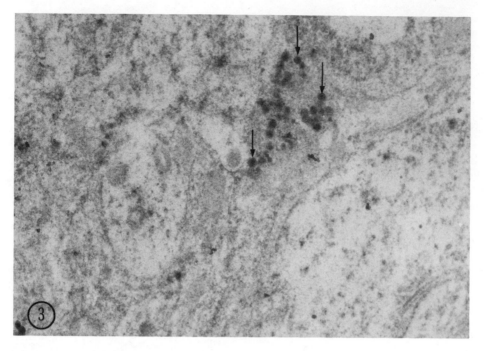

Figure 3.   Immunohistochemical localization of LH–RH in the orga-
            num vasculum of the lamina terminalis (OVLT). A reac-
            tion for LH–RH is present in the secretory granules
            (→) of a nerve ending. The surrounding nervous tissue
            is negative. X 30,000.

    In the organum vasculosum of the lamina terminalis (OVLT), a
strong positive reaction for LH–RH was consistently observed. This
reaction was in the nervous tissue close to blood vessels. Again,
no cell bodies appeared to be labeled. With the electron microscope, LH–RH was mainly found in the granules (of a diameter of
700 A° to 1000 A°) of nerve fibers and/or endings (Fig. 3) and also
in a few cell processes devoided of granules. In the latter case,
the reaction was diffused and did not seem to be associated with
any specific organelle.

    Examination of the serial paraffin sections revealed the pre-
sence of specific reaction in the subfornical organ, the subcommissural organ and the area postrema. A diagram of the periventricular organs is shown in Fig. 4. A common pattern for the distribution of LH–RH was observed in these organs: a strong reaction
was mainly localized in the ependymal and subependymal layers and
also at the vicinity of blood vessels. The nervous tissue at the
proximity of these specialized organs was always completely nega-

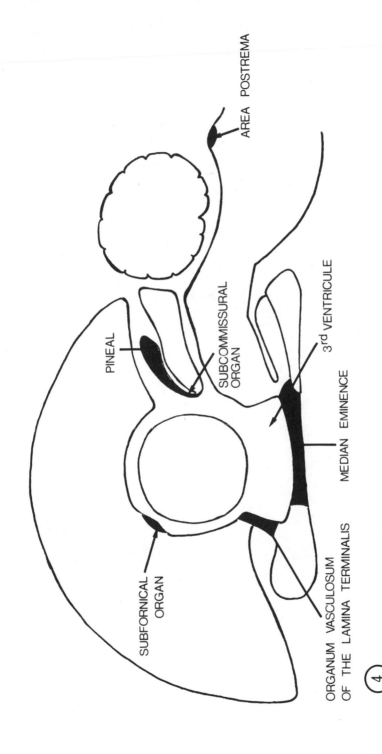

Figure 4. Topographical representation of the major periventricular organs of the rat on a median sagittal section.

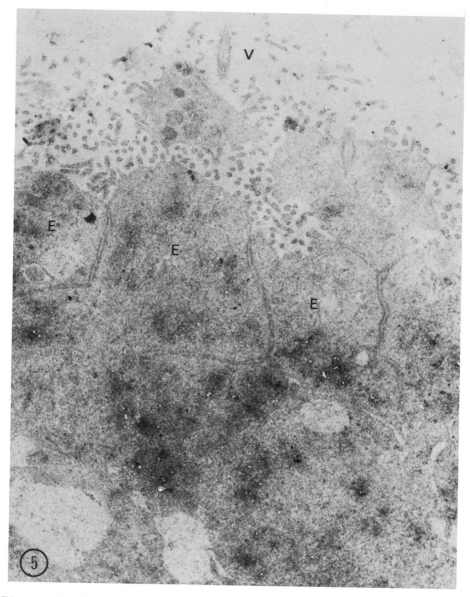

Figure 5. Immunohistochemical detection of LH-RH in the subcommissural organ. A diffuse positive reaction is present
in the cytoplasm of ependymal cells (E). V: third ventricle. X 20,500.

tive. At the ultrastructural level, a diffuse reaction was observed in the cytoplasm of ependymal (Fig. 5) and subependymal cells.

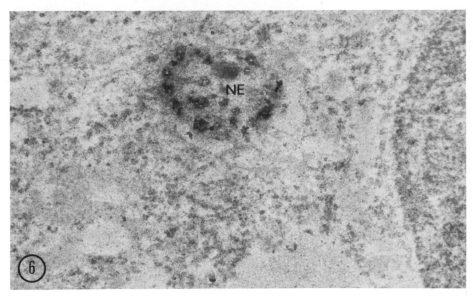

Figure 6.   Immunohistochemical localization of LH-RH in the pi-
            neal gland. Accumulation of PAP molecules indicating
            the presence of LH-RH can be observed over a nerve
            ending (NE). X 37,500

This reaction was not clearly associated with any organelle. In
the subependymal cells, the reaction was often found at one pole
of the cell. Some cell processes were found to be labeled mainly
at the proximity of capillaries.

     In the pineal gland, the reaction for LH-RH occurred around
the blood vessels. This reaction was variable in intensity from
one animal to the other. Ultrastructural study shows a diffuse
positive reaction in the cytoplasm of some cells located at the
proximity of capillaries. The identity of these cells still remains to be clarified. A few nerve endings distributed throughout the gland also showed a positive reaction for LH-RH (Fig. 6).

     From the results of many groups obtained at the light micros-
copic level and from our own observations at both light and electron microscopic levels, it can be generalized that in the hypothalamus, LH-RH is present in the axons but not in the perikarya
of neurosecretory neurons and is not a component of tanycytes.
These LH-RH-containing axons generally terminate close to the
fenestrated capillaries of the pituitary portal plexus. The absence of reaction for LH-RH in perikarya of secretory neurons may
be explained by a low concentration of LH-RH stored in the perikarya. Since a proportion of LH-RH is probably destroyed or lost
during histological procedures, the amount of LH-RH present in

perikarya should become then too low for detection.   It is also
possible that LH-RH is not present in immunoreactive form in the
perikarya and acquires immunoreactivity during its transport along
the axon.   We have recently reported the absence of immunoreactive vasopressin in the perikarya of the secretory cells of supraoptic and paraventricular nuclei, while a strong reaction for
this hormone was observed in the axons and nerve endings (Leclerc
and Pelletier, 1974).   The synthetis of LH-RH within axons endings
should also be seriously considered.

     In the OVLT, our results are in agreement with previous re-
ports demonstrating the presence of LH-RH in the OVLT of guinea
pig and rat by immunofluorescence (Barry et al., 1973)   and immunocytochemistry (Zimmerman et al., 1974).   The presence of LH-RH
in secretory granules suggests that LH-RH is probably released
from the nerve endings into the capillaries.   It is interesting
to note that the diameter of the positive granules is about the
same as those observed to contain LH-RH in the median eminence.
As in the hypothalamic nuclei, no cell bodies were found to be
positive in this organ.

     The presence of LH-RH in the cytoplasm of most ependymal
and subependymal cells in the subfornical and subcommissural organ and area posterna suggests that these cells are capable of
synthesizing and/or concentrating this neurohormone.   The presence of LH-RH in cell processes at the vicinity of the fenestrated
capillaries may also indicate the possibility of exchange between
circulating blood of these specialized organs which lack the
blood-brain barrier.   In the pineal gland, the diffuse positive
reaction for LH-RH in the cytoplasm of cells located in close
proximity of the capilarries also favor the hypothesis of exchan-
ges between this organ and the blood.   We have previously shown
an uptake of radioactivity by the pineal gland after the administration of [^{3}H] LH-RH (Dupont et al., 1974).   The physiological
significance of these findings remains however to be investigated.

LOCALIZATION OF SOMATOSTATIN IN THE BRAIN

     Immunohistochemical localization of somatostatin has also
been investigated with the technique involving use of the peroxidase-anti-peroxidase complex.   As observed for LH-RH, somatostatin was found to be present in the median eminence and also in
OVLT, subfornical organ, subcommissural organ, area postrema and
pineal gland in both rat and guinea pig (Pelletier et al., 1975a;
Dubé et al., 1975).   In a preliminary report, Hökfelt et al.
(1974) using an immunofluorescence technique, have localized somatostatin in the external zone of the median eminence and the
ventro-medial nucleus in the guinea pig brain although they did
not mention any positive reaction in the periventricular organs.

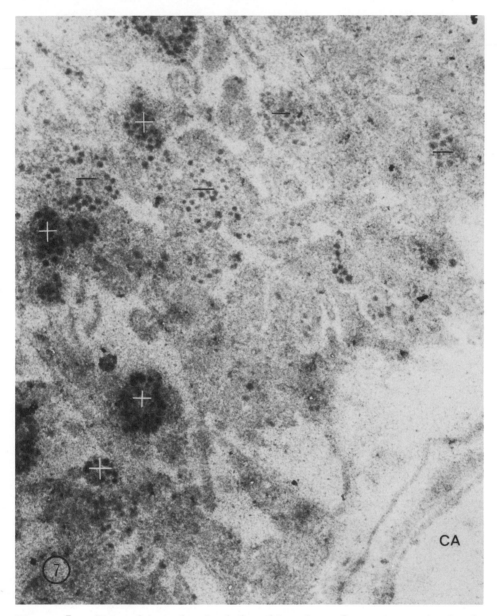

Figure 7.   Immunohistochemical localization of somatostatin in the
median eminence. Many positive (+) nerve endings are
present in the external zone close to fenestrated capillaries. Other nerve endings (-) do not contain somatostatin. CA: capillary. X 23,400.

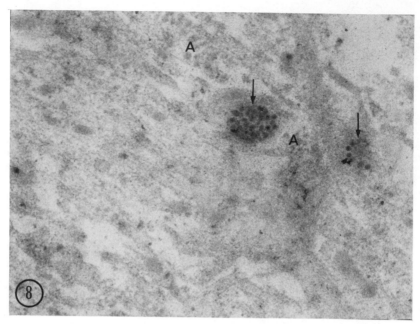

Figure 8.   Internal zone of the median eminence. Two somatostatin
            positive fibers (→) are observed at the proximity of
            negative axons (A).   X 9,000.

     In the median eminence, somatostatin was mainly localized in
the external zone close to capillaries, although some positive
reaction was also consistently observed in the internal zone
(Pelletier et al., 1975a).   No tanycytes showed specific staining.
Somatostatin was found to be distributed evenly throughout the
median eminence from the cephalic to the caudal region.   At the
ultrastructural level (Pelletier et al., 1974b), somatostatin was
found in the secretory granules (about 900 A° to 1100 A° in diameter) of many nerve endings located near the extravascular space
of the fenestrated capillaries (Fig. 7).   A few immunoreactive nerve fibers were also observed in the internal zone of the median
eminence (Fig. 8).   No cell bodies appeared to be reactive.   In the
ventral portion of the arcuate nucleus, positive nerve fibers were
occasionally observed near the lateral parts of the median eminence.

     In the OVLT, immunostaining was present around the capillaries
and larger blood vessels whereas ependymal cells remained unstained.
As demonstrated on serial sections, the localization of somatostatin was completely different from that of LH-RH.   With high resolution immunohistochemistry, somatostatin was detected in secretory granules of many nerve endings.   The diameter of these soma-

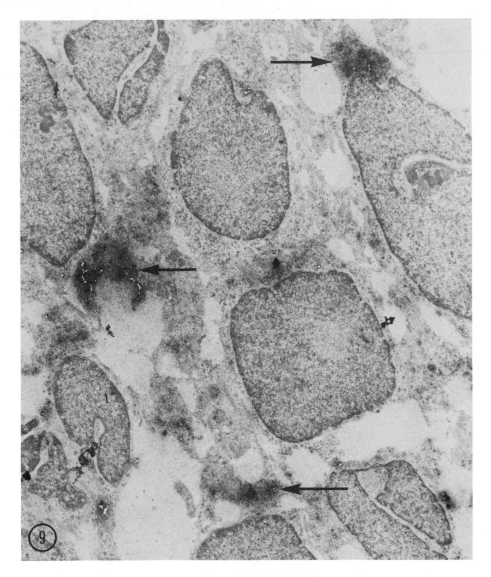

Figure 9. Immunohistochemical detection of somatostatin in the
subcommissural organ. A diffuse positive reaction for
somatostatin is observed in the cytoplasm of many subependymal cells. The reaction is generally present at
one pole of the cell (→). X 10,000.

tostatin-containing granules was of 900 Å to 1200 A°. A few cell
processes were also labeled without any specific localization over
organelles.

In the subfornical organ, subcommissural organ and area postrema, the reaction was similar to that observed for LH-RH. The accumulation of PAP molecules was present over the cytoplasm of ependymal and subependymal cells (Fig. 9) and various cell processes, especially these processes extending close to the endothelial cells of the fenestrated capillaries. In the pineal gland, as previously noted for LH-RH, a diffuse reaction was concentrated mainly in the cytoplasm of cells surrounding the capillaries. A few nerve endings were also found to be stained for somatostatin.

The first immunohistochemical detection of somatostatin in the secretory granules of nerve endings of the median eminence indicates, that at least two hypothalamic hormones, LH-RH and somatostatin, are stored in nerve endings of the median eminence. Since the somatostatin-containing nerve endings are much more abundant than those containing LH-RH and since somatostatin-positive granules are larger than those containing LH-RH (900-1100 A^{o} versus 750-950 A^{o}), it can be concluded that LH-RH and somatostatin are present in different nerve endings. The absence of immunostaining for somatostatin in the perikarya of hypothalamic neurons can be interpreted as a consequence of a low concentration or a lack of immunoreactivity of this neurohormone in the perikarya of secretory neurons.

In the OVLT, the localization of somatostatin in nerve endings suggests that this organ, besides its possible role in the control of gonadotropins secretion, may also play a role in the control of growth hormone secretion. Since the granules which contain somatostatin are slightly larger than those containing LH-RH, the two neurohormones appear to be stored in different nerve endings. Moreover, at the light microscope level, the distribution of immunostaining for these two hormones is completely different. In the other periventricular organs, as previously discussed for LH-RH, the accumulation of somatostatin in cells which are not neurosecretory neurons may represent synthesis and/or uptake of the neurohormone.

LOCALIZATION OF SOMATOSTATIN IN PANCREAS AND STOMACH

In order to attribute some physiological significance to the observed effect of somatostatin on the secretion of insulin and glucagon by the pancreas (Koerker et al., 1974) and gastrin by the stomach (Hayes et al., 1975), the immunohistochemical localization of somatostatin was studied in the pancreas and different portions of the stomach. In the rat pancreas, a positive reaction for somatostatin was observed in a few cells of the Langerhans islets (Pelletier et al., 1975). These positive cells are located at the periphery of the islets and are different from α-cells which secrete glucagon and β-cells responsible for insulin secretion. At the

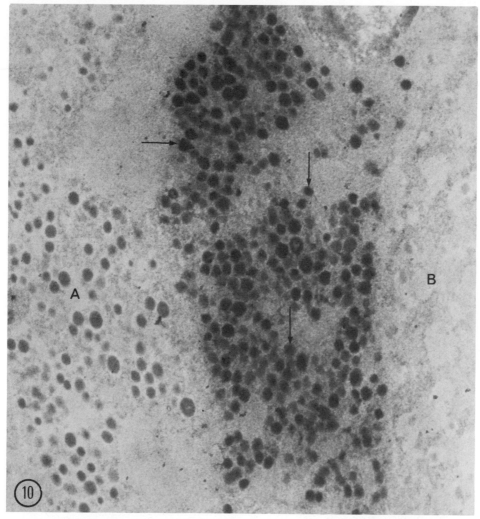

Figure 10.   Immunohistochemical detection of somatostatin in the
endocrine pancreas. A positive reaction is present
in the secretory granules (→) and also to a lesser
degree in the cytoplasm of a cell located at the periphery of a Langerhans islet. Adjacent α-cell (A) and
β-cell (B) are negative. X 23,000.

electron microscope level, the positive reaction demonstrated by
the accumulation of PAP molecules was mainly observed over the secretory granules (Fig. 10). The diameter of the positive secretory granules was about 170-210 nm. The α- and β-cells showed a complete absence of reaction.

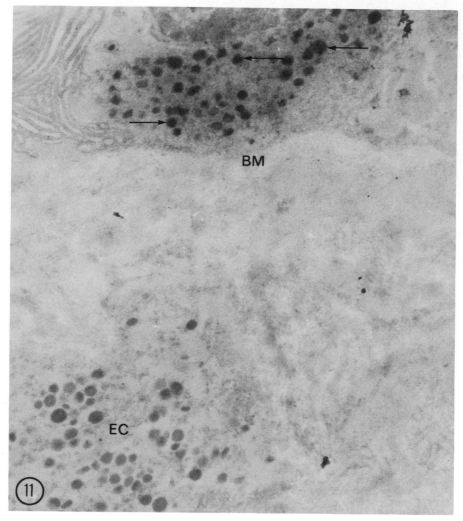

Figure 11.   Immunohistochemical detection of somatostatin in the
             stomach.   Reaction products can be detected over the
             secretory granules (→) and the cytoplasm of an endo-
             crine cell located close to the basement membrane (BM).
             Another endocrine cell (EC) is negative.   X 16,700.

        Our results agree well with the reports of Dubois et al.
(1975) and Polak et al. (1975) which have shown by immunofluorescence the presence of a few somatostatin-positive cells in the
pancreas of man, dog, pig, sheep, rat and chicken.   This first demonstration at the electron microscope level of the presence of

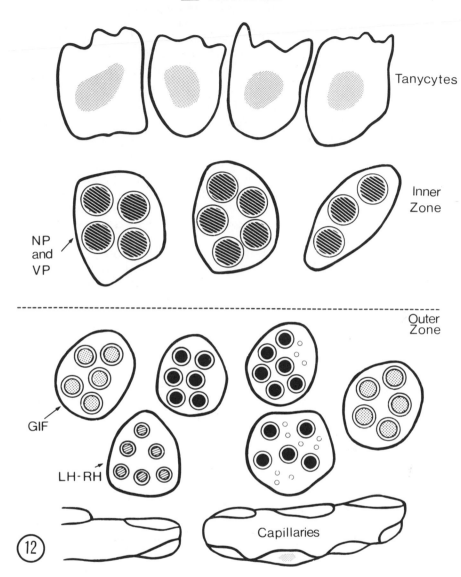

Figure 12. Diagram of the median eminence. LH-RH and somatostatin
(GIF) are present in secretory granules of nerve endings located in the outer zone whereas vasopressin (VP)
and its binding protein neurophysin (NP) are contained
in large granules of axons passing through the inner
zone. LH-RH and somatostatin are released into the
fenestrated capillaries of the pituitary portal plexus
to influence adenohypophyseal secretion.

somatostatin in the secretory granules of a specific cell type of the endocrine pancreas suggests that this peptide may have some physiological importance in the regulation of insulin and gluca- gon secretion. Since the cells (α-cells and β-cells) which are affected by somatostatin do not contain detectable amounts of this hormone, it can be suspected that this other cell type is capable of producing somatostatin which could then be released in order to modulate the secretion of neighbouring α- and β-cells.

The different parts of rat stomach were also examined for the presence of somatostatin. Somatostatin-containing cells were con- sistently found in the mucosa of the pyloric antrum whereas the other portions of the stomach were negative. These positive cells were generally located at the base of pyloric glands and showed a distribution different from gastrin cells which are also more nu- merous. At the ultrastructural level, the reaction product was localized over the secretory granules (150-250 nm in diameter) with some degree of diffusion in the cytoplasm in a cell type which has not been found in contact with the pyloric lumen (Fig. 11). The somatostatin-containing cell found in the stomach appears to correspond very well to the cell type III (intestinal D-cell) of Forsman et al. (1969).

SUMMARY AND CONCLUSION

From the observations of several laboratories at the light microscope level and from our results obtained at the electron mi- croscope level, the following generalizations may be drawn on the localizations of LH-RH and somatostatin. (1) LH-RH and somatos- tatin are contained in axons and nerve endings of the median emi- nence (Fig. 12) and OVLT but not in cell bodies. (2) LH-RH and somatostatin are present in different nerve endings. (3) In the subcommissural organ, subfornical organ and area postrema, these two neurohormones are present in the cytoplasm of ependymal and subependymal cells. (4) In the pineal gland, the neurohormones are mainly concentrated in the cytoplasm of cells situated at the proximity of capillaries. (5) In the endocrine pancreas and gastric mucosa, somatostatin is present in granules of specific secretory cells.

ACKNOWLEDGMENTS

We are grateful to Dr A. Arimura for providing anti-somatos- tatin and anti-LH-RH serums. The peroxidase-anti-peroxidase com- plex was a generous gift from Dr L.A. Sternberger.

REFERENCES

Arimura, A., Sato, H., Coy, D.H. and Schally, A.V. (1975) Proc. Soc. Exp. Biol. Med. 148, 784-788.

Baker, D.L., Dermody, W.C. and Reel, J.R. (1974) Am. J. Anat. 139, 129-134.

Barry, J. and Dubois, M.P. (1973) Ann. Endocr. (Paris) 34, 735-742.

Brownstein, M.J., Palkovits, M., Saavedra, J.M., Bassiri, P.M. and Utiger, R.D. (1974) Science 185, 267-269.

Brownstein, M., Arimura, A., Sato, M., Schally, A.V. and Kizer, J.S. (1975) Endocrinology 96, 1456-1461.

Dubé, D., Leclerc, R., Pelletier, G., Arimura, A., Schally, A.V., (1975) Cell. Tiss. Res., in press.

Dupont, A., Labrie, F., Pelletier, G., Puviani, R., Coy, D.H., Coy, E.J. and Schally, A.V. (1974) Neuroendocrinology 16, 65-73.

Forssman, W.G., Orci, L., Pidet, R., Renold, A.E. and Rouiller, C. (1969) J. Cell. Biol. 40, 698-715.

Hayes, J.R., Johnson, D.G., Koerker, D. and Williams, R.H. (1975) 96, 1374-1376.

Hökfelt, T., Efendic, S., Johansson, O., Luft, R. and Arimura, A. (1974) Brain Res. 80, 165-169.

Ishii, S. (1970) Endocrinology 86, 207-216.

Köerker, D.J., Ruch, W., Chideckel, E., Palmer, J., Goodner, C.J., Ensinck, J. and Gale, C.C. (1974) Science 184, 482-484.

Kordon, C., Kerdelhué, B., Patton, E. and Jutisz, M. (1974) Proc. Soc. Exp. Biol. Med. 147, 122-127.

Krulich, L., Quijada, M., Illmer, P., McCann, S.M. (1971) Proc. Int. Union. Physiol. 9, 326.

Leclerc, R. and Pelletier, G. (1974) Am. J. Anat. 140, 583-588.

Pelletier, G., Labrie, F., Puviani, R., Arimura, A. and Schally, A.V. (1974a) Endocrinology 95, 314-317.

Pelletier, G., Labrie, F., Arimura, A. and Schally, A.V. (1974b) Am. J. Anat. 140, 445-450.

Pelletier, G., Leclerc, R., Dubé, D., Labrie, F., Puviani, R.,
Arimura, A.V., Schally, A.V. (1975a) Am. J. Anat. 142, 297-301.

Pelletier, G., Leclerc, R., Arimura, A. and Schally, A.V. (1975b)
J. Histochem. Cytochem., 9, 699-701.

Polak, J.M., Grimelis, L., Pearse, A.G.E. and Bloom, S.R. (1975)
The Lancet 1, 1220-1222.

Setalo, G., Vigh, S., Schally, A.V., Arimura, A. and Flerko, B.
(1975) Endocrinology 96, 135-142.

Sternberger, L.A. (1974) Immunocytochemistry, Prentice-Hall Inc.,
Englewood Cliffs, N.J.

Zimmerman, E.A., Hsu, K.G., Ferrin, M. and Kozlowski, G.P. (1974)
Endocrinology 95, 1-8.

IMMUNOHISTOCHEMICAL LOCALIZATION OF HYPOTHALAMIC HORMONES

(ESPECIALLY LRF) AT THE LIGHT MICROSCOPY LEVEL

Julien Barry

Laboratoire d'Histologie, Faculté de Médecine

Place de Verdun, 59045   LILLE Cedex   France

INTRODUCTION

Hypothalamic hormones that can now be revealed by immunohistochemical methods may be divided into two groups :
- *post hypophyseal* or *neurohypophyseal hormones* (principally adiuretin-vasopressin, ADH-VP and oxytocin)
- *prehypophysiotropic hormones* (principally LRF, the "Luteinizing Hormone Releasing Factor", McCann *et al* 1960, or LH-RH, the "Luteinizing Hormone Releasing Hormone", and cyclic somatostatin or SRIF, the "Somathormone Release Inhibiting Factor", Krulich *et al* 1967).

We shall not give details of the techniques of histological fixation, microtomy, either with the freezing microtome or after inclusion or immunological reactions(details will be found in the works of authors quoted in the text). The aim of these techniques is to preserve the condition of the tissues and above all to preserve the hypothalamic hormones in immunoreactive form *in situ*, eventually revealing their reactive sites if complexed,in order to obtain their specific demonstration.

At the present time all hypothalamic hormones demonstrated by immunohistochemistry are synthesized by specialized neurons, or more exactly by "neurosecretory cells" in the sense defined by E. Scharrer (ref. in Scharrer and Scharrer 1963).

The quantity of immunoreactive hormone present in the perikaryons, dendrites and axons of these cells varies considerably according to physiological or experimental conditions and species. Immunohistochemistry can reveal only "immunoreactive" segments of these cells, and negative results must therefore be interpreted with great prudence.

IMMUNOREACTIVE ADH-VP AND OXYTOCIN NEURONS

Unlike "prehypophysiotropic"neurons, it was possible
to make histological study of ADH-VP and oxytocin producing neurons
before the chemical formula and synthesis of these hormones were
established by Du Vigneaud *et al* (1953-1954) and Acher and Chauvet
(1954). Bargmann (1949), in fact, using Gomori's technique (1941)
with chromic hematoxylin, was able to show the presence of ADH-VP
and oxytocin producing neurons. These neurons, which are mainly localized in the supraoptic and paraventricular nuclei, give rise to
axons that form the "gomori positive hypothalamo-neurohypophyseal
neurosecretory pathway" and terminate around the capillaries of the
neural lobe. The hormones present in these neurons contain disul-
phur bonds that enable them to be demonstrated by various techniques : 2-2' dihydroxy 6-6' dinaphtyl thioglycolate disulfure
(Barnett and Seligman 1954, Adams and Sloper 1954) : ferric thioglycolate ferricyanure ; Alcian blue performic acid (Adams and
Sloper 1956) ; N-N' dithylpseudoisocyanine chloride (Sterba 1961,
1964).

They are associated with proteins containing abundant
cystin ("neurophysin", Acher *et al* 1955) that are partly responsible for the preceding reactions (Acher 1958). These proteins are
present in the hormonal granules (Ginsburg and Ireland 1963, 1966 ;
Dean and Hope 1966, 1967), and their biochemical study has been carried out in various species : bullock (Rauch *et al* 1969) ; pig
(Uttenhal and Hope 1970 ; Burford *et al* 1971 ; Coy and Wuu 1974) ;
man (Chang and Friesen 1972) ; sheep (Watkins 1972 a) ; rat (Watkins 1972 b ; Pickering *et al* 1974). Researches by Dean *et al* (1968)
provided the first indication of a bond between neurophysin I and
neurophysin II with oxytocin and ADH-VP in the various granules ;
Burford *et al* (1971) also showed the different distribution of neurophysin A and B. Furthermore, Norström *et al* (1974) showed that
there are several intra and extra-granular neurophysin pools in the
neural lobe, with modifications according to age and physiological
state.

Pickering *et al* (1974) characterized two major types
of neurophysin (A and B) and a "minor" neurophysin in the rat.
Neurophysin A (associated with ADH-VP) is absent in homozygotes
of Brattleboro strain (suffering from hereditary hypothalamic diabetes insipidus).

Immunohistochemical Characterization of ADH-VP Neurons

Burlet *et al* (1972, 1973, 1975) characterized ADH-VP
producing cells in rat by means of rabbit antisera to synthetic
lysin-VP linked with rat serum albumin (RSA). The antisera give
complete cross reaction with arginin-vasopressin, which is the biologically active peptide of the rat ; they do not give cross reaction with RSA or oxytocin. Vasopressin cells are found mainly in
the supraoptic and paraventricular nuclei ; they form small groups
in the anterior and posterior nuclei of the fornix, nucleus circu-

laris and nucleus of the medial forebrain bundle; they may also be
isolated. Their axons generally terminate around the capillaries of
the neural lobe; a few terminate around the capillaries of the portal plexus of the infundibulum. Dehydration drains reactive material
from the nerve lobe; hypophysectomy decreases reactive material in
the hypothalamo-neurohypophyseal tract and causes it to accumulate
in the periportal area.

Immunohistochemical Characterization of Oxytocin Neurons
          The immunohistochemical study of oxytocin producing
cells was recently carried out in man and rat (Zimmerman _et al_ 1975).
In normal rat and rat with diabetes insipidus, oxytocin cells are
concentrated in the dorsal area of the supraoptic nuclei and in the
lateral areas of the paraventricular nuclei. In man they are found
in particular in the median dorso-lateral area of the supraoptic nuclei and in the dorsal area of the paraventricular nuclei. Large i-
solated reactive cells are found between these nuclei; furthermore,
oxytocin and nicotine stimulated neurophysin are present in the infundibular nucleus of man deprived of vasopressin and estrogen stimulated neurophysin.

Immunohistochemical Characterization of Neurophysin I and II Neurons
          Alvarez-Buylla _et al_ (1970-1973) showed axoplasmic
transport of neurophysin in cat by means of purified porcine anti-
neurophysin II rabbit antisera, using immunofluorescence on frozen
sections. Watkins and Evans (1972) used porcine anti-neurophysin II
and ovine anti-neurophysin III antisera (which give cross reactions
with rat neurophysins) to show the presence of neurophysin in the
cytoplasm of neurons in the supraoptic and paraventricular nuclei
of rat. Osmotic stimulation causes concomitant reduction in neurophysin and vasopressin. In the guinea pig, ovine anti-neurophysin
II and bovine anti-neurophysin III antisera revealed a single major
neurophysin in the supraoptic and paraventricular magnocellular e-
lements and their axons (Evans and Watkins 1973). In the monkey
and bullock, Zimmerman _et al_ (1973) used bovine anti-neurophysin I
rabbit antiserum to reveal neurophysin I in the cells and axons of
the supraoptic and paraventricular nuclei by labeled immunoperoxidase. In the cow, De Mey _et al_ (1974) used bovine anti-neurophysin
I and II rabbit antiserum labeled with peroxidase-antiperoxidase
complex (PAP) to show the presence of two types of neurons, different morphology and topography, producing neurophysin I and neurophysin II respectively; neurophysin I neurons are more numerous in
the paraventricular nuclei, which also contain neurophysin II neurons. The latter are more numerous in the supraoptic nuclei.
          Using bovine anti-prolactine antiserum containing an-
tineurophysin antibody as contaminant (Dubois, 1974), we have recently shown elements of the hypothalamo-neurohypophyseal neurose-
croty pathway in the squirrel monkey (Barry, 1975, unpublished, fig.
1). At the electron microscope level, immunocytochemistry performed
in the rat showed that neurophysin was localized in the secretory

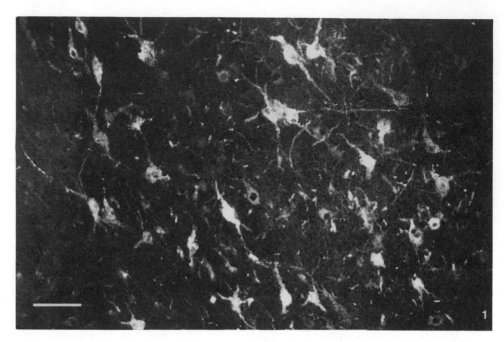

Fig. 1- Immunoreactive neurons of the paraventricular nucleus of
Cebus apella. Antiserum against neurophysin. White bar: 50 microns.

granules of the neurons of supraoptic and paraventricular nuclei, in
axons of the internal zone of the median eminence and the nerve endings of the posterior pituitary (Pelletier *et al.*, 1974c).

IMMUNOREACTIVE "CRF-NEUROPHYSIN" NEURONS

Although decisive results were not obtained by work on
the isolation and purification of "CRF) ("Corticotropin Releasing
Factor": see Schally and Bowers, 1964; Schally *et al* 1968; Burgus
and Guillemin 1970), certain observations have shown the presence of
a "neurophysin-like" substance in the external infundibular area in
monkey (Zimmerman *et al* 1973), rat (Watkins *et al* 1974 ; Vandersande
et al 1974) and cat and dog (Watkins 1975). Adrenalectomy causes
great increase in this substance in rat (Watkins *et al* 1974; Vandesande *et al* 1974) and the appearance of immunoreactive perikaryons
in the suprachiasmatic nuclei (Vandesande *et al* 1974). These facts
suggest that the suprachiasmatic neurons in question may produce a
"CRF neurophysin" type substance. Vasopressin cells were also detected in the suprachiasmatic nuclei (Vandesande *et al* 1975b).

IMMUNOREACTIVE LRF NEURONS

After demonstration of the stimulating action of hypo-

thalamic extracts on prehypophyseal LH secretion (McCann *et al* 1960;
Harris 1960), establishment of the chemical formula of LRF (or LH-RH)
by Matsuo *et al*(1971), Schally *et al* (1971) and Sievertsson *et al*
(1971) and its synthesis, specific immune sera could be prepared. The
use of these antisera since the end of 1972 has made possible the
direct histological study of LRF producing hypothalamic structures
by immunofluorescence or cytoenzymology.

Immunoreactive segments of LRF axons have been easily
characterized in the infundibulum and, eventually, the hypothalamus
of all species studied (Leonardelli *et al* 1973, Mazzuca and Dubois
1973 in guinea pig; Barry and Dubois 1973b and Baker *et al* 1974 in
guinea pig, rat and mouse; Kordon *et al* 1973, Pelletier *et al* 1974a,
King *et al* 1974, Setalo *et al* 1975 and Naik 1975 in rat; Zimmerman
et al 1974 in mouse; Dubois 1973 in ram, bull and pig; De Reviers
and Dubois 1973 in cock; Calas *et al* 197 in duck; Doerr-Schott and
Dubois 1975 in toad).

Only a few investigators, on the contrary, succeeded in
characterizing the perikaryons of LRF neurons in a limited number of
species: guinea pig (Barry *et al* 1973a), mouse (Zimmerman *et al* 1974),
rat (Naik 1975) and toad (Doerr-Schott and Dubois 1975). These works
have been criticized by teams who obtained negative results with
their own material, generally rat (Kordon *et al* 1974, Setalo *et al*
1975). In order to provide fresh data on this subject, we made systematic examination of various species of Mammals (rabbit, cats,
dogs, Korean squirrels) and, more recently, about thirty monkeys of
various species (*Cynomologus, Cynocephalus, Cercopithecus, Papio,
Macacus, Saïmiri* and *Cebus*). We also strictly verified specificity,
completing control by the use of antiserum against unconjugated synthetic LRF (kindly donated by Professor A. Arimura). This antiserum
does not give cross reactions with 17 sunthetic peptides represent-
ing portions of LRF (personal communication by Professeur Arimura),
and may therefore be considered specific or hormonal decapeptide.
All results obtained in guinea-pig, rat and dog were verified with
this antiserum, which were used afterwards in the squirrel monkey
and *Cebus apella* in particular. A report follows of the main results
obtained in all animals were studied personally (totalling several
hundred).

Number and Morphology of Immunoreactive LRF Perikaryons

The total number of immunoreactive perikaryons of LRF
neurons is small, particularly in adult animals of both sexes in most
species and under most physiological or experimental conditions. Perikaryons may therefore escape notice if examinations do not include
systematic examination of seriate sections. For this reason, perikaryons of LRF neurons were first detected (Barry *et al* 1973a) in castrated male guinea-pigs given injections of colchicin in the cerebral
ventricle. Colchicine provides proximal accumulation of immunoreactive
material, probably by inhibiting axonic evacuation and axoplasmic
transport.

There are generally 5 to 15 reactive perikaryons per
hypothalamus in normal adult male guinea pigs (Barry *et al* 1974d),

while the cyclic female generally has none; a few may be found, on
the contrary, at the end of gestation (Barry and Dubois 1974 b).
Perikaryons are more numerous (a few dozen per hypothalamus) in
guinea pig fetus during the last weeks of gestation (Barry and
Dubois 1974 a). A considerable number of reactive perikaryons may
be found in some prepubertal guinea pigs (several hundred per hypothalamus : Barry and Dubois 1974 e). The same applies to male and
female dogs aged 2 to 4 months (Barry and Dubois 1975 b). A small
number of reactive perikaryons are found in the prepubertal female
cat (Barry and Dubois 1975 b) and in various normal adult monkeys
male or female (Barry *et al* 1975 a, particularly *Macacus* and
Cercopithecus ; Barry and Carette 1975 c, *Saïmiri*). The number of
reactive perikaryons may be higher in certain cases, exceeding one
hundred (Barry and Carette 1975 e, *Cebus apella*).

　　　The number of reactive perikaryons may be greatly increased in guinea pigs (up to as many as several hundrer per hypothalamus) by the association of castration and intraventricular injection of colchicin (Barry *et al* 1973 a) or methanol + melatonin
(Barry *et al* 1974 d) and injection of serotonin (Leonardelli *et al*
1974). The use of dopamine and noradrenaline depletors, on the contrary, only increases the perikaryons moderately (approximately 10
to 50 according to animals) (Leonardelli and Dubois 1974 b and c).

　　　Cerebral intraventricular injection of serotonin in the
squirrel monkey and *Cebus apella* causes considerable increase in the
number of reactive perikaryons (up to as many as several hundrer per
hypothalamus : Barry and Carette 1975 c).

　　　Morphology of immunoreactive perikaryons is comparable
in all the species we studied. However, the quantity of reactive material in any one species varies considerably according to the cells
(Barry and Dubois 1974 e), which is quite normal for neurosecretory
cells (Figs 2-6). The shape of the perikaryons varies according to
the incidence of the sections in:guinea pig, cat and dog their di-
mensions are generally 10 to 20 microns ; they can attain about 40
microns in the monkey, with a nucleus of 10 to 14 microns in diameter. The nucleus generally stands out very well against the more or
less brilliant background of the cytoplasm which usually appears to
be finely granular ; this is less distinct in the monkey, and roun-
ded fluorescent droplet-shaped inclusions may be seen. Dendrites
seem very few (2 to 4 average), with few or no ramifications. They
are rarely visible in the guinea pig (except after castration and
methanol + melatonin : Barry *et al* 1974 d), but are easier to observe in the monkey (Figs 2,3,4). Under certain favorable conditions
the root of the axon may be seen, either in the perikaryon or at
the base of a dendrite. They are few images of this kind, as reactive material rarely accumulates in the proximal segment of the axon.

　　　Reactive perikaryons are generally dispersed, but they
may be in groups of 4 or 5, rarely more, or exceptionally in "shoals"
in the middle of axon pathways.

Comparative Topography of Immunoreactive Perikaryons
　　　Reactive perikaryons have characteristic topography in

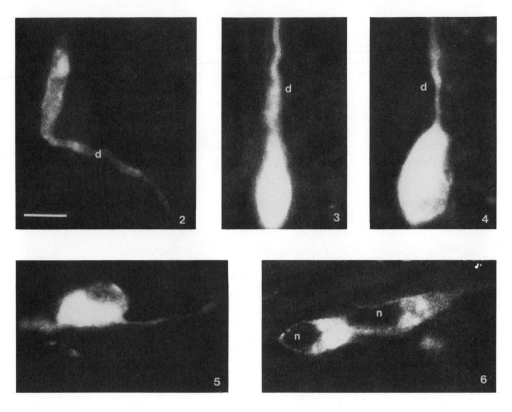

Figs 2-6 -Reactive perikarya of LRF neurons in the premamillary (2)
infundibular (3,4), lamina terminalis (5) and retro chiasmatic a-
reas (6) of the squirrel monkey. d : dendrites ; n : nucleus.
White bar : 10 microns.

all animals of the same species, although it varies according to
the species, sometimes within the same order.

Perikaryons have typical rostral localization in gui-
nea pig (Barry *et al* 1973 a) and cat (Barry and Dubois 1974 a), particularly in the septo-preoptic and anterior hypothalamic areas.
They concentrate electively in the precommissural, supraoptic and
parolfactive areas in guinea pig. Dispersed cells (becoming rarer
in the caudal direction) are found in the retrochiasmatic and tube-
ropremamillary areas.

Reactive perikaryons have a very wide dispersal area
in dog (Barry and Dubois 1974 e) from the parolfactive to the rostral mesencephalic areas. They concentrate electively in the precommissural, supraoptic, infundibular and premamillary areas. Unlike
the guinea pig, a considerable proportion of reactive perikaryons
(about 40 %) is found in the infundibular and premamillary areas.

A few dispersed perikaryons are present in the ventromedian, dorso-
median, posterior hypothalamic and rostral mesencephalic areas.

In *Macacus* and *Cercopithecus* (Barry *et al* 1975 a) most
immunoreactive perikaryons are electively localized in the mediobasal hypothalamic area, accessorily in the anterior and ventromedian hypothalamic areas.

In squirrel monkeys and *Cebus apella* (Fig 7) (Barry
and Carette 1975 c) reactive perikaryons are mainly localized in
the mediobasal area of the hypothalamus (retrochiasmatic area ;
infundibular nucleus, premamillary nucleus) and in the lamina
terminalis.

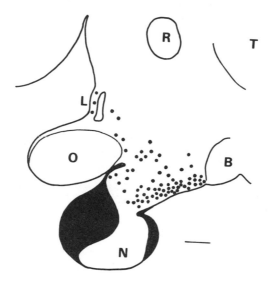

Fig 7- Topographic distribution of reactive perikarya of LRF neurons (black dots) in *Cebus apella* brain, projected on mid-sagittal
plane. B: mamillary body ; L: lamina terminalis ; N: neural lobe
O: optic chiasm; R: rostral commissure ; T: thalamus ; Black bar
: 1 millimeter.

A few isolated cells are found in the anterior hypothalamic and
septopreoptic areas ; unlike the guinea pig and dog, there are
generally few of them.

Some considered the preferential rostral localisation
of reactive LRF perikaryons in the guinea pig (Barry *et al* 1973 a)
incompatible with the idea of "hypophysiotropic area" (Halasz *et al*
1962), the effects of surgical disconnection of the mediobasal hypothalamus in Rodents (Halasz and Gorski 1967) and the persistence of
infundibular immunoreactive material after stereotaxic lesions in
the guinea pig (Barry *et al* 1973 a). However, as we already reported in 1973, a few immunoreactive perikaryons may be found in the

tuber and even in the premamillary area in the guinea pig (Barry
et al 1973 a) ; moreover, administration of metaraminol bitartrate
(monoamine depletor) increases the number of reactive neurons in
this area (Leonardelli and Dubois 1974 c). This increase, however,
is moderate (20 to 50 cells) and represents only a small percentage
of the immunoreactive population that may be demonstrated by other
experimental treatments.

   Results obtained with the dog provide, in fact, the
true response, and for the first time give an almost complete view
of the LRF reactive neuron system. The fact that this system com-
prises two relatively well separated populations, one septopreoptic
and anterior hypothalamic and the other tuberoinfundibular and premamillary, concords quite well with data suggesting double control
(cyclic and tonic) of gonadotropin secretion (Barraclough 1966).
This hypothesis appears to be corroborated by the fact that the topography of LRF reactive neurons in guinea pig, cat and dog is different from that of Primates ; various authors, moreover, have shown
that control of gonadotropin secretion appears distinctly different
in Rodents (Halasz and Gorski 1967) and Monkeys (Karsch et al 1973,
Knobil 1974, Krey et al 1975).

   Zimmermann et al 1974 described reactive neurons in
the infundibular nucleus of the mouse with the aid of immune serum
prepared by Doctor G. Niswender and antiserum labeled with peroxy-
dase, but the specificity of these results was criticized by Setalo
et al 1975. More recently, Naik (1975) also described reactive neurons in the medial and prechiasmatic preoptic hypothalamus in rat
and mouse, as well as in the ventromedian, arcuate and premamillary
nuclei. Lastly, Doerr-Schott and Dubois (1975) found reactive neurons round telencephalic ventricles in various lower Vertebrates
(Xenopus, Triturus, Bufo). We know the latter work in detail, and
it seem very demonstrative. As for the others, we do not have sufficient information about them to make a motivated judgment. Personally we found no immunoreactive neurons in the rat, after examining more than 100 animals killed under various physiological or
experimental circumstances. These results have been confirmed in
this species by various other investigators (Kordon et al 1974 ;
King et al 1974 ; Setalo et al 1975). We likewise found no reactive
neurons in mouse (except one in the precommissural area) after examining the hypothalamus of several dozen animals. However, as we
said before, negative results must always be considered with prudence and should not lead to negation as a matter of course.

Hypothalamo-Infundibular LRF Tract

   Most axons of LRF neurons form part of the hypothalamo-infundibular tract which terminates round the capillaries of the
primary portal plexus. This tract has the same general characteristics in all Mammals we examined, with anterior, lateral and posterior contingents (Fig. 8). The posterior contingent is generally
the most evident owing to the considerable accumulation of reactive
material in this area ; the anterior contingent, on the contrary,

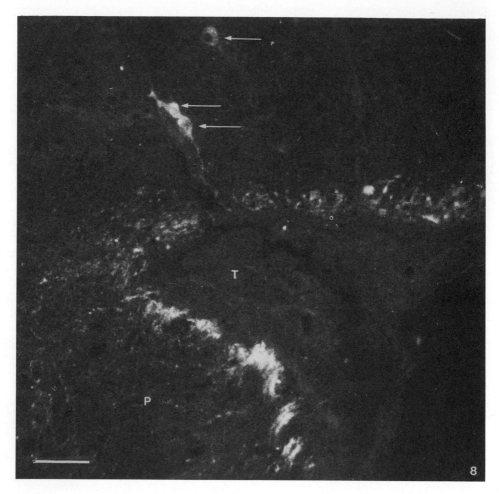

Fig 8-Posterior contingent of the hypothalamo-infundibular LRF tract in *Cebus apella*. P: posterior labium of median eminence ; T: pars tuberalis. The white arrows point to three reactive perikaryons of LRF neurons. Same orientation as fig 7. White bar : 50 microns.

greatly varies in load and has longer radiate terminal collaterals, particularly in guinea pig, rat, mouse and dog. It is difficult to link up the axons of the posterior contingent to the neurons from which they arise in guinea pig and cat, while there is a well indi-visualized "tubero-infundibular" component in the dog. During their passage through the infundibulum, reactive LRF axons follow the external boundary of the fibrillary area ; they emit numerous radiate collaterals which cross the external infundibular area and generally terminate round the capillaries of the intercalary plexus. These collaterals pass the long intrainfundibular loops at a distance in the guinea pig, while they more or less surround some long loops in the monkey.

In the guinea pig, cat and dog (Barry and Dubois 1974 e) and monkey (Barry and Carette 1975 c) some reactive axons cross the entire infundibulum and hypophyseal stem, then penetrate the periphery of the hilum and neural lobe ; they also seem to terminate round the most distal capillaries of the portal system, sometimes even round the capillaries of the neural lobe.

Loading of reactive material begins during the 7th week in guinea pig fetus, in the posterior component of the hypothalamo-infundibular tract ; it later extends to the ventral labium and becomes very important a few days before birth, decreasing abruptly after birth and rising again towards the 10th to 12th day (Barry and Dubois 1974 d). These modifications appear to agree with perinatal variations in plasma LH levels observed mainly in males by Donovan *et al* (1974). Moderate variations are observed later, with important load towards the 6th week and the beginning of the prepubertal period (Barry and Dubois 1974 d).

Moderate variations may be observed in the load of reactive material in the hypothalamo-infundibular tract during guinea pig gestation, with progressive increase towards time of birth, then abrupt fall in level during the hours following the dropping of young (Barry and Dubois 1974 b). During the oestrus cycle in the guinea pig there is important load at the end of the diestrus, with abrupt fall in level during the proestrus ; load is at a minimum during the pre- or peri-ovulatory period, followed by a slight rise during the post-estrus, then progressive increase in load during the diestrus (Barry and Dubois 1974 c). These modifications completely agree with plasma LH variations in the cyclic female guinea pig (Croix *et al* 1975).

Castration of male guinea pig does not greatly modify the load of immunoreactive material, at least during the first weeks   (Barry *et al* 1974). In the long run, neurodepressors (haloperidol, fluphenazine aenanthate), delayed- action testosterone and cyproterone acetate seem to decrease the quantity of infundibular immunoreactive material more or less distinctly (Barry 1974, unpublished). Like modifications in the number of reactive perikaryons under various physiological or experimental conditions, mainly in the guinea pig, the above modifications confirm the fact that the specifically reactive axons and neurons we have described are indeed the elements responsible for synthesis, transport and release of LRF.

Preoptico-Terminal LRF Tract

Reactive axon terminals are observed, sometimes in great numbers, in the area of the supraoptic crest in the guinea

pig (Barry _et al_ 1973 a ; Barry _et al_ 1974 d). These terminals are
not very numerous in cat and dog. In rat and mouse, numerous reactive axons terminate in the vascular organ of the lamina terminalis
(Barry _et al_ 1973 a). Similar aspects were later discerned in the
latter two species by various authors (Kordon _et al_ 1974 ; Zimmermann
_et al_ 1974 ; King _et al_ 1974, Naik 1975). These reactive axons probably correspond partly to certain type II nerve fibres (peptider-
gic ?) discerned by electron microscope by Le Beux (1971, 1972) and
Le Beux _et al_ (1972) in the "medial vascular prechiasmatic gland"
in rat.

In _Cebus apella_ and squirrel monkeys (Barry and Carette
1975c) immunoreactive perikaryons are found in the vascular organ
of the lamina terminalis, sometimes in very large numbers (particularly in the squirrel monkey). These perikaryons give rise to axons
forming an important "preoptico-terminal tract" (Fig 9), most terminals of which are arranged round the capillaries of the primary
plexus of the vascular organ of the lamina terminalis. These nerve
terminals are exactly like the arrangement of pericapillary radiate
collaterals of the infundibulum. A few less numerous axons terminate
either round the subependymal capillaries or between the differen-
tiated ependymal cells of the vascular organ of the lamina terminalis. The latter may be similar elements to those described by Weindl
and Schinko (1974) in the vascular organ of the lamina terminalis of
the hamster by electron microscope. The presence of reactive neurons
or axons in the lamina terminalis sets a certain number of problems
particularly in rat,mouse and squirrel monkey.
Morphological appearances plead in favour of preferential hemocrin
LRF secretion and the constitution of "neuroendocrin cell complexes"
similar to those described by Oksche _et al_ (1974) in the infundibulum. The ependymocytes of the vascular organ in the lamina terminalis may also take part in various processes in the same way as infundibular tanicytes (Knowles 1972, Scott _et al_ 1974, Vaala and
Knigge 1974). Whatever the answer may be, the preoptico-terminal LRF
tract seems likely to be instrumental in the control of sexual functions or behavior in some species.

Immunoreactive Extra-Hypophyseal LRF Pathways
In all species we studied (Barry _et al_ 1973 a ; Barry
_et al_ 1974 d ; Barry and Dubois 1975 a ; Barry and Carette 1975 c)
we found that a certain number of reactive axons are distributed in
various areas of the brain : epithalamus (particularly the median
habenular ganglion in squirrel monkey) ; subfornical organ ; amyg-
dalum ; mediobasal rhinencephalon ; mesencephalon. It is difficult
to study these axons and their terminals because they are very few
and only immunoreactive segments are visible. The most important of
these reactive pathways appears to terminate in the cortico-amygda-
lian nucleus, the habenular ganglion and the reticular formation of
the mesencephalon. These pathways resemble those we described more
than twenty years ago (Barry 1954) for various axons issuing from
magnocellular neurons of the SON and PVN, study of which has recently

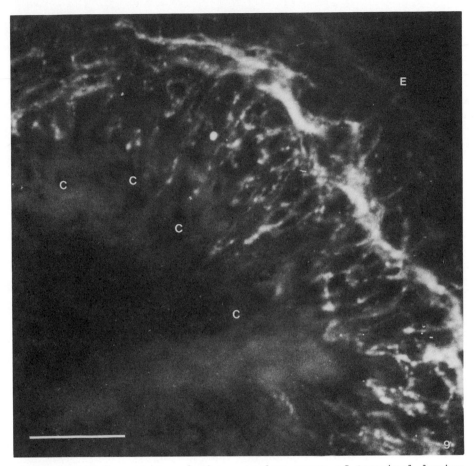

Fig 9-Sagittal section of the vascular organ of terminal lamina in the squirrel monkey. Reactive LRF axons with radiating collaterals ending round the capillaries of the primary plexus. C: capillaries of the subglial layer ; E: ependymal cell lining the ventricular surface of the terminal lamina. Same orientation as fig 7 White bar : 50 microns.

been resumed by Sterba (1974). Various observations (ref in Barry _et al_ 1973 a, 1974 d, Barry and Dubois 1974 b, Barry and Carette 1975 c) suggest that in certain cases these pathways may be instrumental in behavioral processes, retroactive circuits or mechanisms of neuroendocrin integration.

Neurosecretory LRF Synapses

Some axons of the hypothalamo-infundibular tract show images of division and emission of short collaterals along their course (particularly in the anterior hypothalamic area, the supra-

-chiasmatic nucleus and the premamillary region : Barry *et al* 1973 a
Barry and Dubois 1973 b ; Barry *et al* 1974 d). Similar images or
arrangement in "pericellular baskets" may also be seen at the extre-
mity of some "extrahypophyseal LRF pathways". These images recall
the "neurosecretory synapses" we described (Barry 1954) along the
extrahypophyseal pathways issuing from the SON and PVN or in their
terminals ; the existence of these synapses was confirmed in a very
large quantity of material by Sterba (1974)

   The existence of LRF "neurosecretory synapses" suggests
that this hormone is able to behave like a true "neuromodulator" or
"neurotransmitter", in addition to its major prehypophysiotropic action. The results of recent research with microiontophoretic injection of LRF (Moss and McCann 1973, Dyer and Dyball 1974, Kawakami
and Sakuma 1974, Moss *et al* 1975, Renaud *et al* 1975, McCann and
Moss 1975) concord perfectly with this hypothesis.

IMMUNOREACTIVE SOMATOSTATIN NEURONS

   After discovery of a substance inhibiting the secretion of growth hormone in hypothalamic extracts (Krulich *et al* 1967,
SRIF : "Somathormone Release Inhibiting Factor" ; GIF : "Growth Hormone Inhibiting Factor" or Somatostatin) establishment of its chemical formula by Vale *et al* (1972) and its synthesis, specific immune
sera could be prepared.

   Antisomatostatin antibodies enabled localization of the
corresponding hormone in the palisade layer of the median eminence
in various Mammals (bullock, sheep, pig, rat), cock, water salaman-
der and trout, with reactive fibres that may penetrate the pars
tuberalis in the bull and the part distalis in the trout (Pelletier
et al 1974b, 1975; Dubois *et al* 1974, Dubois and Barry 1974). Reactive somatostatine fibres have a different infundibular topography
from that of LRF and "major" neurophysin fibres, and images of SRIF
hydrencephalocrinia may be found in sheep (Dubois *et al* 1974; Dubois
and Barry 1974). A differential hypothalamic distribution of LRF
and somatostatin axons was also found by Alpert *et al* (1975). Hökfelt *et al* (1974) have shown reactive hypothalamic fibres in the
guinea pig, mainly localized in the external infundibular area of
the caudal region of the median eminence. These authors also noted
numerous reactive fibres in the ventromedian nucleus, forming synap-
tic-type systems. At the electron microscope level, Pelletier *et al*
(1974b) have clearly demonstrated that somatostatin is contained in
the secretory granules (about 900A° to 1100 A° in diameter) of many
nerve endings of the external zone of the rat median eminence. I
have recently studies SRIF axons in the dog (Fig. 10) and in *Cebus
apella*(Figs 11, 12). In these two species those axons have a specific topography different from that of LRF and neurophysin axons.

   More recently, Dubois and Kolodziejczyk (1975 a and b)
were able to individualize two reactive cell type in rat:
1- large somatostatin and neurophysin positive cells in the supraoptic and paraventricular nuclei, whose axons are incorporated in
the hypothalamo-infundibular and hypothalamo-pituitary tract. The

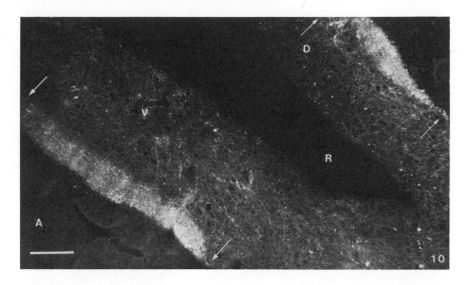

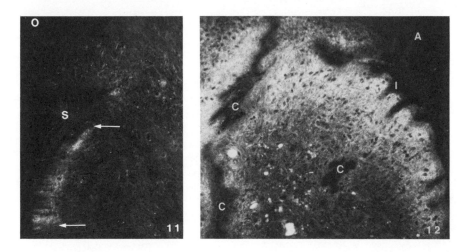

Fig 10- Sagittal section of median eminence in the dog. A: adenohypophysis ; D: dorsal labium of median eminence ; R: infundibular recess ; V: ventral labium of median eminence. White arrows : limit
of the zones of ending of somatostatin axons.

Fig 11, 12 _ Sagittal section of the anterior (11) and posterior part
(12) of median eminence in *Cebus apella*.Zones of ending of somatostatin axons (white arrows, on fig 11). A: adenohypophysis ; C: capillary loops ; I: intercalar plexus ; O: optic chiasm ; S: sulcus
infundibularis.
Same magnification (white bar : 50 microns) ; same orientation as
fig 7.

somatostatin present in these neurons and their extensions may be
associated with neurophysin III;
2- small neurophysin negative cells partly localized around the supraoptic recess, whose axons in the median eminence are distributed
in the palissade layer of the external infundibular area. Although
the problems of extra-nervous localization of hypothalamic hormones
(it might perhaps be better to say "hormones first individualized in
the hypothalamic area") do not explicitly come within the terms of
our subject, we would like to point out in conclusion that reactive
somatostatin cells have been found in the endocrine pancreas, duode-
num, pylorum (Dubois 1975) and stomach, as well as SRIF positive
nerve fibres in rat intestine (Hökfelt *et al* 1975).

CONCLUSIONS

        Recent progress recorded in the field of immunohisto-
chemical characterization of hypothalamic hormones is a striking
confirmation of the concepts of "neurosecretion" and "diencephalic
gland" illustrated by E. Scharrer (for references, see E. and B.
Scharrer 1954), and the works of physiologists, endocrinologists
and biochemists that have gradually extended the theory of central
nervous control of the hypophysis to its present form.
        The differential topography of neurons and prehypophy-
siotropic fibres is coming to light progressively, furnishing neuro
histological information for the first time in a field that was almost unknown a few years ago. Although to our knowledge the use of
anti-TRF antisera ("Thyrotropin Releasing Factor") and anti GH-RH
("Growth Hormone Releasing Hormone") has not yet supplied positive
histological documents, an abundant harvest of new results will
assuredly be gathered in the years to come.

Acknowledgments : I would like to thank Doctor Dubois (INRA-CNRZ
Nouzilly) for the kind donation of anti LH-RF and anti SRIF antisera conjugated with HSA, and Professor A. Arimura (Tulasne University, LA) for synthetic anti LRF antisera conjugated or unconjugated with HSA.
This work was supported by the D.G.R.S.T. (Contract n° 74-7-0518)
the I.N.S.E.R.M. and the Fondation pour la Recherche Médicale
Française.

REFERENCES

Acher, R. and Chauvet, J. (1954) Biochem. Biophys. Acta 14, 421–429

Acher, R. and Fromageot, Cl. (1955) Ergeb. d. Physiol. Biol. Chem. u. Exp. Pharmacol. 48, 286–327.

Acher, R., Manoussos, G. and Olivry, G. (1955) Biochem. Biophys. Acta (Amst.) 16, 155–156.

Adams, C.W.M. and Sloper, J.C. (1955) Lancet 268, 651–652.

Adams, C.W.M. and Sloper, J.C. (1956) J. Endocr. (London) 13, 221–228.

Alpert, C.C., Brawer, J.R., Jackson, I.M.D. and Patel, Y. (1975) Fed. Proc. 34, 239 (abstr. 114)

Alvarez-Buylla, R., Livett, B.G., Uttenhall, L.O., Milton, S.H. and Hope, D.B. (1970) Acta Physiol. Scand. Suppl. 357, 5.

Alvarez-Buylla, R., Livett, B.G., Uttenhall, L.O., Hope, D.B. and Milton, S.H. (1973) Z. Zellforsch. 137, 435–450.

Baker, B.L., Dermody, W.C. and Reel, J.R. (1974) Amer. J. Anat. 58, 129–134.

Bargmann, W. (1949) Z. Zellforsch. 34, 610–634.

Barraclough, C.A. (1966) Recent Progr. Hormone Res. 22, 503–536.

Barrnett, R.J. and Seligman, A.A. (1952) Science 116, 323–327.

Barry, J. (1954) Arch. Anat. Micr. Morph. Exp. 43, 310–320.

Barry, J., Dubois, M.P. and Poulain, P. (1973a) Z. Zellforsch. 146 351–366.

Barry, J. and Dubois, M.P. (1973b) Ann. Endocr. 34, 735–742.

Barry, J. and Dubois, M.P. (1974a) Brain Res. 67, 103–113.

Barry, J. and Dubois, M.P. (1974b) In: Neurosecretion - The final neuroendocrine pathway (F. Knowles and L. Vollrath, eds) Springer-Verlag, Berlin, Heidelberg, New York, pp. 148–153.

Barry, J. and Dubois, M.P. (1974c) Neuroendocrinology 15, 200–208.

Barry, J., Dubois, M.P. and Carette, B. (1974 d) Endocrinology 95, 1416–1423.

Barry, J. and Dubois, M.P. (1974 e) Arch. Anat. Micr. Morph. Exp. 63, 363-374.

Barry, J., Girod, Chr. and Dubois, M.P. (1975a) Bull. Ass. Anat. 59, 103-110.

Barry, J. and Dubois, M.P. (1975 b) Neuroendocrinology "in press".

Barry, J. and Carette, B. (1975 c) Cell Tissue Res. "submitted for publication".

Brazeau, P., Vale, W., Burgus, R., Ling, N., Butcher, M., Rivier, J. and Guillemin, R. (1973) Science 179, 77-79.

Burford, G.D., Ginsburg, M. and Thomas, P.J. (1971) Biochem. Biophys. Acta (Amst.) 229, 730-738.

Burgus, R. and Guillemin, R. (1970) Ann. Rev. Biochem. 39, 499-526.

Burlet, A., Marchetti, J. and Duheille , J. (1972) ⊤ille Med. 17, 1415 (abstr.).

Burlet, A., Marchetti, J. and Duheille, J. (1973) C.R. Soc. Biol. (Paris) 167, 924-927.

Burlet, A., Marchetti, J. and Duheille, J. (1974) In : Neurosecretion - The final neuroendocrine pathway (F. Knowles and L. Vollrath eds) Springer-Verlag, Berlin, Heidelberg, New York, pp. 24-30.

Calas, A., Kerdelhué, B., Assenmacher, I. and Jutisz, M. (1974) C.R. Acad. Sci. (Paris) 278, 2557-2560.

Cheng, K.W. and Friesen, H.G. (1972) J. Clin. Endocr. 34, 165-176.

Coy, D.H. and Wuu, T.C. (1971) Analyt. Biochem. 44, 174-181.

Croix, D. and Franchimont, P. (1975) Neuroendocrinology "in press".

Dean, C.R. and Hope, D.B. (1966) Biochem. J. 101, 17-18.

Dean, C.R. and Hope, D.B. (1967) Biochem. J. 104, 1082-1088.

Dean, C.R., Hope, D.B. and Kazic, T. (1968) Brit. J. Pharmac. 34, 192.

De Mey, J., Vandesande, F. and Dierickx, K. (1974) Z. Zellforsch. 153, 531-544.

De Riviers, M. and Dubois, M.P. (1974) Horm. Metab. Res. 6, 494.

Doerr-Schott, J. and Dubois, M.P. (1975) C.R. Acad. Sci. (Paris) 180, 285-289.

Donovan, B.T., ter Haar, M.B. and Peddie, M.J. (1974) In: Sexual endocrinology of the perinatal period (M.G. Forest and J. Bertrand eds) INSERM, Paris, pp. 161-176.

Dubois, M.P. (1973) J. Reprod. Fertil. 35, 595 (abstr.).

Dubois, M.P. (1975) Proc. Natl. Acad. Sci. (USA) 72, 1340-1343.

Dubois, M.P. and Barry, J. (1974) Ann. Endocrinol. (Paris) 35, 663-664.

Dubois, M.P., Barry, J. and Leonardelli, J. (1974) C.R. Acad. Sci. (Paris) 279, 1899-1902.

Dubois, M.P. and Kolodziejczyk, E. (1975 a) C.R. Acad. Sci. (Paris) "in press).

Dubois, M.P. and Kolodziejczyk, E. (1975 b) International Symp. Hypothalamus and endocrine functions (abstract) Quebec 21-24 sept.

Dyer, R.G. and Dyball, R.E.J. (1974) Nature 252, 486-488.

Evans, J.J. and Watkins, W.B. (1973) Z. Zellforsch. 145, 39-55.

Ginsburg, M. and Ireland, M. (1963) J. Physiol. (Lond.) 169, 114-115.

Ginsburg, M. and Ireland, M. (1966) J. Endocr. 35, 289-290.

Gomori, G. (1941) Amer. J. Path 17, 395-406.

Halasz, B. and Gorski, R.A. (1967) Endocrinology 80, 608-622.

Halasz, B., Pupp, L. and Uhlarik, S. (1962) J. Endocr. (London) 25, 147-154.

Harris, G.W. (1960) In: Control of Ovulation (C.A. Villée, ed.) Pergamon Press, New York, p. 56.

Hökfelt, T., Efendic, S., Johansson, O., Luft, R. and Arimura, A. (1974) Brain Res. 80, 165-169.

Hökfelt, T., Johansson, O., Efendic, S., Luft, R. and Arimura, A. (1975) Experientia 31, 853-854.

Karsch, F.J., Dierschke, D.J. and Knobil, E. (1973) Science 179, 484-486.

Kawakami, M. and Sakuma, Y. (1974) Neuroendocrinology 15, 290-307.

King, J.C., Parson, J.A., Erlandsen, S.L. and Williams, T.H. (1974) Cell Tissue Res. 153, 211-218.

Knobil, E. (1974) Recent Progr. Hormone Res. 30, 1-46.

Knowles, F. (1972) In: Topics in neuroendocrinology. Progr. Brain Res. (J. Ariens Kappers and P. Schadé, eds), vol. 38, Elsevier Publ., Amsterdam, pp. 225-270.

Kordon, C., Kerdelhué, B., Pattou, E. and Jutisz, M. (1974) Proc. Soc. Exp. Biol. Med. 147, 122-127.

Krey, L.C., Butler, W.R. and Knobil, E. (1975) Endocrinology 96, 1073-10°7.

Krulich, L., Lackey, L. and Dhariwal, A.P.S. (1967) Fed. Proc. 26, 316.

Le Beux, Y.J. (1971) Z. Zellforsch. 114, 404-440.

Le Beux, Y.J., Langelier, P. and Poirier, L.J. (1971) Z. Zellforsch. 118, 147-155.

Le Beux, Y.J. (1972) ⁊. Zellforsch. 127, 439-461.

Leonardelli, J., Barry, J. and Dubois, M.P. (1973) C.R. Acad. Sci. (Paris) 276, 2043-2046.

Leonardelli, J., Dubois, M.P. and Poulain, P. (1974a) Neuroendocrinology 15, 69-72.

Leonardelli, J. and Dubois, M.P. (1974b) Ann. Endocr. (Paris) 35, 639-645.

Leonardelli, J. and Dubois, M.P. (1974c) ᴿull. Ass. Anat. 58, 599-609.

Matsuo, H., Baba, Y., Nair, R.M.G., Arimura, A. and Schally, A.V. (1971) Biochem. Biophys. Res Commun. 43, 1334-1339.

Mazzuca, M. and Dubois, M.P. (1974) J. Histochem. Cytochem. 22, 993-996.

McCann, S.M., Taleisnik, S. and Friedmann, H.M. (1960) Proc. Soc. Exp. Biol. ᴹed. 104, 431-434.

McCann, S.M. and Moss, R.L. (1975) Life Sci. 16, 833-852.

Moss, R.L. and McCann, S.M. (1973) Science 181, 177.

Moss, R.L., Kelly, A. and Dudley, C. (1975) Fed. Proc. 34, 219 (abstré 5).

Naik, D.V. (1975) Cell Tissue Res. 157, 423-434.

Norström, A. (1974) In: Neurosecretion - The final neuroendocrine pathway (F. Knowles and L. Vollrath, eds) Springer-Verlag, Berlin, Heidelberg, New York, pp. 86-93.

Pease, D.C. (1962) Anat. Rec. 142, 342.

Pelletier, G., Labrie, F., Puviani, R., Arimura, A. and Schally, A. V. (1974a) Endocrinology 95, 314-317.

Pelletier, G., Labrie, F., Puviani, R., Arimura, A. and Schally, A. V. (1974b) J. Anat. 140, 445-450.

Pelletier, G., Leclerc, R., Labrie, F. and Puviani, R. (1974c) Mol. Cell. Endocrinol. 1, 157-166.

Pelletier, G., Leclerc, R., Dubé, D., Labrie, F., Puviani, R., Arimura, A. and Schally, A.V. (1973) Am. J. Anat. 142, 297-301.

Pickering, B.T., Jones, C.W. and Burford, G.D. (1974) In: Neurosecretion - The final neuroendocrine pathway (F. Knowles and L. Vollrath, eds) Springer-Verlag, Berlin, Heidelberg, New York, pp. 72-85.

Rauch, R., Hollenberg, M.D. and Hope, D.B. (1969) Biochem. J. 115, 473-479.

Renard, L.P., Martin, J.B. and Brazeau, P. (1975) Nature 255, 233-235.

Schally, A.V. and Bowers, C.Y. (1964) Metabolism 13, 1190-1205.

Schally, A.V., Arimura, A., Bowers, C.Y., Kastin, A.J., Sawano, S. and Reeding, T.W. (1968) Recent Prog. Hormone Res. 24, 497-581.

Schally, A.V., Arimura, A., Kastin, A.J., Baha, N., Reeding, T.W., Nair, R.M.G. and Debeljuk, L. (1971) Science 173, 1036-1037.

Scharrer, E. and Scharrer, B. (1954) In: BdVI/5 Handbuch der mikroskopischen Anatomie des Menschen (W. Bargmann, ed.) Springer-Verlag, Berlin, Göttingen, Heidelberg.

Scharrer, E. and Scharrer, B. (1963) In: Neuroendocrinology Columbia Univ. Press., New York, London, 289 p.

Scott, D.E., Dudley, K., Knigge, K.M. and Koslowski, G.P. (1974) Z. Zellforsch. 149, 371-378.

Setalo, G., Vigh, S., Schally, A.V., Arimura, A. and Flerko, B. (1975) Endocrinology 96, 135-142.

Sievertsson, H., Chang, J.K., Currie, B.L., Bogentoft, C., Folkers, K. and Bowers, C.Y. (1971) Fed. Proc. 30, 1193-1195.

Sloper, J.C. (1954) J. Anat. (London) 88, 576-577.

Sterba, G. (1961) Z. Zellforsch. 55, 763-789.

Sterba, G. (1964) Acta Histochem. (Iena) 17, 268-292.

Sterba, G. (1974) In: Neurosecretion - The final neuroendocrine pathway (F. Knowles and L. Vollrath, eds) Springer-Verlag, Berlin, Heidelberg, New York, pp. 38-47.

Sternberger, L.A., Hardy, P.H., Cuculus, J.J. and Meyer, G.H. (1970) J. Histochem. Cytochem. 18, 315-333.

Stoeckard, R., Jansen, H.G. and Kreike, A.J. (1973) Z. Zellforsch. 136, 111-120.

Uttenhall, L.O. and Hope, D.B. (1970) Biochem. J. 116, 899-909.

Vaala, S. and Knigge, K.M. (1974) Endocrinology 15, 147-157.

Vale, M., Brazeau, P., Grant, G., Nussey, A., Burgus, R., Rivier, J., Ling, N. and Guillemin, R. (1972) C.R. Acad. Sci. (Paris) 275, 2913-2915.

Vandesande, F., De Mey, J. and Dierickx, K. (1974) Z. Zellforsch. 151, 187-200.

Vandesande, F., Dierickx, K. and De Mey, J. (1975a) Cell Tissue Res. 156, 189-200.

Vandesande, F., Dierickx, K. and De Mey, J. (1975b) Cell Tissue Res. 156, 377-380.

Vigneaud, V. du, Ressler, J.M., Swan, J.M., Roberts, C.W., Katsoyannis, P.G. and Gordon, S. (1953) J. Amer. Chem. Soc. 75, 4879-4880.

Vigneaud, V. du, Gish, D.T. and Katsoyannis, P.G. (1954) J. Amer. Chem. Soc. 76, 4751-4752.

Watkins, W.B. (1972 a) Biochem. J. 126, 759–760.

Watkins, W.B. and Evans, J.J. (1972) Z. Zellforsch. 131, 149–170.

Watkins, W.B. (1972 b) J. Endocr. 55, 577–589.

Watkins, W.B. (1975) Cell Tissue Res. 155, 201–210.

Watkins, W.B., Schwabedal, P. and Bock, R. (1974) Z. Zellforsch. 153, 411–421.

Weindl, A. and Schinko, I. (1974) In: Neurosecretion – The final neuroendocrine pathway (F. Knowles and L. Vollrath, eds) Springer-Verlag, Berlin, Göttingen, Heidelberg, New York, pp. 327 (abstract).

Zimmerman, E.A., Hsu, K.C., Robinson, A.G., Carmel, P.W., Frantz, A.G. and Tannenbaum, M. (1973) Endocrinology 92, 931–940.

Zimmerman, E.A., Hsu, K.C., Ferin, M. and Kozlowski, G.P. (1974) Endocrinology 95, 1–8.

Zimmerman, E.A., Defendini, R., Sokol, K.W. and Robinson, A.G. (1975) Abstracts 57th Ann. Meet. of the Endocrine Sci. New York, abstr. 95.

Abstracts

ABSTRACTS

1 SPECIFIC PROGESTERONE RECEPTORS IN DMBA-INDUCED MAMMARY TUMORS.
J. Asselin, F. Labrie, P.A. Kelly and J.P. Raynaud. Medical Re-
search Council Group in Molecular Endocrinology, CHUL, Québec,
G1V 4G2, Canada and Centre de Recherches Roussel-UCLAF, Paris,
France.

The growing evidence for a correlation between the hormonal
dependence of neoplastic tissues and the presence of specific
hormone receptors led us to investigate the possible presence
of specific progesterone receptors in dimethyl benzanthracene
(DMBA)-induced mammary tumors in the rat. After homogeneisation
in 3 vol (w/v) of 25 mM Tris-HCl (pH 7.4), 1.5 mM EDTA, 10 mM
thioglycerol and 10% glycerol (buffer A), the 105,000 xg supernatant was used for binding studies with the highly potent synthetic progestin $[^3H]$ R 5020 (17, 21-dimethyl-19-nor-pregna-4,
9-diene-3, 20-dione). Specificity of $[^3H]$ R 5020 binding was
studied by both sucrose gradients and charcoal adsorption. As
evidenced by sucrose gradient analysis, specific binding of $[^3H]$
R 5020 is associated with components migrating at 6-7S and 4-5S.
Unspecific binding of the synthetic progestin at 4S is eliminated by pretreatment with dextran-coated charcoal. $[^3H]$ R 5020
binding is easily displaced by unlabeled R 5020, progesterone,
norgestreal, chlormethindrone and norethindrone. 17β-estradiol,
diethylstilbestrol, testosterone, dihydrotestosterone, dexamethasone and cortisol have little, if any effect on $[^3H]$ R 5020
binding. The potential significance of measurements of the level of progesterone receptors in mammary tumors is indicated
by our recent findings of a marked decrease of the level of this
receptor after ovariectomy, a treatment accompanied by important
regression of the tumors, and by the stimulatory effect of progesterone upon tumor development.

2 CORRELATION BETWEEN LH-RH-STIMULATED PROSTAGLANDIN AND CYCLIC
AMP ACCUMULATION AND LH RELEASE IN ANTERIOR PITUITARY GLAND.
N. Barden, L. Bergeron, A. Bélanger and A. Betteridge. Medical
Research Council Group in Molecular Endocrinology, CHUL, Québec,
G1V 4G2, Canada.

LH-RH increased prostaglandin E concentrations in monolayer
cultures of dispersed anterior pituitary cells. This effect on
PGE levels was apparent after 90 min, reached a maximum after

$2\frac{1}{2}$h, and decreased to basal levels after 4h of incubation. N^6-monobutyryl or 8-bromo-cyclic AMP also increased PGE levels in a manner similar to that of LH-RH. Flufenamic acid or indomethacin prevented completely the LH-RH stimulation of PGE levels. Indomethacin did not inhibit the LH-RH dependent accumulation of cyclic AMP or LH release. Flufenamic or meclofenamic acid, at concentrations > 5µg/ml inhibited the increase in cyclic AMP resulting from LH-RH addition. Low doses of the fenamates decreased the LH-RH dependent rate of LH secretion whilst, at higher concentrations, the rate of LH release recovered and surpassed that due to LH-RH alone. This apparent biphasic effect is explained by the ability of high concentrations of flufenamic or meclofenamic acid alone to stimulate LH release. It is concluded that the increase in PGE levels plays no role in the mechanism of LH-RH stimulated LH secretion, but may be secondary to increases in cyclic AMP.

3 IMMUNOHISTOCHEMICAL LOCALIZATION OF HYPOTHALAMIC HORMONES (ESPECIALLY LRF) AT THE LIGHT MICROSCOPY LEVEL. J. Barry. Laboratory of Histology, Faculty of Medicine, 59045, Lille Cédex, France.

LRF-producing neurons have been identified in mammals by the use of antisera against synthetic LRF conjugated with HSA (prepared by M.P. Dubois). These neurons are widely dispersed from the parolfactive area up to the mesencephalon. They have variable elective concentrations according to the species: septo-preoptic and anterior hypothalamic area in the guinea pig and cat; rostral area on one hand and tuberal area on the other hand in the dog; mediobasal area and lamina terminalis in primates. "Extra-hypophyseal" pathways containing synaptic systems are added to the main "hypothalamo-infundibular" pathway formed by most axons. These observations suggest that in addition to its prehypophysiotropic action, LRF can act as a neurotransmitter or neuromodulator. The specificity of our results was verified by means of antiserum against unconjugated synthetic LRF (provided by Professor A. Arimura). The study of somatostatin-producing neurons was undertaken in monkeys with the aid of antisera against cyclic synthetic SRIF conjugated with HSA (prepared by M.P. Dubois). The use of antisera against synthetic TRF (also prepared by M.P. Dubois) provided only negative results. The differential topography of neurohypophysiotropic and prehypophysiotropic axons was verified by the use of antisera against neurohypophyseal hormones and neurophysins.

4 EFFECT OF PROSTAGLANDINS E_1, E_2 and $F_{2\alpha}$ ON PITUITARY GONADOTRO-
PIN SECRETION IN RHESUS MONKEYS (MACACA MULATTA). S.K. Batta,
B.G. Brackett and G. Niswender. Dept. of Ob/Gyn, School of Medicine, and Dept. of Clinical Studies, School of Veterinary Medicine, University of Pennsylvania, Philadelphia, Pa., and Dept.
of Physiology and Biophysics, Colorado State University, Fort
Collins, Col., U.S.A.

Prostaglandins (PGs) are reported to modulate ovulation in
various animal species. The mechanism of action of PGs in this
process has not been well elucidated. Attempts have been made
to determine whether PGs act on the hypothalamo-hypophysial axis
by altering gonadotropin secretion to affect the maturation and
rupture of ovarian follicles. To test this hypothesis, rhesus
monkeys were bilaterally ovairectomized. Three to 5 weeks later,
for 2 days prior to the experiment, the monkeys were primed with
100 µg/day of estradiol benzoate. Under pentobarbital sodium
anaesthesia (35 mg/kg), one jugular vein and one carotid artery
were cannulated. Both femoral veins were cannulated, one for
withdrawal of blood, the other for infusion of saline. Injections of PGE_1, PGE_2 and $PGF_{2\alpha}$ (1 mg and 5 mg) were made intraar-
terially while blood was collected at various intervals from
the jugular and one femoral vein. Plasma samples were assayed
in duplicate by radioimmunoassay using LER-M-970D standards
for LH and FSH. Estradiol treatment significantly lowered the
post-ovariectomy-elevated LH and FSH levels in plasma. Preliminary data indicate that PGE_1 and PGE_2 had a dose-related stimulatory effect on the release of LH and a variable but stimulatory effect on FSH release. Plasma LH levels peaked in 4-5 minutes after the injection, then tapered off to basal values in
60 minutes. PGE_2 had a marginally stronger effect on LH secretion as compared to PGE_1, while $PGF_{2\alpha}$ had little or no effect on
pituitary gonadotropin secretion. Under the experimental conditions reported here, it appeared that PGs do play a quantitative
role in the release of pituitary gonadotropins in primates.

5 INHIBITION BY LH-RH ANTAGONISTS OF LH-RH-INDUCED CYCLIC AMP ACCU-
MULATION AND LH RELEASE IN RAT ANTERIOR PITUITARY GLAND IN VITRO.
M. Beaulieu, F. Labrie, D.H. Coy, E.J. Coy, and A.V. Schally.
Medical Research Council Group in Molecular Endocrinology, CHUL,
Québec, G1V 4G2, Canada and V.A. Hospital and Tulane University
School of Medicine, New Orleans, La. 70146.

3 x 10^{-9}M LH-RH leads to a 300 to 400% stimulation of adenohypophyseal cyclic AMP accumulation in rat anterior pituitary
tissue in vitro. At a 100-molar excess, [Des-His^2, D-Leu^6] LH-
RH inhibited cyclic AMP accumulation to 58.1 ± 1.7% of the level
obtained with LH-RH alone while levels of 41.9 ± 7.0 and 24.4 ±
3.6% were obtained at 300- and 1000-molar ratios, respectively.
At molar ratios of 300 and 1000, [D-Phe^2, D-Leu^6] LH-RH led to
an inhibition of cyclic AMP accumulation and LH release to res-

pectively 44.6 ± 6.9 and 41.2 ± 4.6 and 26.1 ± 0.9 and 20.7 ± 1.1% of the levels obtained with LH-RH alone. A similar correlation between inhibition of LH release and cyclic AMP accumulation was obtained with Des-His[2], D-Leu[6] LH-RH. D-Phe[2], D-Phe[6] LH-RH was even more potent, a significant inhibition of LH-RH-induced cyclic AMP accumulation being found at a molar ratio of 30. These data illustrate that LH-RH antagonists always show a close parallelism between inhibition of LH release and cyclic AMP accumulation, thus adding   strong support to the already obtained evidence for a role of cyclic AMP as mediator of LH-RH action in the anterior pituitary gland.

6 PROLACTIN ELEVATION WITHIN 14 DAYS OF CONCEPTION IN HYPERPROLAC-
TINEMIC PATIENTS TREATED WITH 2α BROMOERGOCRYPTINE. M. Ben-David
S. Yarkoni and Z.P. Polishuk. Departments of Pharmacology and
Obstetrics and Gynecology, Hebrew University, Hadassah Hospital
Medical Center, Jerusalem, Israel.

Seven hyperprolactinemic patients with primary or secondary sterility were treated with 2α bromoergocryptine (Sandoz, Basle), 2.5 mg b.i.d., to suppress serum prolactin levels and to allow ovulation and fertility. Serum prolactin, LH and FSH were determined by homologous double-antibody radioimmunoassays. The prolactin RIA showed no crossreactivity with HCS, HCG or HGH. Serum prolactin levels were rapidly suppressed reaching normal values within 1 to 3 days of treatment. Menstrual cycles which were presumed ovulatory reappeared in all patients. Four patients conceived within three months of treatment. Treatment was discontinued as soon as pregnancy was suspected (about 16 days after the LH peak). In the patients where pregnancy was determined by a positive HCG titer serum prolactin levels were profoundly elevated starting 10 to 14 days after the LH peak, while patients were still receiving bromoergocryptine. No prolactin elevation was observed in 3 treated patients who did not conceive. In another patient with slightly high basal prolactin level who received no treatment and became pregnant, a significant serum prolactin elevation was detected 8 days after the LH peak. In conclusion, we suggest that the events of early pregnancy constitutes a powerful stimulus for prolactin release in hyperprolactinemic states.

7 COMPARISON OF THE POTENCY OF TRH, ACTH4-10, AND RELATED PEPTIDES
TO REVERSE PENTOBARBITAL-INDUCED NARCOSIS AND HYPOTHERMIA. G.
Bisette, C.B. Nemeroff, P.T. Loosen, A.J. Prange Jr., G.R. Breese
and M.A. Lipton. Biological Sciences Research Center, University of North Carolina, School of Medicine, Chapel Hill, North
Carolina 27514.

Various peptide hormones appear to exert behavioral and pharmacologic effects apart from their classical endocrine actions.

TRH (pGlu-His-Pro-NH$_2$), for example, antagonizes the sedation and hypothermia produced by barbiturate and other depressant drugs, and de Wied has shown that ACTH4-10 and certain related substances inhibit extinction of a pole-jumping avoidance response. In the latter paradigm, TRH showed slight but definite activity. This concatenation of findings provided the motivation for testing ACTH4-10 and related substances in the pentobarbital antagonism paradigm, in which TRH has been found potent. Male Swiss Webster mice (22-30 g) were pretreated with TRH (p-Glu-His-Pro-NH$_2$), ACTH$_{4-10}$, related peptides or vehicle (0.9% saline) two minutes before the intraperitoneal injection of sodium pentobarbital (50 mg/kg). Periodic assessment of rectal temperature and duration of sedation were recorded. TRH (1 mg/kg) was the most potent antagonist of pentobarbital-induced sedation and hypothermia. ACTH4-10 was inactive in this paradigm; ACTH4-7 and Met (O),8-D-Lys,9-Phe-ACTH$_{4-9}$ both reduced barbiturate-induced sleeping time (p<0.001) and hypothermia (p<0.05). Two tripeptides (pGlu-His-Trp-NH$_2$ and pGlu-His-Phe-NH$_2$), which bear similarity to sequences found both in TRH and ACTH4-10, were inactive. The present data, considered with the other findings cited above, suggest that TRH and ACTH fragments and analogs show relative but incomplete specificity in behavioral and pharmacologic tests. This project was supported by Grant #MH-11107, HD-03110, MH-00013, MH-16522, AA-02-334, and the Alfred P. Sloan Foundation.

8 INHIBITION OF PENTOBARBITAL-INDUCED RELEASE OF GH AND PRL BY TRH. R. Collu, M.J. Clermont, J. Letarte, G. Leboeuf and J.R. Ducharme Div. Endocrinol. and Metab. Dept. of Ped., Hôpital Ste-Justine and Université de Montréal, Québec, Canada.

TRH has recently been reported to exert effects on the central nervous system which are independent of its pituitary-thyroid actions. In particular, TRH can antagonize the behavioral and temperature-reducing effects of pentobarbital in rodents. The present study was undertaken to verify whether TRH could antagonize also the pentobarbital-induced release of GH and PRL in rats. Male Sprague-Dawley rats (250-300 g) were injected at 0 min with TRH either intraperitoneally (IP) or into a lateral ventricle of the brain (IVT) while control animals (S) were injected with saline. At 5 min, the animals were anesthetized with pentobarbital (50 mg/kg, IP) and then decapitated at 20 min. Some rats received at 0 min LH-RH, MIF, triiodothyronine (T$_3$) or TRH analogs instead of TRH. Some animals injected with saline both at 0 min and at 5 min and decapitated at 20 min constitute the non-anesthetized controls (NAC). The effects of TRH were also verified in thyroidectomized and propranolol-treated animals. Pentobarbital induced a significant rise in plasma GH and PRL levels. This rise was completely blocked by TRH (10 mg/kg, IP): (GH, ng/ml, M ± SE: NAC 58 ± 25; S 162 ± 43; TRH 21 ± 6; P<0.01. PRL

ng/ml, M ± SE: NAC 30 ± 6; S 62 ± 8; TRH 6 ± 1; P<0.01). TRH
injected IVT (10 µg/rat) was equally effective. LH-RH and MIF
(10 mg/kg, IP) and two TRH analogs (10 µg/rat, IVT) were ineffective. Pentobarbital-induced GH rise was blocked also in thyroidectomized animals. T_3 (50 µg/rat, IP) was able to block GH
but not PRL rise induced by the anesthesia. Propranolol (10 mg/
kg, IP) administered simultaneously with TRH (10 mg/kg, IP) prevented its blocking effect on the pentobarbital-induced rise of
GH but not the one exerted on the pentobarbital-induced rise of
PRL. These data indicate that TRH can antagonize the pentobarbital-induced secretions of GH and PRL by a specific pharmacological
action that seems partly independent from the pituitary-thyroid
axis, and necessitates, at least for its effect on GH secretion,
the integrity of β-adrenergic receptors. These investigations
were supported by M.R.C. of Canada Grant MA-4691.

9 THE EFFECT OF AN INHIBITORY ANALOGUE OF LH-RH ON GONADOTROPIN
SURGE, OVULATION AND ESTROUS CYCLE OF RATS. A. de la Cruz,
D.H. Coy, J.A. Vilchez-Martinez and Andrew V. Schally. Depart-
ment of Medicine, Tulane University School of Medicine, Endo.
& Polypep. Labs., Veterans Administration Hospital, New Orleans,
La., U.S.A.
    We have previously reported that [D-Phe^2, D-Leu^6] LH-RH, an
inhibitory analogue of luteinizing hormone-releasing hormone
(LH-RH), suppressed the preovulatory surge of LH in proestrous
hamsters and partially blocked ovulation (de la Cruz et al.,
PSEBM: 149, 576, 1975). Recently, we have synthesized [D-Phe^2,
Phe^3, D-Phe^6] LH-RH (DC-3-113), another antagonist of LH-RH
which suppressed LH and FSH release in male rats in response to
LH-RH for at least 4 hours. Three sc injections of 1 mg of this
analogue into proestrous rats completely suppressed ovulation
on the next morning. A single sc injection of 1.5 mg/rat (7.4
mg/kg) of this analogue suppressed ovulation by 86.4% and blocked
almost completely the preovulatory surge of LH and to a lesser
extent that of FSH. Monitoring of subsequent estrous cycles and
ovulation after treatment with 1.5 mg/rat of the analogue indicated that ovulation was delayed by 24, 48 and 72 hours in a
group of 31 animals treated with the analogue, but not in 10
diluent-treated animals. Moreover, the maturity and capacity
of fertilization of these retarded ova remains to be elucidated.
These preliminary results suggest that this compound or related
ones may be useful in the development of a new method of birth
control.

10 RELEASE AND SYNTHESIS OF PROLACTIN BY RAT PITUITARY CELL STRAINS
ARE REGULATED INDEPENDENTLY BY THYROTROPIN-RELEASING HORMONE.
P.S. Dannies, and A.H. Tashjian Jr.   Harvard School of Dental
Medicine, Laboratory of Pharmacology, 188 Longwood Avenue, Boston
MA. 02115, U.S.A.

   Thyrotropin-releasing hormone (TRH) stimulates the release and
synthesis of prolactin (PRL) in GH-cells, clonal strains of rat
pituitary cells which synthesize PRL and growth hormone but not
thyrotropin.   TRH stimulates PRL release within 1 hr, while increased PRL synthesis is first detected at 3-4 hr and reaches a
maximum after 1-2 days.   The responses of prolactin release to
increasing concentrations of TRH or analogs of TRH are not the
same as the prolactin synthesis responses.   The concentrations of
tripeptide required for half-maximal stimulation of PRL synthesis and release and the ratios of the concentrations required
for synthesis and release vary considerably.   Some examples are
given in the Table below.

PEPTIDE	RELEASE [peptide] for $\frac{1}{2}$ max (nM)	SYNTHESIS [peptide] for $\frac{1}{2}$ max (nM)	[PEPTIDE] for synthesis for release
pGlu-His-ProNH$_2$ (TRH)	0.3	3	10
pGlu-N^t-MeHis-Pro-NH$_2$	0.5	0.5	1
pGlu-dHis-Pro-NH$_2$	25	100	4
pGlu-His-Pro-NHCH$_3$	4	50	12
pGlu-His-Pro	200	4000	20
Pro-His-ProNH$_2$	1250	250	0.2

   These experiments are performed in serum-free medium, and we have
shown that TRH is stable in this medium even during incubation
with GH-cells (Hinkle et al. J. Biol. Chem. 249:3085, 1974).
Studies with the analogs listed and other analogs indicate that
changes in the N-terminal pGlu and His residues affect PRL release more than synthesis and that changing the C-terminal ProNH$_2$
residue may affect PRL synthesis more than release.   The analog
with Pro in place of the N-terminal pGlu causes a half-maximal
stimulation of PRL synthesis at 250 nM (see table); at this concentration there is no detectable stimulation of PRL release.
We conclude that in GH-cells PRL release and synthesis are independent processes which are mediated by two distinct hormone-
receptor interactions.

11 OPPOSITE EFFECTS OF THYROID HORMONE AND ESTROGENS ON TSH AND PRL
    RESPONSES TO TRH. A. De Léan, J. Drouin, L. Ferland and F. Labrie
    Medical Research Council Group in Molecular Endocrinology, CHUL,
    Québec, G1V 4G2, Canada.
        This study was aimed at investigating the correlation between
    changes of the level of pituitary TRH receptor sites and the
    plasma TSH and PRL responses to TRH. Treatment of adult male
    or female rats with estradiol benzoate (EB) (25 μg/day) led to
    a 200 to 300% increase of the concentration of pituitary TRH
    binding sites while the affinity of the receptor for the neurohor-
    mone remained unchanged (Kd=3-4 x 10^{-8}M). Half-maximal increase
    of the number of TRH binding sites is measured at 4 days of
    treatment with EB. In order to study the responses to TRH in
    vivo, adult normal or propylthiouracil (PTU)-treated rats were
    injected daily for 9 days with EB (50 μg), T_4 (10 μg) a combi-
    nation of both hormones or the vehicle alone (1% gelatin-0.9%
    NaCl) and the plasma TSH and PRL responses to TRH measured by
    blood sampling at six intervals up to 60 minutes under Surital
    anesthesia. EB treatment led to a 60 (normal rats) to 100%
    (PTU-treated animals) reversal of the almost complete inhibition
    observed with T_4 alone. In fact, in intact rats treated with
    the vehicle, EB, T_4 or EB + T_4, the maximal plasma TSH values
    after TRH were 2205 ± 125, 2560 ± 158, 185 ± 49 and 1217 ± 160
    ng/ml plasma, respectively. In rats made hypothyroid with PTU,
    the peak plasma TSH values in similarly treated groups were
    3586 ± 269, 4375 ± 241, 558 ± 90 and 3907 ± 368 ng/ml plasma,
    respectively. EB alone led only to a slight stimulation of the
    TSH response to TRH. The reversal of T_4 inhibition by EB was
    dose-dependent. TRH injection led to a similar increase of
    plasma PRL (30 to 50 ng/ml) in normal and hypothyroid rats al-
    though the basal levels were higher in PTU-treated animals. T_4
    treatment was followed by a 50 to 60% inhibition of the plasma
    PRL response in EB-treated hypothyroid rats but had only a 20
    to 25% inhibitory effect in control animals. The present fin-
    dings show that the amplitude of the TSH and PRL responses to
    TRH can be modulated by the respective stimulatory and inhibitory
    influences of estrogens and thyroid hormone and suggest that the
    level of TRH receptor sites in the respective cell types may well
    play an important role in the control of activity of both thyro-
    trophs and mammotrophs in the anterior pituitary gland.

12 INHIBITORY EFFECT OF ANDROGENS ON THE LH RESPONSIVENESS TO LH-RH
    IN ANTERIOR PITUITARY CELLS IN PRIMARY CULTURE. J. Drouin, R.
    Veilleux and Fernand Labrie. Medical Research Council Group in
    Molecular Endocrinology, CHUL, Québec, G1V 4G2, Canada.
        The direct feedback effect of androgens on gonadotrophin re-
    lease at the pituitary level was studied using primary cultu-
    res of rat anterior pituitary cells. It was found that after
    preincubation of cells for about 36 hours in the presence of

3×10^{-9}M testosterone (T), the 50% effective dose (ED_{50}) of stimulation of LH release by LH–RH was increased by an order of magnitude from about 10^{-10}M to 10^{-9}M. In the same experiment, the ED_{50} of stimulation of FSH release by LH–RH was not affected by T, an ED_{50} value of 2×10^{-10}M being found in the presence and absence of T. Dihydrotestosterone (DHT) and T led to the same maximal inhibition of the LH responsiveness to 10^{-10}M LH–RH but DHT was 3 times more potent than T, their ED_{50} values being of 1.6×10^{-10}M and 5×10^{-10}M, respectively. Measurement of the LH cell content at the end of the incubation demonstrated a decreased responsiveness of LH–RH-induced LH release without any change in hormone synthesis. In fact, an increased LH cell content was found when decreased release had occured, the sum of hormone release and cell content remaining constant. Δ^4-androstenedione can also inhibit the LH responsiveness to LH–RH although this steroid with an ED_{50} value of only 10^{-8}M is approximately 20 times less potent than T. Dehydroepiandrosterone at concentrations up to 10^{-5}M does not change the LH responsiveness to LH–RH. The observed effects of androgens on the LH responsiveness to LH–RH could be secondary to changes of the number of receptor sites for LH–RH in the LH-secreting cells.

13 IMMUNOHISTOCHEMICAL STUDY OF THE ONTOGENY OF SOMATOSTATIN IN THE RAT AND PHYLOGENY OF THIS NEUROHORMONE. D. Dubé, R. Leclerc and G. Pelletier, Medical Research Council Group in Molecular Endocrinology, CHUL, Québec, G1V 4G2, Canada.

In order to gain a better knowledge of the initial action of hypothalamic hormones on anterior pituitary function, we carried out immunohistochemical studies of the localization of somatostatin, the neurohormone which inhibits the release of growth hormone. Localization of somatostatin was studied in brain of developing rat and adult guinea pig, frog and trout. Brains were fixed either by immersion or by cardiac perfusion with 4% paraformaldehyde in cacodylate buffer (0.1M). The immunohistochemical technique involves successive use of rabbit anti–somatostatin serum (supplied by A. Arimura), goat anti–rabbit IgG and soluble peroxidase-anti-peroxidase complex. In adult rats, the reaction was localized on almost half the granules fibers of the external zone of the median eminence. These fibers contained granules of 900 to 1100 Å in diameter. Many nerve endings in the vascular organ of the lamina terminalis and cells of the subcommissural organ and pineal gland were also immunoreactive. In developing rats, the reaction was not detected with certainty until 5 days after birth and appeared localized in two main fiber bundles lateral to the infundibular recess. These bundles seemed to originate from the arcuate nucleus. The intensity of the reaction increased at 9 and 15 days of age and at 30 days was similar to the reaction observed in adults, no reaction was present in the median eminence of 16, 19, 20 and 21 day old foetuses nor in

newborn and 3 day-old rats. The significance of a cytoplasmic
reaction in some cells of the internal and tuberal regions of the
median eminence observed at the electron microscope level in newborn and older rats is still unclear. A positive reaction was
also detected in the external zone of guinea pig and frog
median eminence as well as in fibers of trout neurohypophysis.
These observations seem to indicate that, in the rat, somatostatin appears relatively late in development. However, it
appears early in the vertebrate phylogenetic scale.

14 SOMATOSTATIN-CONTAINING PERIKARYA IN THE RAT HYPOTHALAMUS: THEIR
DISTRIBUTION ACCORDING TO SIZE, LOCALIZATION AND BINDING WITH
NEUROPHYSIN. M.P. Dubois and E. Kolodziejczyk. *I.N.R.A. – Sta-
tion de Physiologie de la Reproduction, 37380 Nouzilly, France
**Lab. d'histology (Prof. Maillet) Fac. de Médecine 37000 Tours
France.

Somatostatin-containing cells were evidenced by immunocytolo-
gical methods in the hypothalamus of the rat. Immunoreactive
perikaryans appeared in two patterns: 1) a magnocellular system
(about 23 M in diameter), part of supraoptic and paraventricular
nuclei (SON, PVN); somatostatin was present altogether with
neurophysin (NP) in these cells; 2) a parvocellular system
(about 12 M in diameter), a part of which was localized near by
the walls of the supraoptic recessus of the IIIrd ventricle,
this group was NP negative; the other part included small cells
of PVN and SON where serial sections failed to reveal NB with
certainty because of the small size of the cells. Suprachiasmatic nucleus was somatostatin negative. Nervous fibers somatostatin positive coming from SON and PVN were part of the hypothalamo-infundibular and hypothalamo-pituitary tracts whereas fibers
coming from the parvocellular system NP negative were assumed
to reach the median eminence and distributed themselves in the
palissadic layer of the external zone where the repartition of
NP and somatostatin was distinct. According to the binding
[NP I/oxytocin] and [NP II/vasopressin] it is suggested that
somatostatin may be linked with NP III in the structures where
somatostatin and NP are associated.

15 EFFECTS OF SYNTHETIC AND PURIFIED RELEASING FACTORS ON ISOLATED
PITUITARY HORMONE GRANULES. R. Dular and F. LaBella. Depart-
ment of Pharmacology and Therapeutics, University of Manitoba,
Winnipeg, Canada.

Bovine anterior pituitary secretory granules containing prolactin (PRL) and growth hormone (GH), but only traces of other
hormones, were prepared by centrifugation in isotonic sucrose
(LaBella et al., Endocrinology 89: 1094, 1971). Aliquots of
granule suspension, about 2 mg protein, were added to 2 ml of
10 mM Tris-HCl buffer (pH 7.4) containing 154 mM NaCl, 5 mM KCl,

0.5 mM $MgCl_2$ and 2 mM $CaCl_2$, and incubated at 37º for 10 to 30
min. Incubation was terminated by centrifugation at 24,000 xg
for 7 min. Hormones released into the medium were estimated by
solid phase radioimmunoassay. Synthetic TRH, in concentrations
of 1 and 10 ng/ml, stimulated the release of PRL by 30 and 112%,
respectively, without any appreciable effect on release of GH,
and at 1000 ng/ml, inhibited PRL secretion by over 50%. In
several experiments using different preparations of granules,
SRIF (1 to 1000 ng) consistently inhibited release of GH, whereas
release of PRL was stimulated in some cases and inhibited in
others. We have observed enhanced release of PRL with SRIF in
bovine pituitary cell monolayers. SRIF, 10 µg/ml, consistently
inhibited release of both GH and PRL. Partially purified pro-
lactin-release inhibiting (PIF) or prolactin releasing (PRF)
factor (Dular et al., Endocrinology 95: 563, 1974) had marked
effects on PRL release. PIF, 0.25 µg protein, caused 50% inhibition of PRL and 30% stimulation of GH release. Higher concentrations (3 µg protein/ml) inhibited release of both PRL and GH.
PRF, 1 µg protein/ml, stimulated release of PRL by 100%. Rat
hypothalamic extract (0.2 mg protein) had variable effects on
release of GH and PRL from one preparation of granules to another,
as we have observed for responses of pituitary tissue in vitro.
Synthetic LH-RH had no effect on release of GH and PRL (Supported
by the Medical Research Council).

16 PURIFICATION AND CHARACTERIZATION OF PIF FROM PIG HYPOTHALAMI.
A. Dupont, T.W. Redding, A. Arimura and A.V. Schally. Medical
Research Council Group in Molecular Endocrinology, CHUL, Québec,
G1V 4G2, Canada and Tulane University School of Medicine and
V.A. Hospital, New Orleans, Louisiana 70112.
    Prolactin-release inhibiting factor (PIF) activity in frac-
tions of acetic acid extracts of 470,000 pig hypothalami was
followed by inhibition of prolactin release in vitro from rat
pituitaries incubated in KRBG. These extracts were purified by
gel filtration on Sephadex G-25 and the PIF-active fractions were
extracted with phenol. Phenol extracts were then chromatogra-
phed on carboxymethyl-cellulose (CMC). The materials with PIF
activity emerged in several fractions. One of the PIF fractions
appeared to have a neutral or a negative charge, in contrast to
catecholamines which were more strongly retained on CMC. This
PIF-active material was found to contain only 0.28 ng/µg of norepinephrine (NE) and 0.3 ng/µg of dopamine (DA). After repurifi-
cation by gel filtration on Sephadex G-25 (R_f 0.43), the PIF-active fraction had 0.6 ng/µg of NE, DA being undetectable. Perphenazine (1.25 x 10^{-7}M), which inhibited the response up to
100 ng/µg of NE and of DA, did not suppress the PIF activity of
10 µg of that fraction. The PIF-active material was then subjected to countercurrent distribution (CCD) in 0.1% acetic acid:
1-butanol:pyridine=11:5:3. In this system, the PIF active frac-

tion displayed a different coefficient of partition (K=0.2) from
catecholamines (K=0.6). In continuous free flow electrophoresis
at pH 6.3, the material migrated to the anode. The material was
then further concentrated by CCD in 1-butanol:acetic acid:H_2O=
4:15. In conclusion, we have purified a fraction with PIF activity having different physico-chemical characteristics (Molecular weight, charge, K in CCD) from NE and DA. The catecholamines
analyses were performed by Dr. J. Clemens and Dr. C. Shaar. This
work was supported by a Medical Research Council of Canada fel-
lowship (to A.D.), and USPHS grant AM 07467, and the Veterans
Administration (to A.V.S.).

17 DEVELOPMENT OF THE HYPOTHALAMIC-PITUITARY-THYROID AXIS IN THE
NEONATAL RAT. J.H. Dussault and F. Labrie. Service d'endocrinologie, CHUL, Québec, G1V 4G2, Canada.

The hypothalamic content of thyrotropin releasing hormone
(TRH), the pituitary concentration of thyrotropin stimulating
hormone (TSH), and the serum concentrations of TSH, thyroxine
(T_4) and triiodothyronine (T_3) have been determined at different
intervals during the first 50 days following birth in the rat.
From a minimum concentration of 1 pg/μg protein at birth, the
hypothalamic concentration of TRH increased to a maximum of 5 to
6 pg between 16 and 28 days of age. Serum and pituitary TSH
concentrations increased to maximum levels by the end of the
first post-natal week; the elevated hormonal levels were then
maintained up to the end of the third post-natal week. Circulating thyroid hormone concentrations were very low at birth.
T_4 increased rapidly between days 4 and 16 to reach a peak
concentration of 6 μg/100 ml while T_3 followed a parallel pattern
with a peak concentration of 108 ng/100 ml obtained only at
day 28. Although serum hormone concentrations may not strictly
be equated to secretion, one is tempted to compare the post-
natal period with mid-gestation in human where a surge in T_4 and
TSH is encountered. The delayed T_3 elevation compared to the
T_3 surge is possibly due to the nonmaturation of the enzyme
system responsible for conversion of T_4 to T_3 in the newborn
rat as well as in human. These data obtained in the rat indicate that components of the hypothalamic-pituitary-thyroid-axis develop simultaneously during the post-natal period, and that this
model might be applied to the development of the same axis in
human.

18 NEONATAL DETERMINATION OF ADULT AMYGDALA-HYPOTHALAMIC CONNEXIONS
    R.G. Dyer, F. Ellendorff and N. MacLEOD. A.R.C. Institute of
    animal physiology, Babraham, Cambridge, CG2 4AT, England.
        Neonatal exposure to gonadal hormones can influence endocrine
    sex in adult rats and such treatment produces a morphological
    change to the synaptic arrangement of the preoptic area (G.
    Raisman & P. Field, Aggression 52, 42, 1974). To analyse sy-
    naptic transmission in normal males, diestrus females, males
    castrated on day 1 (fales) and females neonatally injected with
    testosterone propionate (T.P. 1.25 mg/rat), we recorded action
    potentials from over 600 cells in the rostral hypothalamus of
    51 rats. The neurones were classified by their response to sti-
    mulation in the medial basal hypothalamus (MBH; R.G. Dyer, J.
    Physiol., 234, 421, 1973) and synaptic pathways from the amyg-
    dala activated by stimulation of the cortico-medial zone (CMA).
    In cells antidromically identified as projecting to MBH (N=151),
    the effect of CMA stimulation on firing rate was (partly) de-
    pendent on endocrine sex. Thus 10 out of 41 (24%) neurones in
    diestrus females responded to CMA stimulation compared with 29
    out of 52 (56%) in males (P<0.01). The fales (9 out of 29
    responding - 31%) were also significantly different from males
    (P<0.05) whereas the T.P. females occupied an intermediate posi-
    tion (12 out of 29 responding - 41%). Our work shows that neo-
    natal exposure to hormone permanently modifies neural transmis-
    sion in the forebrain.

19 EFFECT OF LH-RH ANTAGONISTS IN VITRO AND IN VIVO. L. Ferland,
    F. Labrie, D.H. Coy, E.J. Coy and A.V. Schally. Medical Research
    Council Group in Molecular Endocrinology, CHUL, Québec, G1V 4G2,
    Canada and Tulane University School of Medicine and V.A. Hospi-
    tal, New Orleans, Louisiana 70112.
        Improved inhibitors of LH-RH are those which, beside removal
    of the histidine residue at position 2 of LH-RH, include repla-
    cement of glycine at position 6 by a D-amino acid. A still
    better modification is replacement of the histidine residue at
    position 2 by D-phenylalanine. Analogs containing these modifi-
    cations were tested for their ability to inhibit the stimulation
    of LH release in vitro and in vivo. When tested in pituitary cells
    in culture, [Des-His^2] LH-RH, [Des-His^2, D-Leu^6] LH-RH, [Des-His^2,
    D-Phe^6] LH-RH, [D-Phe^2] LH-RH, [D-Phe^2, D-Leu^6] LH-RH and [D-
    Phe^2, D-Phe^6] LH-RH inhibit 50% of LH release induced by LH-RH
    at molar ratios (MR$_{50}$s) of 3000, 500, 60, 1000, 150 and 25 res-
    pectively. [D-Phe^2, D-Phe^6, Phe^7] LH-RH, [D-Phe^2, Phe^3, D-Phe^6]
    LH-RH and [D-Phe^2, Phe^5, D-Phe^6] LH-RH have MR$_{50}$ values of 400,
    100 and 75, respectively. When evaluated in vivo, some of the
    mentioned analogs inhibit LH-RH action at molar ratios lower than
    observed in vitro. At a 300 molar ratio, [Des-His^2, D-Ala^6]
    LH-RH, [Des-His^2, D-Leu^6] LH-RH and [D-Phe^2, D-Leu^6] LH-RH lead
    to approximately a 90% inhibition of the plasma LH rise induced

by LH–RH. [D–Phe[2], Phe[5], D–Phe[6]] LH–RH, at a 500–molar ratio, inhibits the plasma LH rise induced by LH–RH 75% up to 5 hours after its injection. When administered at 12:00 hours at the dose of 2 mg, this analog inhibits the spontaneous proestrous LH surge and ovulation by 85 and 75%, respectively.

20 IN VIVO AND IN VITRO ACTIVITY OF ANALOGS OF SOMATOSTATIN ON GH AND TSH RELEASE. L. Ferland, J. Drouin, R. Veilleux, F. Labrie, D.H. Coy, E.J. Coy and A.V. Schally. Medical Research Council Group in Molecular Endocrinology, CHUL, Québec, G1V 4G2, Canada and Polypeptide Endocrine Laboratory, V.A. Hospital and Tulane University School of Medicine, New Orleans, La.

In order to evaluate the in vivo potency and duration of action of somatostatin and its analogs a model based on inhibition of plasma GH levels stimulated by sodium thiamylal (50 mg/kg, B.W., i.p.) and morphine (3 mg/animal, s.c.) was developed. A significant inhibitory effect of somatostatin (45% inhibition) is observed 15 min after a sc injection of 1 µg of the peptide while a near maximal effect (90-95% inhibition) is found at a dose of 25 µg. [Tyr[1]] somatostatin, [D-Ala[1]] somatostatin, [N-acetyl-Cys[3]] somatostatin and [N-benzoyl-Cys[3]] somatostatin have activities undistinguishable from somatostatin itself while [D-Lys[4]] somatostatin and [des-amino[1]-des-carboxy[14]] somatostatin have approximately 10% the activity of the natural hypothalamic peptide. Estimation of the relative affinities of somatostatin and its analogs on pituitary receptors was obtained by measuring their effects on GH and TSH release in pituitary cells in monolayer culture. The following data are expressed as % of the activity of somatostatin itself.

Peptide	Relative potency on hormone release (%)	
	GH	TSH
Somatostatin (S)	100	100
[Tyr[1]] S	100	–
[D-Ala[1]] S	100	–
[Des-amino[1]] S	30	20
[Des-carboxy[14]] S	20	10
[Des-amino[1], des-carboxy[14]] S	100	100
[D-Lys[4]] S	3	3
[D-Lys[9]] S	0.02	–
[N-acetyl-Cys[3]] S	100	–
[N-benzoyl-Cys[3]] S	50	–

21   CONTROL OF GONADOTROPHIN RELEASE IN HYPERPROLACTINAEMIC WOMEN.
      M.R. Glass, R.W. Shaw, R. Logan Edwards, W.R. Butt, D.R. London.
      Women's hospital and Queen Elizabeth Hospital, Birminghan, U.K.
      The modulatory effects of oestradiol and progesterone on the
      gonadotrophin response to LH-RH was studied in women with hyper-
      prolactinaemia (>30 μg/l) selected by the absence of pituitary
      tumour and by their normal, or exaggerated, LH response to LH-
      RH. 15 out of 16 women showed the absence of a positive feed-
      back response to oestradiol benzoate. All the subjects had a
      normal negative feedback receptor as judged by an initial fall
      in gonadotrophin levels after oestradiol as well as an increase
      in oestradiol levels during clomiphene. Those who did not sub-
      sequently release LH after oestradiol also failed to ovulate on
      clomiphene. When, on a separate occasion, hyperprolactinaemic
      women were given oestradiol benzoate (2.5 mg) immediately after
      a study of the gonadotrophin response to LH-RH, a second LH-RH
      stimulation performed 44 hours later produced an LH response
      greater than before the oestrogen administration. This is the
      pattern found in the normal woman. These findings support the
      view that the inability of hyperprolactinaemic women to ovulate
      is due to a failure to respond to the oestrogenic positive
      feedback signal at the level of the hypothalamus.

22   STUDIES CONCERNING THE ROLE OF RENIN IN THE HYPOTHALAMO-HYPOPHY-
      SEAL COMPLEX. I. Haulica, A. Stratone, D. Branisteanu, V.
      Rosca, M. Coculescu and Gh. Balan. Department of Physiology,
      Institute of Medicine, Iasi, Romania.
      Using the Boucher (1967) micromethod for separating and mea-
      suring the renin activity in rat hypothalamus and hypophysis,
      it was observed that the renin content of hypophyseal glandular
      tissue is about 5 times higher than in hypothalamus (96.8 ± 21
      as compared to 20 ± 8.9 ng ang./g/h). In turn, hypophysis
      showed 3 times higher values in the posterior lobe than in the
      anterior one. While hyperosmosis induced by intravenous admi-
      nistration of 10% NaCl significantly changed the renin content
      of the hypothalamo-hypophyseal complex in terms of its increase
      at the hypothalamic level and its decrease in hypophysis, the 12
      hours contention stress did not influence renin activity in the
      two studied structures. In the rats with congenital insipid dia-
      betes, the renin-like activity is significantly depressed in
      both hypothalamus and hypophysis. The results obtained are dis-
      cussed according to the possible participation of the renin-an-
      giotensin system in the ADH secretion modulation, with the cor-
      responding consequences upon the local and general hydroelec-
      trolytic regulation.

23   INHIBITION AND REGRESSION OF DMBA-INDUCED RAT MAMMARY TUMORS
      BY RU-16117, A NEW ANTI-ESTROGEN. P.A. Kelly, F. Labrie, J. Asse-
      lin and J.P. Raynaud. Medical Research Council Group in Mole-
      cular Endocrinology, CHUL, Québec, G1V 4G2, Canada and Centre
      de Recherches Roussel-UCLAF, Romainville, France.
          When started at the same time as DMBA treatment, daily injec-
      tions of 8 or 24 µg of 11 α-methoxy ethinylestradiol (RU-16117)
      into rats completely inhibited mammary tumor development up to
      130 days after administration of the carcinogen. A daily in-
      jection of 2 µg caused a 50% reduction in tumor incidence when
      compared to control rats, as well as a reduction in tumor number
      and tumor size. Specific binding of [^{3}H] estradiol (E_2), [^{3}H]
      5020 (7, 21-dimethyl-19-nor-pregna-4, 9-diene-3,20-dione, a syn-
      thetic progestin) and ^{125}I-oPRL to the tumors from rats recei-
      ving 2 µg RU-16117 per day were reduced when compared to tumors
      from control animals. RU-16117 was also capable of causing the
      regression of established DMBA-induced tumors. In these experi-
      ments, starting three months after DMBA administration, animals
      were injected daily for 4 weeks with either 2,8 or 24 µg of RU-
      16117 or 0.1, 0.5, 2.5 or 12.5 µg of 17β-E_2. Another group of
      animals were ovariectomized (OVX). A marked reduction of tumor
      incidence was observed at 8 and 24 µg of RU-16117 with the pat-
      tern of regression obtained with 24 µg being almost superimpo-
      sable to that observed after ovariectomy. Specific binding of
      [^{3}H] E_2 to tumors from rats treated with 24 µg of RU-16117/day
      or OVX was significantly reduced when compared to control rats
      while binding of [^{3}H] 5020 was very low in the tumors remaining
      in these two groups of animals at the end of the experiment
      (4 weeks). The present data clearly show that RU-16117, at re-
      latively low doses, not only completely prevents the appearance
      of mammary tumors after DMBA administration but also induced
      a tumor regression similar to that observed after ovariectomy.

24   DEGRADATION OF LUTEINIZING HORMONE-RELEASING HORMONE BY HYPOTHA-
      LAMIC ENZYME(S). Y. Koch, T. Baram, M. Fridkin*, and P. Chob-
      sieng. Departments of Hormone Research and of Chemistry*, The
      Weizmann Institute of Science, Rehovot, Israel.
          Synthetic luteinizing hormone-releasing hormone (LH-RH) lost
      both its immunoreactivity and hormonal activity on incubation
      with hypothalamic or cerebrocortical slices or homogenates. This
      inactivation was shown to be due to degradation of the decapepti-
      de by soluble enzyme(s) present in the 100,000 xg supernatant
      fraction of the homogenates. The supernatant derived from one
      rat hypothalamus was capable of destroying within 5 min 1 µg of
      exogenous LH-RH, i.e. an amount equivalent to about 200 times
      the endogenous content of LH-RH. Evidence was obtained that
      endogenous LH-RH, before its secretion, is protected from enzy-
      mic breakdown. The hexapeptide pGlu-His-Trp-Ser-Tyr-Gly was
      identified as the major-radioactive breakdown product of [pGlu-3-

^{3}H] LH-RH, and tentative evidence for the formation of the tetra-
peptide Leu-Arg-Pro-Gly-NH$_2$ was obtained by sequential electrophoresis and paper chromatography. These findings suggest that
the Gly-Leu bond may be the preferred site of cleavage. LH-RH
analogs having D-amino acids at position 6, i.e. [D-Ala^6] LH-RH
and [D-Leu^6] LH-RH, were 37% and 34% degraded, under conditions
where LH-RH was 55% degraded. High concentrations of crude preparations of Kallikrein inactivator (Trasylol), prevented the
enzymic degradation of LH-RH. Attempts are being made to isolate the enzyme inhibiting fraction.

25 NEUROTRANSMITTERS AND CONTROL OF PITUITARY FUNCTION. C. Kordon.
Unité de Neurobiologie de l'INSERM (U 109), 2 ter, rue d'Alésia
75014 Paris.
    Hypothalamic serotonin (5-HT) has paradoxical effects upon
phasic release of FSH and LH in the female rat. Pharmacological, micropharmacological and surgical approaches suggest that
the classical inhibitory action of the amine affects directly
tubero-infuncibular neurons, whereas a distinct, facilitatory
interference of 5-HT takes place at a higher level of gonadotropic release-regulating structures and possibly involves the
suprachiasmatic nucleus. 5-HT has also a permissive action
upon the release of prolactin induced by mammary stimulation in
lactating animals. The succion reflex electively stimulates
release of 5-HT within the medio- and the anterobasal hypothalamus. Other serotonin-containing projections are not affected,
and the duration of this activation is strictly correlated with
the capacity of the stimulus to release prolactin. Hypothalamic
dopamine concentrations are also affected by lactation. The
respective roles of both amines in physiological regulation of
gonadotropic and prolactin secretion will be discussed.

26 IMMUNOHISTOCHEMICAL LOCALIZATION OF β-LPH, β-FSH and β-LH IN THE
PITUITARY GLAND. R. Leclerc, G. Pelletier, R. Puviani, M. Chré-
tien and M. Lis. Medical Research Council Group in Molecular
Endocrinology, CHUL, Québec, G1V 4G2, Canada and Institut de
Recherches Cliniques de Montréal, Montréal, Québec.
    Although identification of the adenohypophyseal cell type se-
creting both ACTH and β-MSH has been achieved, it has not been
clearly established if the same cell is also responsible for the
production of β-LPH, a possible precursor of β-MSH. In order to
clearly identify the β-LPH-producing cells, we have localized
this hormone in pituitaries of rat, pig, sheep, beef, monkey
and man with an immunoperoxidase technique involving use of the
peroxidase-anti-peroxidase complex. ACTH was also localized in
contiguous sections. Control reactions were achieved by incubating the specific antiserum with an excess of the corresponding
antigen. In the rat, β-LPH was always found in all cells of the
pars intermedia and in a few cells of the pars distalis. In

rat pars distalis, β-LPH was localized at the electron microscope
level in the stellate cells which correspond to melano-cortico-
tropic cells. In other species, the distribution of β-LPH and
ACTH containing cells was also similar. However, some cells
reacted more intensively with anti-β-LPH serum than with anti-
ACTH serum. All cells of the pars intermedia showed a positive
reaction to both ACTH and LPH but, probably due to a poor fixation, the immunoreactivity was weak in pig, sheep and beef.
From this work, it may be concluded that: 1o all cells of the
pars intermedia contain both β-LPH and ACTH, 2o the same cells
in the pars distalis produce both hormones although some cells
could contain more β-LPH than ACTH. Although it is generally
thought that FSH and LH are produced by the same cell type, dissociation of the secretion of these two hormones in some experimental conditions suggests that FSH and LH could be stored in
different cell types. Since α-chain of these two hormone are similar, we have used antibodies against β chains of both LH and
FSH in order to identify specifically hypophyseal cells containing these two hormones. The immunoperoxydase technique was
applied on consecutive semithin sections of male rat pituitary.
Round cells situated near capillaries appear to contain both
hormones. Experiments are in progress to identify β-FSH and
β-LH-containing cells under differents physiologic states in
the female rat.

27 SYNTHESIS AND BIOLOGICAL ACTIVITY OF CAMEL AND BOVINE β-MELANO-
    TROPINS. S. Lemaire, D. Yamashiro and C.H. Li. Hormone Research
    Laboratory, University of California, San Francisco, California
    94143, U.S.A.
        Two natural occuring melanotropins, camel β C_2-MSH and bovine
    β_b-MSH, have been synthesized by improved solid-phase procedures.
    The coupling reaction of Boc-amino acids was achieved by using
    their performed symetrical anhydrides. The synthetic hormones
    were purified by gel filtration on Sephadex G-10 and G-25,
    chromatography on carboxymethylcellulose and partition chroma-
    tography on Sephadex G-25 with final yields of 56% and 35% for
    β_{C2}-MSH and β_b-MSH, respectively. They were then shown to be
    identical to their natural hormones in amino acid analysis, paper
    electrophoresis, disc electrophoresis, thin layer chromatography,
    enzymic digests, and bioassays. This work was supported in part
    by USPHS Grant GM-2907.

28   GROWTH HORMONE RELEASE BY MtT-F4 RAT PITUITARY TUMOR IN VITRO.
     EFFECT OF SOMATOSTATIN AND CYCLIC AMP. M. Lis, T. Motomatsu
     and M. Chrétien. Clinical Research Institute, Montréal.
         Fluoride-stimulated adenylate cyclase was studied in isola-
     ted tumor cells of transplantable rat pituitary tumor MtT-F4 in
     vitro. The intracellular cyclic AMP is lower in the cells
     incubated in the presence of synthetic somatostatin. Contrary
     to the findings reported for normal pituitary, however, the
     immunoreactive growth hormone release did not change when soma-
     tostatin phosphodiesterase inhibitors or dibutyryl cyclic AMP
     were added to the incubation medium.

29   LONG-TERM ORGAN CULTURE OF RAT ANTERIOR PITUITARY GLANDS. J.E.
     Martin and D.C. Klein. Section on Physiological Controls, La-
     boratory of Biomedical Sciences, National Institute of Child
     Health and Human Development, National Institutes of Health,
     Bethesda, Maryland 20014.
         A pituitary organ culture system has been developed in which
     cellular integrity and responsiveness to luteinizing hormone
     releasing factor (LRF) are maintained for at least 4 days. An-
     terior pituitaries from 5-day-old female Sprague-Dawley rats were
     cultured individually at $37^{\circ}C$ in an atmosphere of 95% O_2-5% CO_2
     in chemically defined medium. Histologic examination of 5-day-
     old pituitaries cultured for 96 hr in control medium revealed
     no evidence of tissue necrosis. By contrast, adult rat anterior
     pituitary glands were necrotic after only 24 hr of incubation.
     The neonatal pituitaries were treated for 24 hr with synthetic
     LRF, and medium and pituitary LH concentrations were measured by
     radioimmunoassay. On the first day of culture, LRF caused a
     dose-related release of LH. The minimal effective dose was bet-
     ween 10^{-10} and $10^{-9}M$ LRF; near-maximal LH release was attained
     with $10^{-6}M$ LRF which induced a 12-fold increase in medium LH over
     control values. Release was evident 3 hr after stimulation with
     $10^{-9}M$ LRF. The response to LRF and the LH content of unstimu-
     lated glands increased markedly during the 4-day incubation.
     The simplicity, sensitivity, reproducibility, and long-term
     viability of this anterior pituitary organ culture system make
     it a valuable tool for the study of pituitary physiology.

30   REGULATION OF ORNITHINE DECARBOXYLASE ACTIVITY IN THE RAT PITUI-
     TARY. P. May, G.N. Burrow and S.W. Spaulding. Departments of
     Medicine and Laboratory Medicine, Yale University School of Medi-
     cine, New Haven, Connecticut.
         Ornithine decarboxylase (ODC) activity parallels the synthe-
     sis of polyamines which may be important in the control of RNA
     synthesis and tissue growth. Polypeptide hormone which induce
     cell growth stimulate ODC activity. Accordingly, we have
     undertaken a study of factors which regulate the synthesis and/or

release of TSH in the pituitary gland. Two hundred male Sprague
Dawley rats were used for all experiments and were divided into
four categories: 1) Normal 2) Methyl xanthine-injected (150 μ
moles) 3-isobutyl-1 methyl xanthine injected i.p. 5 hours before
sacrifice) 3) PTU treated - 0.05% PTU in drinking water for 18
days 4) PTU and T4 treated - PTU same as group #3, but with
50 μg T4 injected i.p. daily for 4 days. There were 2 rats in
each group. Rats were sacrificed by decapitation and the pituitary glands were extracted for ODC activity. Results are expressed as percent increase in ODC activity over controls per
mg pituitary tissue of the treated rats (groups 2, 3, 4). The
results are as follows: MeXanthine treated - 350% increase of
ODC activity over normal; PTU treated - 130% increase of ODC
activity over normal; PTU and T4 treated - 40% increase of ODC
activity over normal. These results suggest that enhanced TSH
synthesis in the rat pituitary gland is associated with increased ODC activity and that this action may be mediated by cAMP.

31   AN ASSAY FOR CATECHOL ESTROGENS BASED UPON THEIR ENZYMATIC O-
      METHYLATION. G.R. Merriam, F. Naftolin and K.J. Ryan. Labora-
      tory of Human Reproduction & Reproductive biology, Harvard
      Medical School, Boston & Department of Obstetrics and Gynae-
      cology, Royal Victoria Hospital, Montreal.
         Catechol estrogens (CE's) such as 2-OH estrone and 2-OH
      estradiol, are natural metabolites of estrogens in rats and hu-
      mans, and are formed at especially high rates in the hypothala-
      mus. Administered CE's increase LH and FSH in male rats, sug-
      gesting their possible involvement in physiological gonadotro-
      pin regulation. Since CE's are easily degraded, their assay
      has been difficult. We have used their ready methylation by
      catechol-o-methyl transferase (COMT) as the basis of a simple
      and rapid microassay for CE's and for measuring their rate
      of formation in tissues such as hypothalamus. Methylene chlo-
      ride extracted samples are incubated under N_2 with excess se-
      mipurified rat liver COMT, mg^{++} , EGTA, and $[^3H]$ S-adenosyl
      methionine as the methyl donor; the $[^3H]$2-and 3-methoxy
      products are extracted into heptane and counted. Standard
      curves are linear. Sensitivity to 2-OH estrone, the principal
      CE, is <0.4 pmole. There is 20% cross-reactivity to 2-OH es-
      tradiol, whose reaction products can be easily separated by
      paper chromatography, but none to 2-OH estriol or catecholamines
      whose methylated products are not extractable by heptane.
      Assays of 3rd trimester pregnancy plasma yield values of 1mg/ml
      in good agreement with prior estimates. Using estradiol as subs-
      trate and supplying cofactors for its 2-hydroxyation, the rate
      of formation of CE's in tissue extracts can be assessed by im-
      mediately O-methylating CE's as they are synthesized. Kinetics
      of these reactions have been determined.

32   EFFECT OF SOMATOSTATIN AND THYROTROPIN-RELEASING HORMONE (TRH)
      ON PROLACTIN (PRL) AND GROWTH HORMONE (GH) RELEASE IN GH_1 PITUI-
      TARY TUMOR CELLS IN CULTURE. O. Morin and F. Labrie. Medical
      Research Council Group in Molecular Endocrinology, CHUL, Québec,
      G1V 4G2, Canada.

      When anterior pituitary cells in primary culture obtained
      from intact adult female rats are used, somatostatin inhibits
      the basal release of both GH and PRL as well as the TRH-induced
      PRL release. In order to minimize problems related to hetero-
      geneity of the cell types present in normal pituitary tissue,
      the effect of somatostatin and TRH was next studied in pitui-
      tary tumor cells secreting exclusively PRL and GH. In these
      tumor cells, somatostatin was found to inhibit the basal relea-
      se of both GH and PRL to 25-35% of the control rate up to 6
      hours of incubation, a maximal inhibitory effect being already
      measured after 1 hour. Half-maximal inhibition (ED_{50}) of PRL
      and GH release was measured at $2 \times 10^{-9}M$ somatostatin. TRH
      leads to a 2- to 3-fold stimulation of PRL release 5 minutes
      after addition of TRH, the effect remaining constant up to
      60 minutes of incubation, TRH stimulates also GH secretion,
      a half-maximal stimulation of both GH and PRL secretion being
      measured at $10^{-9}M$ TRH. The TRH-induced release of both GH and
      PRL is inhibited by somatostatin at an ED_{50} of $2 \times 10^{-9}M$.
      Theophylline (1 mM) and N^6-monobutyryl cyclic AMP (2.5 mM) sti-
      mulate both GH and PRL release, the stimulation being also inhi-
      bited by somatostatin. The present data show that somatostatin
      inhibits while TRH stimulates both PRL and GH release in tumoral
      pituitary cells, the interaction between the two peptides being
      of a non-competitive type. The stimulation of PRL and GH re-
      lease by theophylline and N^6-monobutyryl cyclic AMP suggests
      a role of cyclic AMP as mediator of the action of these two
      hypothalamic peptides.

33   REGULATION OF PLASMA FSH LEVELS BY OVINE TESTICULAR EXTRACT (OTE)
      N.R. Moudgal, S.G. Nandini and H. Lipner. Laboratory of Endo-
      crine Biochemistry, Dept of Biochemistry, Indian Institute of
      Science, Bangalore-560012, India.

      FSH in the male is lowered by an "inhibin"-like material pre-
      sent in aqueous testicular extracts. Although this observation
      has been confirmed in several laboratories, no simple sensitive
      assay is yet available. We have standardized a model system for
      the bioassay of inhibin activity. Male rats were castrated on
      day 34 (p.m.) and administered OTE on day 35 (a.m.). Blood
      samples were collected prior to and after injection. Suppression
      of FSH was evident within 3 to 6 hr. A single, maximal dose of
      OTE suppressed FSH level by 50%, while with successive maximal
      doses, the suppression was only 75%. OTE is thus unable to
      suppress FSH levels below a minimal basal value. The OTE effect
      is dose-dependent, persists for 12 hr, and disappears by 36 hrs.
      OTE does not suppress LH levels. Following castration, the

sensitivity to OTE suppression gradually decreases and the animal becomes refractory beyond 48 hr, suggesting possible involvement of a steroid in a sensitization step. The active principle in OTE is a heat stable, non-dialysable and lyophilizable material precipitated by high salt concentration and is free of steroids. Extracts of rat testis, like OTE, exhibit inhibin-like activity suggesting the material to be species non-specific. Work supported by grants from Indian Council of Medical Research, India, and United States Educational Foundation, India.

34   LH-RH NEUROSECRETORY CELLS AND THE ROLE PLAYED BY THE EPENDYMA IN REGULATION OF GONADOTROPHIN SECRETION. D.V. Naik. Department of Anatomy, Faculty of Medicine, University of Sherbrooke, Sherbrooke, Québec, Canada.

Naik (1975 a, b) has already achieved precise immunohistochemical localization of LH-RH neurons and their axonal pathways in hypothalami of rats (Cell. Tiss. Res. 157, 423, 437). Now, localization of LH-RH in the median eminence (ME) of rat during different phases of estrus cycle, with special emphasis on the arcuate neurons and the ependymal cells, has been done by immunofluorescence and immunoelectron microscopy, with rabbit anti-LH-RH serum supplied by Drs. Givner and Hirsch, Ayerst Research Laboratories, Montreal. Immunoelectron microscopic LH-RH localization in arcuate neurons varied markedly in different phases of estrus cycle. Late diestrus showed a very active Golgi complex with maximum LH-RH positive granules around it and scattered granules in the cytoplasm. Rest of the cycle showed fewer LH-RH granules with a less active Golgi complex. Specialized ependymal cells bordering the 3rd ventricle in infundibular recess, also showed varied LH-RH positive reaction during different phases of estrus cycle. This LH-RH localization was not granular like that in the neurons and the nerve profiles, but it was clumped and pleomorphic, suggesting that ependymal cells do not synthesize LH-RH. Ependymal cells on the surface of the ventricle wall were phagocytic. Immunofluorescent studies showed that during late diestrus, LH-RH positive material had started increasing in the lumen of the infundibular recess and was found maximum at early proestrus phase. Maximum increase in the fluorescence of the ependymal cells during proestrus was accompanied by a marked decrease of fluorescence in the cerebro spinal fluid (CSF) of the 3rd ventricle. Ependymal cells and the lumen of the infundibular recess showed very weak fluorescence during estrus to early diestrus phases. However, in males, fluorescent material at the above sites did not show any noticeable change. These findings were also confirmed by immunoelectron microscopy. With the present and previous work, it is concluded that neurons in different nuclei synthesize LH-RH and transport it to the ME portal system primarily through the nerve fibers and secondarily by the ventricular route. It is also suggested that ependymal transport of LH-RH to the ME por-

tal system is cyclic and thus controls the gonadotrophin secretion. (Supported by MRC Canada, MA-5160).

35   THERAPEUTIC USE OF LH-RH IN THE HUMAN FEMALE. S.J. Nillius and
     L. Wide. Department of Obstetrics & Gynaecology and Clinical
     Chemistry, University Hospital, Upsala, Sweden.
         The exciting possibility of using synthetic LH-releasing hor-
     mone (LH-RH) instead of human gonadotrophins for induction of
     follicular maturation and ovulation was studied in 13 amenor-
     rheic women who had no evidence of endogenous ovarian activity.
     LH-RH, 500 µg every eight hours, was administered intramuscular-
     ly or subcutaneously during 16 treatment cycles. Follicular ma-
     turation was produced after 9-23 days treatment in all but 2
     cycles. Ovulation was also induced in 7 patients who were trea-
     ted with LH-RH alone. However, the progesterone values during
     the luteal phases in four of these induced cycles were rather
     low, suggesting insufficient corpus luteum function. LH-RH
     was therefore combined with HCG during seven treatment cycles.
     Six of these cycles were ovulatory with normal luteal phase pro-
     gesterone values. Thus, it seems possible to replace human
     gonadotrophins with LH-RH for induction of follicular maturation
     and ovulation in some women with amenorrhea. LH-RH may prove
     to have advantages over human gonadotrophins for induction of
     ovulation. It is known that gonadal steroids can modulate the
     pituitary responsiveness to LH-RH. The interrelationship
     between the pituitary and the ovaries, which is present in
     patients treated with LH-RH, can be regarded as an internal
     control mechanism which may automatically prevent hyperstimula-
     tion of the ovaries during prolonged treatments with LH-RH.

36   GROWTH HORMONE SECRETION BY HUMAN SOMATOTROPIC ADENOMAS IN VITRO:
     EFFECT OF SOMATOSTATIN (SRIF). F. Peillon, P.E. Garnier, J.L.
     Chaussain, A. Brandi, P. Rivaille. Facultés de Médecine Pitié,
     Cochin, Saint-Antoine, Paris, France.
         SRIF was demonstrated to decrease blood growth hormone (GH)
     levels in acromegalic patients. In order to investigate the
     pituitary effects of SRIF in these patients, five somatotropic
     adenomas were collected after surgery and fragmented. 1 mm^3
     fragments were incubated in medium M 199 with 5 or 10 µg/ml of
     pure synthetic SRIF during 4 hours, and compared to control
     fragments incubated under identical conditions without SRIF.
     Medium was then collected and assayed for GH radioimmunoactivity
     (IRGH). Fragments of two others adenomas were incubated 1, 2, 3
     and 4 hours with and without SRIF, IRGH content assayed, and GH
     molecular heterogeneity studied on Sephadex G 200. Incubated
     fragments were studied by electron microscopy. A significant de-
     crease of IRGH (30 to 60% when compared to controls) was observed
     in media of the SRIF-incubated fragments. IRGH content was also

lower in SRIF-incubated and the heterogeneity pattern of GH
was not modified by SRIF. Electron microscopy demonstrated a
constant decrease (30 to 50%) of the number of secretory granules in the cells of the SRIF-incubated fragments, without any
lysosomal formation, the morphology of the remaining granules
being different from that in control fragments. These data
lead to hypothesize an inhibitory effect of SRIF upon GH synthesis by the cells of somatotropic adenomas in vitro.

37   DOPAMINE INFUSION ACUTELY INHIBITS THE TSH AND PROLACTIN RESPON-
      SE TO TRH. S.W. Spaulding, G.S. Besses, G.N. Burrow and R.K.
      Donabedian with the assistance of T. Pechinski. Departments
      of Medicine and Laboratory Medicine, Yale University School of
      Medicine, New Haven Connecticut.
         Previous work has shown that chronic L-dopa therapy blunts
      the TSH response to TRH in euthyroid subjects. L-dopa might act
      directly on the pituitary or might first be converted to an
      active metabolite. We therefore tested the effects of the acu-
      te administration of dopamine on the TRH-mediated release of
      prolactin and TSH. Ten normal males were given 100 µg TRH and
      samples obtained for serum TSH and prolactin. After a period
      of at least one week, the TRH test was repeated while the sub-
      jects were receiving L-dopamine infusion. Baseline prolactin
      and TSH were slightly, but significantly lowered by dopamine.
      The mean TSH response to TRH during dopamine infusion was
      significantly suppressed at all times. The mean peak TSH
      response was 14.6 ± 2.6 µU/ml (SEM) during the control period
      and 4.8 ± 0.7 µU/ml during dopamine infusion (P<0.01). The
      mean prolactin response was completely suppressed by dopamine,
      never significantly above baseline. The demonstration that
      chronic administration of L-dopa inhibits the TSH response to
      TRH while acute L-dopa administration does not, suggests that
      L-dopa may have to be converted to an active metabolite. Sin-
      ce neither norepinephrine nor adrenergic blockade alter the
      TSH response to TRH, the active metabolite would apparently
      have to be at an earlier step. This study suggests that dopa-
      mine is the active metabolite, and thus dopaminergic neurons
      may act hormonally through the pituitary portal system to
      play a role in the regulation of TSH and prolactin secretion.

38   ON THE MECHANISM OF AMENORRHEA INDUCED BY NEUROLEPTICS AND AL-
      PHAMETHYLDOPA. G. Tolis and T. Kolivakis. Departments of
      Medicine & Psychiatry, Royal Victoria Hospital, Mc Gill Univer-
      sity, Montréal, Québec.
         Five women presented with amenorrhea-galactorrhea following
      chronic ingestion of phenothiazines (n=3) and alphamethyldopa
      (n=2). Physical examination and skull X-ray were within normal
      limits. Serum prolactin levels (normal: less than 30 ng/ml)
      were elevated ranging from 45-162 ng/ml, were suppressed less

than 50 percent in response to 0.5 g levodopa and increased following the I.V. administration of 500 µg thyrotropin releasing factor (TRF, Abbott). Basal serum FSH and LH levels were within the normal range but showed no pulsatile pattern when measured every 20 minutes for 3-6 hours. Pituitary gonadotropin reserve was adequate as tested by the increments in serum FSH and LH following the S.C. administration of 100 µg of gonadotropin-releasing factor (LRF, Ayerst). This suggested a suprahypophyseal origin of the altered gonadotropin secretion. Discontinuation of the above medications resulted in reappearance of pulsatile gonadotropin secretion and ovulatory menses. It is suggested that the above mentioned medications lead to amenorrhea by influencing not the tonic but the pulsatile center of gonadotropin release at a surprahypophyseal level.

39 THE POSSIBLE INVOLVEMENT OF CYCLIC AMP IN THE FEEDBACK MECHANISM OF SEX HORMONES. B.A. Weissman and D.F. Johnson. NIAMDD, NIH, Bethesda, Maryland.

Gonadal steroids, estrogens as well as androgens, induce cyclic AMP formation in immature rat hypothalamus in vivo and in vitro. Monoamines may be involved in the above mentioned pathway, as amine antagonists can block the effect of gonadal steroids. Diethylstilbesterol (DES) has been shown to be the most potent adenylate cyclase activator in both sexes. The effects of DES can be blocked by the anti-estrogen, clomiphene. From a variety of adrenergic and dopaminergic antagonists tested, only propranolol, a β-blocker, exhibited a 50% reduction of DES-elicited cyclic AMP accumulation in hypothalami from male rats. Stimulation of the cyclic AMP generating system in the female hypothalamus could be blocked by either α or β-adrenergic blockers. 17β-estradiol shows a very similar effect in both sexes. In the male rat hypothalamus dihydrotestosterone resembles 17β-estradiol (a 50% increase in cyclic AMP levels). Disruption of the tissue integrity abolished the effect of 17β-estradiol ($2 \times 10^{-5}M$) and DES ($2 \times 10^{-5}M$) while DES ($10^{-4}M$) had only a marginal effect. Theophylline completely blocked DES-elicited accumulations of cyclic AMP in the sliced hypothalami and reduced the levels of the latter in incubated intact female hypothalamus. Our data illustrates that preincubation of male rat hypothalami with DES potentiates dopamine as well as norepinephrine responses. It is suggested that DES, the synthetic estrogen, has a dual mechanism; a) stimulation of the adenylate cyclase via estrogen-receptor interaction, and b) a non-specific component involving adenosine release. It is suggested that cyclic AMP formation as a result of high gonadal steroids concentration in the hypothalamus will in turn inhibit the synthesis and/or the release of gonadotrophin releasing hormones.

40   APPLICATIONS OF OXYTOCIN RADIOIMMUNOASSAY.   N. Wilson and
V. Yakoleff Greenhouse.   Department of Physiology, Faculty of
Medicine, University of British Columbia, Vancouver, B.C.
      A radioimmunoassay was developed using an antiserum primarily
directed againt the C-terminal tripeptide of the oxytocin molecule. ^{125}I-oxytocin was prepared using the thallium chloride
iodination method (Commerford, Biochem. 10: 1993, 1971; Getz,
Altenburg and Saunders, Bioch. Biophys. Acta 287: 485, 1972).
Extraction of animal and human plasma, as well as the radioimmunoassay incubation conditions were as described by Robertson
(J. Clin. Invest. 52:2340, 1973).   The assay sensitivity was in
10 - 100 fmoles/ml range.   Measurements of human plasma in
this radioimmunoassay system showed that while unextracted plasma levels remain undetectable, the extraction procedure resulted
in measurable (100 - 200 fmoles/ml range) levels of an immunoreactive oxytocin-like substance.   Measurement of oxytocin plasma
levels in human females following the administration of exogenous oxytocin, also resulted in higher oxytocin values in the
extracted as compared to the unextracted plasma samples.   Application of our oxytocin immunoassay to the measurement of oxytocin content of the rat posterior pituitary glands gave values
of 481.2 ± 39.15 pmoles per gland (n=10) for rats decapitated
without anesthesia, and 486.9 ± 35.7 pmoles per gland (n=7) for
animals decapitated under urethane anaesthesia.   Electrical stimulation in the region of paraventricular nucleus reduced oxytocin content of pituitary glands by at least 20%.

CONTRIBUTORS

N.A. ABRAHAM, Ayerst Research Laboratory, St.Laurent, Que.

M. AMOSS, Salk Institute, La Jolla, California

AKIRA ARIMURA, Tulane University School of Medicine and
        Veterans Administration Hospital, New Orleans, Loui-
        siana, U.S.A.

NICHOLAS BARDEN, Medical Research Council Group in Mole-
        cular Endocrinology, Centre Hospitalier de l'Univer-
        sité Laval, Quebec, Canada

JULIEN BARRY, Laboratoire d'Histologie, Faculté de Méde-
        cine, Place de Verdun, 59045 Lille Cedex, France

MICHELE BEAULIEU, Medical Research Council Group in Mo-
        lecular Endocrinology, Centre Hospitalier de l'Uni-
        versité Laval, Quebec, Canada

G.M. BESSER, The Medical Professorial Unit, St. Bartho-
        lomew's Hospital, London, England

H.G. BOHNET, University of Manitoba, Winnipeg, Manitoba

PIERRE BORGEAT, Medical Research Council Group in Mole-
        cular Endocrinology, Centre Hospitalier de l'Uni-
        versité Laval, Quebec, Canada

J. BORRELL, Departments of Endocrinology and Pharmacolo-
        gy, University of Milano, Italy

MARIE-MADELEINE BOUTON, Centre de Recherches Roussel-
        UCLAF, France

PAUL BRAZEAU, Research Institute, Montreal General Hos-
        pital, Montreal, Quebec

MARVIN BROWN, Salk Institute, La Jolla, California

R. BURGUS, Salk Institute, La Jolla, California

LANA CHAN, Salk Institute, La Jolla, California

JAMES A. CLEMENS, The Lilly Research Laboratories (Eli
        Lilly and Co.), Indianapolis, Indiana 46206

DAVID H. COY, Department of Medicine, Tulane University
    School of Medicine and Veterans Administration Hos-
    pital, New Orleans, Louisiana, U.S.A.

ESTER J. COY, Department of Medicine, Tulane University
    School of Medicine and Veterans Administration Hos-
    pital, New Orleans, Louisiana, U.S.A.

ANTONIO DE LA CRUZ, Department of Medicine, Tulane Uni-
    versity School of Medicine and Veterans Administra-
    tion Hospital, New Orleans, Louisiana, U.S.A.

ANDRE DE LEAN, Medical Research Council Group in Molecu-
    lar Endocrinology, Centre Hospitalier de l'Univer-
    sité Laval, Quebec, Canada

JACQUES DROUIN, Medical Research Council Group in Mole-
    cular Endocrinology, Centre Hospitalier de l'Uni-
    versité Laval, Quebec, Canada

ALAIN ENJALBERT, Unité de Neurobiologie, INSERM, Paris,
    France

C.P. FAWCETT, The University of Texas Health Science
    Center at Dallas, Southwestern Medical School, Dal-
    las, Texas

LOUISE FERLAND, Medical Research Council Group in Mole-
    cular Endocrinology, Centre Hospitalier de l'Uni-
    versité Laval, Quebec, Canada

HENRY G. FRIESEN, University of Manitoba, Winnipeg, Ma-
    nitoba

JOHN E. GERICH, Metabolic Research Unit and Department
    of Medicine, University of California, San Francis-
    co, California

MANFRED GOTZ, Ayerst Research Laboratories, St.Laurent,
    Quebec, Canada

ROGER GUILLEMIN, Salk Institute, La Jolla, California

P.G. HARMS, The University of Texas Health Science Center
    at Dallas, Southwestern Medical School, Dallas,
    Texas 75235

MICHELINE HERY, Unité de Neurobiologie, INSERM, Paris,
    France

H.H. HUANG, Department of Physiology, Michigan State
    University, East Lansing, Michigan

HANS IMMER, Ayerst Research Laboratories, St.Laurent,
    Quebec

ROBERT J. JAFFE, Reproductive Endocrinology Center, De-
    partment of Obstetrics and Gynecology, University
    of California, San Francisco, California 94143

PAUL A. KELLY, Medical Research Council Group in Molecu-
    lar Endocrinology, Centre Hospitalier de l'Univer-
    sité Laval, Quebec, Canada

WILLIAM R. JR. KEYE, Reproductive Endocrinology Center,
    Department of Obstetrics and Gynecology, University
    of California, San Francisco, California

CLAUDE KORDON, Unité de Neurobiologie, INSERM, Paris,
    France

FERNAND LABRIE, Medical Research Council Group in Mole-
    cular Endocrinology, Centre Hospitalier de l'Uni-
    versité Laval, Quebec, Canada

NICK LING, Salk Institute, La Jolla, California

JOSEPH B. MARTIN, Division of Neurology, Department of
    Medicine, Montreal General Hospital, Mc Gill Uni-
    versity, Montreal, Quebec

LUCIANO MARTINI, Departments of Endocrinology and Phar-
    macology, University of Milano, Italy

SAMUEL McCANN, The University of Texas Health Science
    Center at Dallas, Southwestern Medical School,
    Dallas, Texas

JOSEPH MEITES, Department of Physiology, Michigan State
    University, East Lansing, Michigan

ODETTE MORIN, Medical Research Council Group in Molecu-
    lar Endocrinology, Centre Hospitalier de l'Univer-
    sité Laval, Quebec, Canada

V. NELSON, Ayerst Research Laboratories, St. Laurent,
    Quebec

SVEN JOHAN NILLIUS, Department of Obstetrics and Gyneco-
     logy, University Hospital, Uppsala, Sweden

S.R. OJEDA, The University of Texas Health Science Center
     at Dallas, Southwestern Medical School, Dallas,
     Texas

GEORGES PELLETIER, Medical Research Group in Molecular
     Endocrinology, Centre Hospitalier de l'Université
     Laval, Quebec, Canada

DANIEL PHILIBERT, Centre de Recherches Roussel-UCLAF,
     France

F. PIVA, Departments of Endocrinology and Pharmacology,
     University of Milano, Milano, Italy

JEAN-PIERRE RAYNAUD, Centre de Recherches Roussel-UCLAF,
     France

G.D. RIEGLE, Department of Physiology, Michigan State
     University, East Lansing, Michigan

CATHERINE RIVIER, Salk Institute, La Jolla, California

JEAN RIVIER, Salk Institute, La Jolla, California

JEAN-GUY ROCHEFORT, Department of Clinical Pharmacology,
     Ayerst Research Laboratories, Montreal, Quebec,
     Canada

ANDREW V. SCHALLY, Department of Medicine, Tulane Univer-
     sity School of Medicine and Veterans Administration
     Hospital, New Orleans, Louisiana

LUIS SCHWARZSTEIN, G.E.F.E.R. (Grupo de Estudios en
     Fertilidad y Endocrinologia de Rosario), Rosario,
     Argentina

K. SESTANJ, Ayerst Research Laboratories, St. Laurent,
     Quebec

D.K. SUNDBERG, The University of Texas Health Science
     Center at Dallas, Southwestern Medical School,
     Dallas, Texas 75235

GEORGE TOLIS, Department of Endocrinology, Royal Victo-
     ria Hospital, Montreal, Quebec

WILEY VALE, Salk Institute, La Jolla, California

JACQUES VAN CAMPENHOUT, Department of Obstetric and
     Gynaecology, Hopital Notre Dame, Montreal, Quebec
     Canada

BERNARD VANNIER, Centre de Recherches Roussel-UCLAF,
     France

JESUS A. VILCHEZ-MARTINEZ, Department of Medicine,
     Tulane University School of Medicine and Veterans
     Administration Hospital, New Orleans, Louisiana

J. VILLARREAL, Salk Institute, La Jolla, California

J.E. WHEATON, The University of Texas Health Science
     Center at Dallas, Southwestern Medical School,
     Dallas, Texas

JOHN O. WILLOUGHBY, Division of Neurology, Department of
     Medicine, Montreal General Hospital, McGill Univer-
     sity, Montreal, Quebec, Canada

JOHN R. YOUNG, Reproductive Endocrinology Center, Depart-
     ment of Obstetrics and Gynecology, University of
     California, San Francisco, California

Acetylcholine, 297
ACTH
  ACTH 4-10, 478
  and prostaglandins, 22
  releasing factor for, 405-407
Acromegaly, 115-117
Antiestrogens, 327, 490
2-Bromo-2-ergocryptine (CB-154)
    44, 267
Calcium, 410, 411
Clonidine, 42
Circumventricular organs,
    436-440, 442-444
Corticosterone, 307-308
Culture, pituitary, 398-399
Cyclic AMP
  and LH-RH, 148, 477
  and prostaglandins, 163-164,
    475-476
  and somatostatin, 158
Dexamethasone, 456, 413
Diabetes Mellitus, 120, 132-137
Dopamine, 284-287, 402
  agonists, 287-290
  antagonists, 291-293
Ergot alkaloids, 269, 478
Estrogens
  effect on
    LH-RH, 103-104, 208-234
    prolactin, 267-268, 330-331,
    4
    prolactin receptors,
      325-333
    TSH, 155, 482
  plasma binding, 172, 173
  receptors,uterus, 173

receptors, hypothalamus, 178-182
  and LH and FSH, 192-197
    213-251
  and TSH, 482
Estrous cycle
  and inhibitory analogs of LH-RH,
    480
  and L-Dopa, 9-12
  and progesterone, 12
  in old rats, 7
Follicle-stimulating hormone (FSH)
  female rats, 4, 5
  localization, immunohistoche-
    mistry, 491
  release
    and amygdala, 40, 44
    and estradiol, 192-197,
      213-251
    and prostaglandins, 23, 25
    and serotonin, 52-54
    and testosterone, 198-206
  response to LH-RH, 66-69, 75,
      76, 88, 108, 196-198
Gastrin, 118, 119
Glucagon, 119, 122, 130-134
Glucose, 132-137
Growth hormone (GH)
  pulsatile secretion, 304-314
    and dexamethasone, 413
  receptors, 322
  release
    and prostaglandins, 24
    and somatostatin, 121
    and TSH, 413
Growth hormone release-inhibiting
hormone (GH-RIH) See somatostatin

Human chorionic gonadotropin
    (HCG), 104-107
Immunoelectron microscopy,
    433-448
Immunofluorescence, 451-466
Implantation, 391-393
Indomethacin, 30-33
Insulin, 128-131
β-Lipotropic hormone, 491
Luteinizing hormone (LH)
    female rats, 4, 5
    release
        and amygdala, 40, 44
        and estradiol, 192-194,
            213-250
        and prostaglandins, 23, 25
        and serotonin, 52-54
    response to LH-RH, 6, 66-69,
        75, 78, 88, 108, 196-
        198, 342
    and testosterone and DHT,
        198-206
Luteinizing hormone-releasing
    hormone (LH-RH)
    antibodies against, 389-393
    characterization, 362-368
    degradation, 490
    follicular growth, 100-102
    FSH, LH, 213-251, 493-497, 200-
        206, 367, 388-389
    hypogonadism, 66-70
    inhibitory analogs, 342-353,
        319-320, 377-387, 475-
        480
    localization, immunohistoche-
    mistry, 433-440, 454-464, 476
    oligospermia, 83-87
    ovulation, 99-100
    secondary amenorrhea, 69, 102-
        106
    superactive analogs 81-83, 89,
        339-342, 414-419
Mammary tumors, 271, 272, 475,
    490
β-Melanotropins, 492
11β-Methoxy ethinyl estradiol
    (R 2858), 175, 178, 182, 194
Morphine, 381-382
MSH inhibiting factor (MIF) 356-
    358

Neurophysins, 447, 453-454
Norepinephrine, 297
Ovulation
    timing, 2-4
    induction, 97-100
    suppression, 350-352, 480
Oxytocin, 452-453
Pentobarbital, 478, 479
Phenoxybenzamine, 41
Pregnancy, 94, 95
Progesterone
    plasma binding, 183
    receptors, mammary tumors, 475
    receptors, various tissues,
        184-185
    release and LH-RH, 95, 103-104
Prolactin
    and gonadotropin release, 489
    breast cancer, 271-272
    female rats, 5
    galactorrhea, 271
    heterogeneity, 258-260
    inhibiting factor, 403-404
    pituitary tumors, 269-270
    receptors, 323-333
    release
        and ergot derivatives, 478
        and prostaglandin, 23, 27
        and serotonin, 56-58, 491
        and suckling, 57
        and TSH, 481
Propanolol, 41
Prostaglandins
    and cyclic AMP, 475-476
    and LH secretion, 160-163,
        475-476, 477
    and PRL secretion, 160-163
    and TSH secretion, 160-163, 411
Prostigmine, 45
Renin, 489
Serotonin, 56-58, 293-296, 491
Somatostatin (growth hormone-re-
    leasing-inhibiting hormone)
    analogs, 374-378, 381-385, 421-
        424, 488
    and acromegaly, 115-117
    and diabetes mellitus, 132-138
    and glucagon secretion, 134-138
    and GH secretion, 157-159
        381-385, 394, 484, 488

and non-pituitary tumors, 118
and TSH secretion, 157-159,
        408-410, 487
antibodies against, 157-158,
        393-394
cyclic AMP, 149
localization in brain, immuno-
    chemistry, 440-444, 464-466,
        483-484
localization in pancreas and
    stomach, immunohistochemistry,
        444-448
protamine-zinc, combination with,
        379, 383-385
purification, 400-401
synthesis, 373
Stress, 394
Testosterone
and amygdala, 487
and FSH and LH, 198-206
and prolactin receptors, 327-
        329
response to LH-RH, 67-68, 76, 79,
        81, 82
Theophylline, 411
Thyrotropin-releasing hormone (TRH)
        148, 151
and GH, 413
and pentobarbital narcosis and
    hypothermia, 478, 479
and prolactin, 481, 482, 484
and TSH, 411
binding sites for, 152-154
characterization, 356, 362
ontogeny, 486
Thyrotropin-Stimulating Hormone
        (TSH)
release
    and estrogens, 155
    and prostaglandins, 20-23,
        411
    and somatostatin, 119
    and theophylline, 411
    and TSH, 411
Thyroxine, 152-154, 411, 482
Uterus, 175
Vasopressin, 447, 452
Ventro-medial nucleus, 312-313